CLINICAL IMMUNOLOGY
A Physician's Guide

SECOND EDITION

CLINICAL IMMUNOLOGY
A Physician's Guide

SECOND EDITION

Maxwell Asher Richter,
Ph.D., M.D.

Professor, Department of Pathology
School of Medicine, University of Ottawa
Director, Immunology Laboratory, and
Consultant, Allergy and Clinical Immunology,
Ottawa Civic Hospital
Career Investigator,
Medical Research Council, Canada

WILLIAMS & WILKINS
Baltimore/London

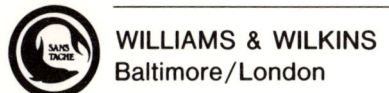

428 E. Preston Street
Baltimore, MD 21202, U.S.A.

Made in the United States of America

Library of Congress Cataloging in Publication Data

Richter, Maxwell Asher
Clinical immunology—a physician's guide.
First ed.: A physician's guide to the theory and practice of clinical immunology.
Bibliography: p.
Includes index.
1. Immunology. 2. Immunologic diseases.I. Title. [DNLM: 1. Allergy and immunology.
2. Immunity. 3. Immunologic diseases. QW 504 R536c]
QR181.R49 1982 616.07'9 81-7475
ISBN 0-683-07255-2 AACR2

Composed and printed at the
Waverly Press, Inc.
Mt. Royal and Guilford Aves.
Baltimore, MD 21202, U.S.A.

First Edition, published 1980, by the University of Ottawa Press, was titled *A Physician's Guide to the Theory and Practice of Clinical Immunology.*

In seeking wisdom,
The first step is silence,
The second is listening,
The third is remembering,
The fourth is practicing,
The fifth—teaching others.

RABBI SOLOMON IBN GABIROL
(1021-1052 A.D.)

Dedication

This book is dedicated to my wife, Iris Lipfeld, as thanks for her unlimited patience with me during our 23 years of marriage, and to my children, Margaret Anne and Andrew Clark, in the hope that it may help to answer the question which they have posed to me on countless occasions with sincerity and a tinge of sympathy, "What do you do at work, Daddy?".

It is also dedicated to my long-time teacher, professor and later colleague, Dr. Bram Rose, M.D., Ph.D., F.R.C.P., F.R.S. (C.)., Professor of Medicine, McGill University, and founder and Director of the Division of Immunochemistry and Allergy, Department of Experimental Medicine, McGill University Clinic, Royal Victoria Hospital, Montreal, with whom I had the privilege of being associated for a period of 18 years. This was the first laboratory in Canada dedicated to furthering our understanding of diseases considered to have an immunologic etiology and pathogenesis.

This book is also dedicated to Dr. Felix Haurowitz, M.D., D.Sc., teacher extraordinaire of biochemistry, immunology, cell biology, physiology, and chemistry. The year which my wife and I spent (I as a postdoctoral fellow) at the University of Indiana, Bloomington, Indiana (1958–1959) is indelibly fixed in my mind. Dr. Haurowitz demonstrated to me the uncanny ability to combine a gentle nature, a humble disposition, a wry sense of humor, a piercing mind, and a fountain of knowledge in a manner which was most disarming but which left a permanent imprint on me.

Preface to the Second Edition

The primary aim of this book is to seduce the medical practitioner to immerse himself in immunology in as painless a manner as possible, in order to attain a grasp of the fundamentals of immunology and then to entertain a differential diagnosis of an immunologically mediated disease with the same confidence as he would diagnose a gastrointestinal, endocrine, or renal disease. Of course, this does not guarantee immediate benefits to patients with immunologically mediated diseases. Nevertheless, it is imperative to recognize that proper diagnosis must necessarily precede the cure. Specific chemotherapy can only be instituted once the etiology and pathogenesis of the disease are understood. It is the author's hope that this book will enlighten the physician to the "pros and cons" of clinical immunology sufficiently to enable him to see the light without getting burned.

Emphasis is placed upon an understanding of the immune system in man. Addressed are the frequently asked but rarely answered questions: (1) What are the conditions which favor a humoral (antibody) response to one antigen but a cell-mediated response to another? (2) What are the transplantation antigens and why do they exist at all? (3) Why is a fetal allograft not rejected by the mother while all other allografts are uniformly and rapidly rejected? (4) Is there a relationship between autoimmune disease, cancer, immunodeficiency disease, and transplantation immunity? (5) What is the precise relationship between allergy and immunity in practical, as well as theoretical, terms? (6) What are the appropriate laboratory tests which should be requested, in their order of priority, to confirm or reject a diagnosis of an immunologically mediated disease? The interpretations for the different laboratory assays normally available in a clinical immunology service are presented.

I have expanded the chapters dealing with basic immunology. This does not mean that they are complete, for it is still my intention to present the material in a manner and depth commensurate with the needs of the practicing physician rather than the research immunologist. The chapters on immunodeficiency diseases and suppressor cells and suppressor factors have been much enlarged to take new developments into account. Cell-mediated immunity has been delegated its own chapter. New chapters have been added dealing with nonspecific immune mechanisms, the role of nutrition in the immune response, and immunity of the aged. As in the first edition, highly controversial issues have been omitted since they only muddy the waters, confuse the reader, and do not really add to the knowledge which can be applied at the bedside.

Preface to the First Edition

During the past decade medical curriculae have undergone extensive surgery and revision in order to attain the objective to decrease to a minimum the time the medical student is exposed (others use the term subjected) to didactic teaching. In this institution, as in many others, the teaching or learning phase of the curriculum has been drastically shortened from the customary 4 years (prior to 1967) to a brief period of slightly longer than 2 years. This is a paradoxical situation if one considers the immense yearly increase of knowledge in the theoretical, technological, and applied spheres which must be transmitted to the student in addition to the generally unchanging content of the primary preclinical subjects (anatomy, histology, embryology, physiology, biochemistry, microbiology, pathology, and pharmacology) which constitute the basis for an understanding of the practice of medicine. Instead of increasing the time allotted to the teaching of medicine, the student now spends the last 2 years of the 4-year medical course as a junior clerk exposed to the totally unstructured activities on the wards, no longer totally a student but a junior member of the "team." The period of time the medical student spends as a true apprentice is unduly, if not irresponsibly, short. There can be no doubt that economic factors (the cost of teaching a medical student per year) have played a not insignificant role in the attempt to graduate medical students at the least possible cost, which translates to the shortest time possible. However, these maneuvers may indeed be suspect, as they leave the student confused and unsure about his grasp of medicine upon graduation from medical school.

The problem facing curriculum committees is how to allot less time to adequately cover more ground. The situation is especially desperate with respect to the newer, often not yet integrated, disciplines such as radiology, geriatrics, neonatology, immunology, and genetics. These can only be incorporated into the time frame of the established curriculum at the expense of the other time-honored disciplines.

Having been allotted but a few hours to teach immunology to the first- and second-year medical students, the author quickly realized that the short time available would only permit presentation and discussion of the subject matter on a very superficial level and would necessitate total disregard of established areas which are even minimally controversial. The task is further aggravated by the fact that immunology has grown exponentially since the 1950s, both in its scope and relevance to the clinical disciplines. The author, therefore, concluded that one possible solution to this dilemma was to write a book (it's as good an excuse as any).

I set out with the modest objective to write a short, easily comprehensible, and well-illustrated book with which to introduce the reader to the principles and practice of basic and clinical immunology. However, during the writing of the book I discovered, as I am sure other writers have in the past, that it is much easier to write a long book than it is to write a short book. I found that I had to actively suppress my inherent desire to constantly expand each section as I wrote it. The deletion of several passages from the final draft almost left me in tears. This problem is probably a reflection of one of the basic laws of nature which states that the size of a book necessary to present the subject matter of the discipline is directly related to the lack of precise knowledge in that discipline. In other words, bigger does not necessarily mean better or wiser. The corollary to this law is that precise, unequivocal knowledge of a field can usually be summarized in a single short sentence or paragraph. For example, consider Einstein's law on the interconversion of mass and energy, $E = MC^2$. This short, seemingly simple equation summarizes many volumes of texts in physics written prior to its enunciation by Einstein.

It has been my observation that students, upon initial exposure to immunology, become confused with respect to their understanding of the mechanism of the antigen-antibody reaction, the different in vitro and in vivo manifestations of the antigen-antibody reactions and their sequelae, the relationship of allergy with immunology, the relationship between the humoral and cell-mediated immune responses, and the appropriate use of the clinical immunology laboratory in the diagnosis of diseases with suspected immunologic etiology and/or pathogenesis. Definitions for the term allergy are presented in often imprecise and diametrically opposed terms in different texts. I have, therefore, focused upon these areas, as I have consistently felt that the medical student must possess an unqualified understanding of them as they constitute the foundation for an appreciation of the deleterious and often life-threatening consequences of the immune reaction in vivo and for the ability to anticipate them. One objective of the author is to have the reader realize that good research quickly gets translated into diagnostic and therapeutic procedures in the practice of medicine.

I have briefly discussed the background of a number of major discoveries and have placed them in a historical perspective with regard to existing knowledge. I believe that an awareness of the historical development of the discipline and the problems confronting investigators at different times provides the student with the necessary perspective to appreciate current developments. I wish to impress upon the reader that, although major research discoveries are not made in a vacuum, nevertheless the absence of a precedent requires that the innovative investigator possess intellect, insight, foresight, and intestinal fortitude far in excess of the average. The history of immunology is, therefore, really a collection of biographies of the greats in the field beginning with Jenner, Pasteur, Koch, Ehrlich, von Behring, Metchnikoff, Virchow, von Pirquet, Shick, Landsteiner, Bordet, Portier, and Richet. They laid the foundation of the discipline of immunology.

I have only presented synopses of certain well-defined and time-honored basic topics, such as the chemistry of antigens and antibodies, since these are discussed in simple and unambiguous terms in most textbooks of pathology, microbiology, or immunology. On the other hand, I have deliberately avoided in-depth discussion of the precise clinical application of immunology to the management of transplanted and cancer patients. These two highly visible areas, transplantation and cancer immunology, are in a constant state of flux and no consensus presently exists as to the underlying immunologic mechanisms and the most appropriate modes of therapy. I have instead attempted to define the raison d'etre for the transplantation antigens and the proposed role of the immune system in the control of cancer within the context of the phylogeny of the immune response. A unified theory has been proposed to integrate autoimmune disease, transplantation immunity, and cancer immunity. I have also attempted to answer that oft-repeated question—why is the embryo not rejected by the mother?

I have refrained from the ego-satisfying activity of documenting this book with mountains of references. Some writers may consider abundant documentation a reflection of their extensive knowledge of their discipline; however, the effort seems hardly worthwhile since students rarely, if ever, have the time or inclination to read the relevant books let alone look up references. Instead, I have included the names of a number of investigators whose theories or findings have left an impact on the discipline. To the many contemporary investigators whose names were omitted but who may subjectively feel entitled to be referred to in a textbook of this type, please be assured that I thought of you all as I left your names out.

This book is not intended to displace any other textbook from the student's required or recommended reading list. Its primary purpose is to introduce the student to the field and to stimulate further reading of more advanced texts.

I have attempted to distill my experiences, knowledge, appreciation, and love of immunology acquired over the past 26 years into a few pages. I hope that it will, at the least, make the reader aware of the immunologic etiology of disease when confronted with the need for an inspired differential diagnosis and, at the best, that it may sufficiently stimulate a number of readers to entertain the thought of embarking on a career in immunology. But most of all, I will have accomplished my objective if the reader, after spending not more than 4 to 6 hours reading this book, will feel a contentment and sense of satisfaction overcoming him, much like the feeling experienced in guessing the name of the villain in an Agatha Christie mystery novel before actually being informed of his identity in the text.

Acknowledgments

I would like to thank my secretary, Miss Linda Rogers, interpreter extraordinaire of illegible scrawl, for the typing of the contents of this book. The book would not have been published were it not for her skills in deciphering the symbols of my handwritten text and transposing them to typewritten form. In spite of many attempts on my part, I was unable to confuse her sufficiently to deter the emergence of a typed, coherent version of my scribble. Since I rarely remember what I hand her to type, it may very well be that the final form of the text is actually Miss Rogers' version of the present state of immunology and not mine. However, the reader ought not to be deterred by this disclosure, as I could not have written it better.

I also wish to thank Mrs. Rosaline Bassett, who volunteered, unwittingly, to type select passages of the manuscript. Her continued enthusiasm to type from my scribble may reflect the activity of a gene, the study of which in terms of its inheritance pattern may produce useful knowledge for those concerned with the hiring of medical secretaries.

I am indebted to Miss Andrea Cross, medical illustrator at the Ottawa Civic Hospital; Messrs. Brian Hutt, Stuart Joyce, Bill Elford, and Harry Turner of the Audio-Visual Department, Ottawa Civic Hospital; M. Peter Medcalf, Director, Audio-Visual Department, Ottawa Civic Hospital; Emile Purgina and Anne Donaldson, principal medical illustrator and graphist, respectively, Visual Aids Department, University of Ottawa; and Mr. Stanley Klosevych, Director of Audio-Visual Services, University of Ottawa, Faculty of Medicine, for their unqualified assistance in the drawing and preparation of the diagrammatic representations.

Finally, I would like to express my thanks to Doctors Gilles Hurteau, Dean, and Donald Layne, Vice-Dean, Faculty of Medicine, University of Ottawa, and Mr. Peter Carruthers, Executive Director, Mr. Sydney Anderson, the past Assistant Executive Director, and Mr. Stuart Haslett, Assistant Executive Director, Ottawa Civic Hospital, for their financial assistance, without which this book could not have been published.

Contents

PREFACE TO THE SECOND EDITION ix

PREFACE TO THE FIRST EDITION xi

ACKNOWLEDGMENTS xv

CHAPTER 1.
INTRODUCTION 1

CHAPTER 2.
IMMUNOLOGY: A HISTORICAL PERSPECTIVE .. 4

CHAPTER 3.
THE CHEMISTRY OF ANTIBODIES 12

CHAPTER 4.
THE CHEMISTRY OF ANTIGENS 25

CHAPTER 5.
THE CELLULAR BASIS OF ANTIBODY FORMATION 30

CHAPTER 6.
CELL-MEDIATED IMMUNITY 58

CHAPTER 7.
IMMUNE REACTIONS USED TO ASSESS THE IMMUNOCOMPETENT STATE 70

CHAPTER 8.
SUPPRESSOR CELLS AND SUPPRESSOR ANTIBODIES 124

CHAPTER 9.
THE CLASSIFICATION AND IMMUNOLOGIC FUNCTIONS OF THE CIRCULATING LYMPHOCYTES, MONOCYTES, AND NEUTROPHILS 148

CHAPTER 10.
IMMUNODEFICIENCY DISEASES 161

CHAPTER 11.
IMMUNOLOGIC TOLERANCE 183

CHAPTER 12.
AUTOIMMUNITY AND AUTOIMMUNE DISEASES 191

CHAPTER 13.
NUTRITION AND IMMUNITY: THE ROLE OF PROSTAGLANDINS 200

CHAPTER 14.
IMMUNOPATHOLOGY 208

CHAPTER 15.
THE HUMORAL VERSUS THE CELL-MEDIATED IMMUNE RESPONSE 243

CHAPTER 16.
ALLOGRAFT REJECTION, PREGNANCY, CANCER, AND THE IMMUNE RESPONSE 248

CHAPTER 17.
IMMUNITY AND THE AGED 275

CHAPTER 18.
NONSPECIFIC MECHANISMS IN IMMUNITY 283

CHAPTER 19.
THE CLINICAL IMMUNOLOGY LABORATORY 286

CHAPTER 20.
FUTURE EXPECTATIONS 308

EPILOGUE 313

RECOMMENDED READING 316

INDEX 321

CHAPTER 1

Introduction

By historical definition, the immune response (immunity, from the Latin immunis, a term introduced by Julius Caesar meaning exempt from) has been associated with resistance to invasive pathogenic microorganisms. The science of serology is an outgrowth of investigations aimed at clearly identifying the invasive agent and quantifying immune reactions in vitro. The raison d'etre for identifying the invasive pathogen was to enable the physician to intervene chemotherapeutically via the administration of specific antisera prepared in animals (horses, cows, goats, sheep, rabbits). The investigations of Pasteur, Koch, von Behring, Calmette, Guerin, and others culminated in the production of attenuated and inactivated bacteria and detoxified toxins which could be safely administered as vaccines via the parenteral route without complications. Until World War II, prophylactic immunization with vaccines and the judicious use of specific antisera constituted the major (and *only*) treatment for infectious disease. The introduction of antibiotics in the treatment of infectious diseases signaled an end to the utilization of specific antisera as chemotherapeutic agents and reduced the dramatic aspects of serology.

It subsequently became apparent that antibodies are not always directed toward extrinsic pathogenic agents and are not necessarily synonymous with resistance. Not only may an immune response be elicited to autologous tissue antigens, culminating in a state of autoimmune disease, but antibodies and immune complexes may themselves induce diseases.

Allergies to pollens, dust, such drugs as local anesthetics or antibiotics, insect bites, foods and food additives, cosmetics, lotions, and sprays are all instances of immune responses directed toward innocuous, noninvasive, nonpathogenic, nonvirulent, and nonreplicating extrinsic agents. The immune reaction and the highly potent mediators activated from serum protein precursors or released from cells as a consequence of the reaction (histamine, serotonin, acetylcholine, anaphylatoxin, kinins, lymphokines) create a derangement of the normal homeostatic balance so as to constitute a life-threatening situation.

The immune reaction is also implicated in, if it is not in fact totally responsible for, the rejection of an allograft such as skin, kidney, or heart.

The immune response to tumor-specific antigens is considered to constitute a major mechanism for the eradication of an existing tumor and for the prevention of metastases. Naturally occurring lymphoid cells capable of interacting with and killing mutant (premalignant?) cells are considered to constitute the initial defense to tumorigenesis (immunologic surveillance).

Individuals with a congenital absence or abnormal development of the immune system display an abnormally high susceptibility to infections with respect to normally nonvirulent and minimally pathogenic microorganisms. The result is that such affected individuals succumb at an early age with bacteremia and septicemia, facilitated by an immunodeficiency state.

Although immunology is replete with numerous terms that are often ill-defined, none is more misunderstood than the term allergy. Since its introduction into the immunologic vocabulary by von Pirquet in 1911, different meanings have been attributed to it, with the result that it is often abused and misused and the reader is left in a confused state of mind.

One school of immunology categorizes all immunologic reactions that occur in vivo and induce disease as "allergic reactions." This approach is regrettable since a host of totally different diseases, characterized by marked differences in etiology, immunologic reactants involved, pathogenesis, and treatment, are all included under the single umbrella term "allergy." Well-intentioned but immunologically unaware practitioners, as well as nonmedically trained immunologists, might conclude that all the diseases classified in this category must be closely related and ought to be treated identically. Of course, such a view is totally incorrect and must be actively discouraged. Furthermore, the term allergy takes on a different and more specific meaning from that presented above when used, appropriately, by the allergist and clinical immunologist. The allergist especially considers hay fever, asthma, seasonal rhinitis, and urticaria to constitute the prototypes of the allergic state. Clinically, these conditions display many common characteristics and it is probably more than just fortuitous that they are all IgE-mediated conditions and are all treated in a similar fashion.

The reader should understand, in unequivocal terms, that many of the diseases with an immunologic etiology represent only the incidental in vivo manifestations of otherwise normal immune reactions. The immune reactions do not in themselves provoke pathologic sequelae in the manner whereby, under other circumstances, the immune reactions convey immunity. It is the mediators released from sensitized cells or activated following interaction of the immune complexes with normal serum constituents (complement) which induce pathology and clinical disease.

A second school of immunology classifies the diseases with a proven or suspected immunologic etiology in a pragmatic fashion, with the emphasis placed primarily upon the nature of the immunologic reactants involved and the mechanisms underlying the induction of the diseases and their management. This school is not bound to the vague classification originally proposed on the basis of very limited and inadequate knowledge of the discipline which was accepted unquestioningly for decades. This new classification stems from the influence exerted by clinically oriented immunologists, during the renaissance of the discipline in the late 1950s and early 1960s, who were primarily concerned with establishing formalized treatment protocols for the diseases under their professional jurisdiction. All of the immune reactions that occur in vivo which induce disturbances of homeostasis resulting in tissue damage and/or loss of function and/or release of potent pharmacologically active agents are classified under the umbrella term "immunopathology." The designation "allergy" is confined to only those diseases mediated by IgE antibodies. In accordance with this classification, allergic diseases are all related in terms of etiology, pathogenesis, and treatment. Other immunologically mediated diseases, where the initial and sustaining insults are perpetrated by the immune reaction or where the immune reaction contributes secondarily to the clinical picture, are classified as autoimmune diseases, immune complex diseases, and cell-mediated (hypersensitivity) diseases. The diseases within each of these categories are characterized more by their common features than by their differences.

In this author's view, this latter approach toward the classification of immunologically mediated diseases is more rational and pragmatic and it is adhered to in this text. The reader will be exempted from needlessly experiencing the "schism or gap effect" which he would encounter were he first exposed to basic textbooks, which still adhere to the former classification and terminology, and only later be required to apply his immunologic skills at the bedside.

CHAPTER 2

Immunology: A Historical Perspective

The late Dr. Jules Freund once remarked that immunology may have a relatively short past but it has a long history (Table 2.1). What he alluded to is that it has been known for at least several millenia that an individual who recovers from an infection exhibits resistance to subsequent reinfection (with the same pathogen). Indeed, it was common knowledge to the ancient Greeks that an individual who contracted a disease and survived seldom contracted that disease again during his lifetime. The Chinese 1,000 years ago recognized that the inhalation of smallpox crusts by previously unexposed people prevented the occurrence of this dreaded disease. Later, the Turks introduced the art of variolation (variola: smallpox), or the intradermal application, of powdered scabs from individuals who had recovered from smallpox. Lady Montague, the wife of the British Ambassador to Constantinople, should be credited with being the first in the Western World to become aware of this form of deliberate exposure to a disease agent and to recognize its clinical implications. However, not being a physician, she was apparently laughed at when she tried to encourage the practice of variolation upon her return to England during the 1780s. It was, therefore, left to Edward Jenner, then a medical student, either having been aware of Lady Montague's preaching or by his own devises, to become recognized as the discoverer (rediscoverer would be more appropriate) of immunization to smallpox in the Western World and to establish the basis for modern immunology. Jenner observed that young countrywomen, who often worked as milkmaids, invariably contracted cowpox, a very mild disease, but rarely came down with smallpox, a very deadly disease, in spite of raging epidemics. In a systematic study he showed that transfer of cowpox crusts intradermally to normal individuals would protect them from smallpox. Like many other milestone findings which would follow Jenner's and lay the foundation of immunology as

Table 2.1
Periods Characterized by Advancements in Immunology

Period	Critical Advances
Pre-1790s	Prehistory Immunity to diseases recognized but not understood
1790s–1880s	Immunity Discovered 1. Relation between immunization (infection or intentional exposure) and immunity defined 2. Bacterial antigens isolated and identified 3. Active immunization accepted as prophylactic treatment for infections 4. Passive immunization or serum therapy accepted as treatment for infections
1890s–1940s	Applied Immunology 1. Phagocytosis discovered 2. Antibodies discovered 3. Complement discovered 4. Humoral (antibody) and cell-mediated immune mechanisms identified and described 5. Anaphylaxis discovered 6. Serum sickness discovered 7. Immunohematology is born (blood group substances, Rh factor) and attains maturity 8. Serologic procedures attain high level of sophistication 9. Mechanism of the antigen-antibody reaction defined 10. Lymphocyte identified as the source of antibodies 11. Age of antibiotics dawns
1950s–1970s	Immunopathology and Clinical Immunology 1. Immunologic tolerance 2. Transplantation immunity 3. Autoimmune diseases 4. Cancer immunology 5. Immunodeficiency diseases 6. Clonal selection theory of antibody formation 7. Allergy as a form of immunity 8. Classification of diseases as a consequence of excessive, inadequate, or inappropriate immune response 9. Structure of the antibody molecule defined and heterogeneity of antibodies (immunoglobulins) established 10. Role of T cells and B cells in the immune response 11. Lymphokines discovered 12. Suppressor cells and suppressor factors discovered 13. Antibiotics used indiscriminately in treatment of infectious and noninfectious diseases 14. Appearance of antibiotic-resistant pathogenic microorganisms

Table 2.1—continued
Periods Characterized by Advancements in Immunology

Period	Critical Advances
1980s–	Postantibiotic Era; Natural Immunity Revisited; Cancer and Allograft Rejection Prevented 1. Immunization to pathogenic organisms greatly improved and safer as a result of efforts to purify major antigens and immunize with appropriate adjuvants 2. Reliance on antibiotics lessens 3. Role of nutrition on the specifically (antigen) inducible and "naturally occurring" immune systems 4. Gerontologic immunity 5. Control and induced regression of certain cancers by prophylactic immunization with cancer-specific antigens 6. Prevention of allograft rejection by induction of immunologic tolerance to specific transplantation antigens

we know it today, it is interesting to note that the element of specificity, the very foundation of the science of immunology, was lacking in Jenner's epoch-making proposal to immunize to smallpox. Jenner proposed immunization not with the specific highly virulent infectious smallpox but with a different, far less virulent, cowpox. The protection afforded cowpox-vaccinated individuals to the dreaded smallpox is today attributable to the antigenic cross-reactivity of these two viruses.

However, the immunization to smallpox proposed by Jenner was based strictly on circumstantial findings and empirical observations, since the mechanism of the immune response was a complete mystery. Jenner's findings must be considered, in perspective, to represent but an anecdotal episode in the evolution of immunology. Further progress in immunology had to await advancements in its two parent disciplines, bacteriology and pathology. By the late 1870s, bacteriology had made great strides and was attaining maturity, credibility, and respectability. Bacteriologists were providing the immunologist with the basic bacterial vaccines to administer. Pathologists provided, through the systematic study of inflammation, the basic understanding of the body's response to invasion by pathogenic microorganisms (Fig. 2.1). Pasteur had demonstrated that microorganisms can cause disease, and he proposed and proved the germ theory of disease. His investigations were so methodically and systematically carried out that even his most violent antagonists could not refute or discredit him. Pasteur was truly the first of the great experimental immunologists. He succeeded in producing attenuated (or non-

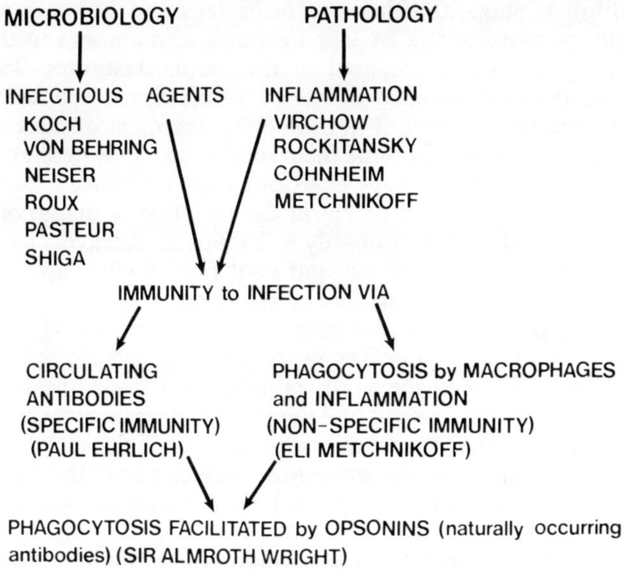

Figure 2.1 *The development of the discipline of immunology in the middle of the 19th century as a result of (synergistic) contributions from bacteriology and pathology.*

disease-producing) forms of highly virulent bacteria as a result of long-term culture under varying conditions, in preparing nontoxic preparations of bacteria by chemical manipulation, and in devising the rabies vaccine which was to remain essentially unaltered until the 1970s. It was Pasteur who introduced the terms "vaccine" (the infectious agent to be administered) and "vaccination" to commemorate Jenner's intradermal application or variolation with cowpox crusts (vacca is Greek for cow). (Today the terms vaccination and immunization are used synonymously.)

Within a 10-year period following acceptance of Pasteur's findings, the field of microbiology was literally a thriving "growth" industry. Many of the present pharmaceutical giants can trace their humble beginnings to the Pasteur era. Pasteur Institutes were established world-wide, and these were followed by Serum Institutes. Bacteria were systematically either detoxified, inactivated, killed, or attenuated, and powerful bacterial toxins were isolated and detoxified by chemical means. These were used for vaccination or **active immunization**. The scientists who are credited with the majority of these accomplishments, in addition to Pasteur, are Koch, von Behring, Roux, Yersin, Kitasato, Ehrlich, Shiga, and Neisser. The bacteria and the toxins were usually prepared at the Pasteur Institutes, and antisera to these agents were usually prepared at the Serum Institutes. These specific antisera, prepared in horses, sheep, goats, and rabbits, constituted the primary, if not the only, treatment of infectious disease until antibiotics made their appearance. This treatment is referred to as **serum therapy** or **passive immunization**.

The next major development in the evolution of immunology took place in the 1880s primarily as a result of endeavors by two individuals—Eli Metchnikoff and Paul Ehrlich—to understand the mechanism of elimination of an invasive agent (Fig. 2.1). Metchnikoff observed that certain mobile cells in the body could quickly engulf foreign bodies introduced through the skin and wall them off from the body proper. He termed these cells **phagocytes** (phagos, to eat) and the process as **phagocytosis**. This **phagocytic theory** as the primary protective mechanism to outside invaders was propounded while Metchnikoff was at the Pasteur Institute. It was violently opposed by the **humoral** (or **serum antibody**) **theory** of resistance which had as its protagonist a giant in the field, Paul Ehrlich, then working in Frankfurt. Ehrlich considered that antibodies, formed in response to antigens, were the primary providers of immunity to pathogens, and he viewed the interaction of antigen with antibody as a "key-in-a-lock" mechanism. He believed that there must be configurational complementariness between the antigen and the antibody at their sites of interaction. Among his many accomplishments which have weathered the century since their disclosure were quantitative assays for toxin neutralization and toxin standardization, the proposal of receptors on antibody-forming cells capable of interacting with specific chemical groupings on the antigen (which he termed the side-chain or receptor theory, which is still valid today), the founding of chemotherapy, and the synthesis of the first specific nontoxic, chemotherapeutic agent, salvarsan, for the treatment of syphilis.

The often intense debates and violent controversies which raged throughout the world between the Metchnikoff phagocytic theory school and the Ehrlich humoral theory school during the 1890s were finally reconciled and resolved at the turn of the 20th century by the findings of Sir Almroth Wright that serum factors are capable of reinforcing and markedly enhancing the bacteria-destructive capabilities of phagocytic cells. This property of the serum he called **opsonic** (opsono, to prepare food for), the substance in the serum **opsonin**, and the engulfing process by the phagocytic cell **opsonization**. We now know that opsonins are, in reality, specific antibody molecules present in low concentration in serum even in the absence of deliberate immunization (Fig. 2.1).

While the Metchnikoff and Ehrlich schools were at each others' throats, Bordet had discovered elexine, or **complement** as it was referred to by Ehrlich, and von Pirquet and Schick described the first immunologically induced iatrogenic (physician-induced) disease, serum sickness. This disease is a consequence of an inappropriate immune response to a chemotherapeutic agent, usually horse antiserum used in passive immunization containing antibodies directed toward a particular pathogen. It is only inappropriate from the immunologists' or chemotherapists' point of view. It is quite consistent with a normal immune response to a foreign agent insofar as the immune system is concerned. Serum sickness is today referred to as an immune-complex disease. At about the same time, Portier and Richet described another new disease with an apparent immunologic etiology and pathogenesis, often life-threatening in character. The symptoms appeared following a second administration of an otherwise innocuous extract of a sea anemone. They referred to this disease as **anaphylaxis** (ana, counter to; phylaxis, protection), in contradistinction to prophylaxis (pro, in favor of; phylaxis, protection). In an attempt to bring a semblance of order to an apparently chaotic situation, von Pirquet proposed the term **allergy**, which he defined as an altered reactivity of the host which could prove beneficial (resistance to infectious agents) or detrimental (serum sickness, anaphylaxis). von Pirquet referred to the beneficial state as **immunity** and the detrimental state as **hypersensitivity**. The reader will immediately realize that, in practice, we have today altered the original definitions of these terms. Immunity is now the all-embracing term which defines the altered state of reactivity of the host following antigenic stimulation. The term allergy (or hypersensitivity) is reserved for one of the clinicopathologic states categorized as a Type I (IgE-mediated) reaction. Thus, immunity characterizes the two fundamentally opposed states, both of which are antibody dependent—**resistant immunity** and **pathologic immunity**.

By the turn of the 20th century, the blood groups had been discovered by Landsteiner, a finding which permitted transfusions to be carried out safely for the first time. Immunization constituted the primary, if not the only, protection to infectious disease. Immunization could be induced by deliberate introduction of the specific antigen (**active immunity**) or as a result of the administration of specific antibody-containing xenogeneic antisera (**serum therapy** or **passive immunity**). Along with specific public health measures, such as the separation of drinking water from sewage, prophylactic immunization did much to reduce the incidence of morbidity and mortality due to infections. Public health measures and immunization procedures probably did more to improve the quality of life and extend the life-span than any other advances in medical science.

By the late 1920s, sulfonamides made their appearance as chemotherapeutic agents. Following the discovery by Fleming of penicillin, the first of the major antibiotics (and still the safest and most widely used), it became apparent that active and passive immunization to infectious agents and the sophisticated and extensive serologic service required for successful passive immunization might be considered obsolete, to be replaced by antibiotic therapy. Further research into antibiotic research was halted during World War II, but by the 1950s a number of new, very effective antibiotics—such as streptomycin, chloramphenicol, the tetracyclines, and erythromycin—had made their appearance and were being produced on a massive scale.

Thus, by the mid-1950s, immunology as it had been taught and practiced as a discipline concerned primarily with immunization as the means to induce enhanced resistance to invasion by pathogenic microorganisms appeared to be moribund as immunization became less fashionable and antibiotics became the treatment of choice for infectious disease. However, just in the nick of time, relevant discoveries in clinical medicine not only helped to resurrect immunology but gave it a totally new outlook and appearance. Medawar, Brent, and Billingham demonstrated that the allograft rejection reaction can be explained and predicted on the basis of an immunologic response by the host toward constituents of the allograft (now referred to as **transplantation antigens**); Felton discovered the phenomenon of **immunologic tolerance** (which he referred to as immunologic paralysis); the Kleins were actively engaged in cancer research using immunologic theory and techniques. Their work gave birth to the field of **cancer immunology**. Miller, Good, Waksman, and their colleagues presented unequivocal evidence which established an immunologic role for the thymus, and they demonstrated a relationship between thymic function and defective immune responsiveness. These findings gave birth to the subdiscipline of **immunodeficiency diseases**.

Autoimmune diseases attained respectibility if not credibility, and a great deal of notoriety, as diseases with no known etiology suddenly were thrust into the sphere of the immunologist. Coons had developed the immunofluorescence assay to facilitate the detection of antibody-producing cells, a technique which was to be used very successfully to diagnose a number of autoimmune diseases; and a number of investigators, especially Bram Rose and his associates and Arbesman and his colleagues, demonstrated that conventional antibodies do indeed characterize the allergic state. Porter and Edelman delineated the structure of the basic immunoglobulin unit, the IgG molecule, and the Ishizakas demonstrated that antibodies of a new subclass of immunoglobulins, IgE, are responsible for the liberation from the mast cells of symptom-causing mediators in clinical allergy following exposure to the allergen. Thus, immunology became much more concerned with disease states than with the immunochemical nature of antigens, antibodies, complement, and the nature of the immune reaction in vivo, which constituted the major areas of immunologic investigation prior to the 1950s. A subdiscipline of immunology, **immunopathology**, became one of the more active areas of investigation by the 1960s and gave rise to the practice of **clinical immunology**. The milestone discovery by Claman and his colleagues of T cell-B cell interaction in the humoral (antibody) immune response, and the discovery of the lymphokines which are mediators secreted from sensitized cells stimulated by the specific antigen, prepared the groundwork for the discovery and understanding of the various types of **primary immunodeficiency diseases** first postulated in the mid-1960s. The discovery of **suppressor cells** in the late 1960s as regulators of the immune response provided a new dimension toward the understanding and treatment of immunodeficiency and autoimmune diseases. Organ transplantation (kidney, heart, lung), which was a figment of the imagination in the 1950s and considered to be only a remote possibility in the early 1960s, became a reality in the 1970s. In the field of oncology, the application of immunologic principles resulted in the demonstration of circulating tumor-specific antigens in patients afflicted with aggressively growing tumors. Recurrence of the tumor in a treated patient can be monitored by analysis for the circulating tumor-specific antigen. However, as the decade of the 1970s came to a close, it became apparent that all is not milk and honey. The treatment of patients with immunodeficiency diseases is more apparent than real, and the treatment of patients with cancer, autoimmune diseases, and allografts (to inhibit rejection of the allografts) is still dependent upon the administration of powerful, highly toxic, nonspecific "all purpose" drugs.

If history records that the 1960s and 1970s bore witness to the explosion in the number of diseases with an immunologic etiology and pathogenesis, the 1980s and 1990s will hopefully bear witness to improvements in the treatment and prevention of these diseases.

CHAPTER 3

The Chemistry of Antibodies (or *Anti*-foreign *Bodies*)

Tiselius and Kabat, in the late 1930s, introduced the technique of electrophoresis to permit the separation of protein molecules on the basis of net electric charge at a particular pH and buffer composition and concentration. When human serum undergoes electrophoresis in barbital buffer pH 8.6, the serum proteins migrate as five distinct, identifiable bands.

The proteins in the most rapidly migrating band were shown to be soluble in 50% saturated ammonium sulfate solution and, therefore, were named albumin to maintain a consistency in the nomenclature of the serum proteins. The proteins in each of the remaining four bands were shown to precipitate in the 50% saturated ammonium sulfate solution and, therefore, in accordance with tradition, they were all named globulins. The most rapidly migrating of these was given the prefix α_1 and the slowest migrating proteins were given the prefix γ or gamma. The five migrating bands of proteins were, therefore, designated albumin(s), α_1, α_2, β, and γ globulins (Fig. 7.6). Fortuitously, all antibodies were found to migrate only with the gamma globulins when subjected to electrophoresis under standard conditions. At first (in the early 1950s), it was assumed that the gamma globulins were homogeneous; however, it quickly became apparent that heterogeneity, rather than homogeneity, is the rule.

By the early 1960s, three classes of gamma globulin molecules had been identified. These were classified as γG, γM, and γA. Following immunization, antibodies could be detected in all of these classes of gamma globulins. A study commissioned by the World Health Organization in the 1960s suggested that the prefix "immunoglobulin" or Ig be used to designate any family or class of serum proteins exhibiting antibody activity. Since only the gamma globulin classes possessed antibody activity, these were named IgG, IgM, and IgA. Shortly thereafter a new class of gamma globulins was discovered, and it was promptly named

IgD. Unfortunately, this class of gamma globulins did not live up to its name, as no antibody activity could be found associated with it. The most recent class of gamma globulins, the IgE, was discovered by K. and T. Ishizaka, who showed conclusively that immunoglobulins in the IgE class are responsible for the initiation of the allergic reaction. There are, therefore, five distinct and immunologically defined classes of immunoglobulins—IgG, IgM, IgA, IgD, and IgE (Table 3.1).

The basic structural unit of an immunoglobulin consists of two light (L) peptide chains and two heavy (H) peptide chains held together by disulphide bonds (Fig. 3.1). This four-chain structure is common to all immunoglobulin molecules. The light chains on the different immunoglobulin molecules are antigenically identical; however, the heavy chains are antigenically different for each of the immunoglobulin classes, thus imparting to them their antigenically distinctive properties.

Pepsin digestion of the IgG molecule results in the recovery of a large antigen-binding fragment, referred to as the $F(ab)_2$ fragment (Fig. 3.1). The designation $F(ab)_2$ refers to the fragment of IgG which displays the antigen-binding property of the antibody molecule. Each IgG molecule has two antigen-binding sites located at the amino terminal ends of the $F(ab)_2$ fragment through which interaction with the antigen is accomplished. Both the untreated antibody molecules and the $F(ab)_2$ fragments are able to precipitate or agglutinate with the antigen, providing they are present in sufficiently high concentration.

Papain digestion of the IgG molecule results in the liberation of three fragments—two F(ab) and one Fc (Fig. 3.1). Each F(ab) fragment has only one antigen-binding site and, therefore, cannot precipitate or agglutinate with the antigen, irrespective of its concentration. It behaves serologically as a hapten (see Chapters 4 and 5). The designation Fc was given to the crystallizable residual non-antigen-binding fragment of the IgG molecule following papain digestion.

Each of the light (L) and heavy (H) chains of the IgG immunoglobulin molecule is characterized by regions which have constant amino acid sequences and regions which have variable amino acid sequences. These regions are referred to as the constant (C) and variable (V) domains on the L and H chains (Fig. 3.1). Within the variable domains there exist segments which have such markedly variable amino acid sequences from one immunoglobulin molecule to the next that they are referred to as hypervariable regions. It can be calculated that the number of possible different amino acid sequences which can affect the 8 to 10 amino acids at the N-terminal region of the Fab segment

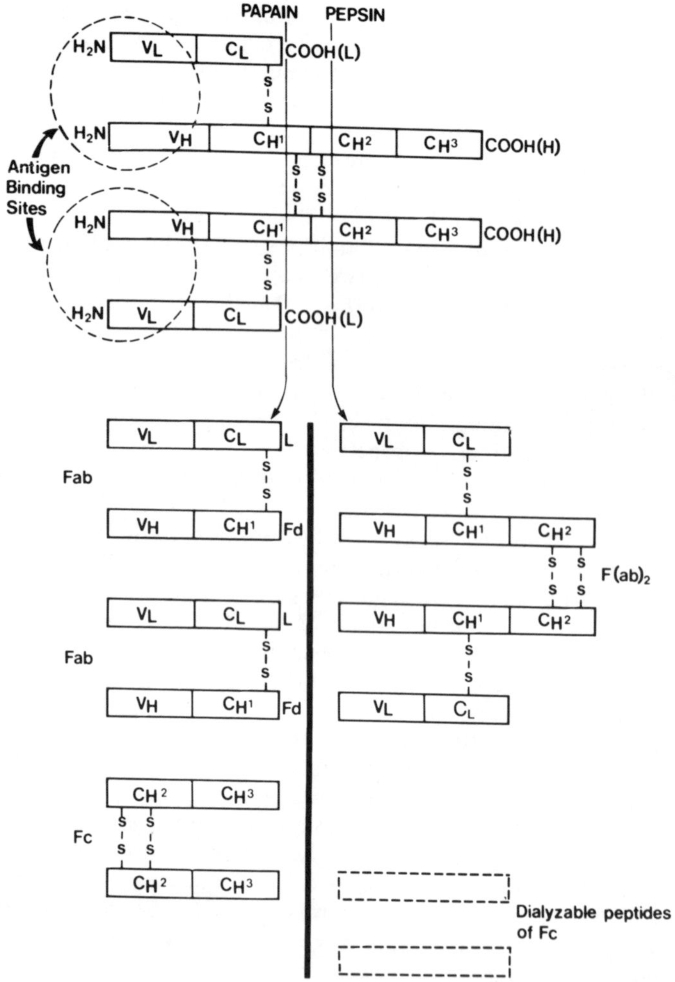

Figure 3.1 *A diagrammatic representation of the IgG immunoglobulin molecule: the location of the antigen-binding sites and the differing effects of degradation by papain and pepsin.*

of the immunoglobulin molecule, that region of the molecule which constitutes the antigen-binding site, greatly exceeds the number of antigenic determinants so far encountered in serology.

There is a certain homology, or similarity in composition, within various regions of the heavy (H) chains of the immunoglobulins in the different immunoglobulin classes which suggests

Table 3.1
Properties of the Circulating and Secretory Immunoglobulins

Immunoglobulin Class	Concentration	Type of Light Chain (mol wt 25,000)	Type of Heavy Chain (mol wt 50,000)	No. of Four-chain Units in Immunoglobulin Molecule	Biologic Function	Complement-fixing Ability
	mg%					
Total Ig	800–2,00					
IgG	600–1,600	k or λ	λ	1	Circulating antibodies (protective) Tissue fluid antibodies (protective)	Yes
IgA	150–400	k or λ	α	1 in serum 2 in secretions	Antibodies in secretion	No
IgM	50–200	k or λ	μ	5	Circulating antibodies (protective)	Yes
IgD	2–10	k or λ	δ	1	?	No
IgE	0.2–1.0	k or λ	ϵ	1	Antibodies which mediate the allergic reaction	No

similar origins for the different immunoglobulins. Nevertheless, the marked differences in composition which characterize the variable regions of the heavy chains of the different immunoglobulin classes impart distinct antigenicity to them when they are injected into the xenogeneic animal (Fig. 3.2). Thus, the immune system of a rabbit or goat, injected with the heavy (H) chains of the different human immunoglobulins, can differentiate between them and synthesize antibodies directed specifically toward the variable regions of the IgG, IgM, IgA, IgD, and IgE heavy (H) chains. These antibodies are, therefore, specific for the IgG, IgM, IgA, IgD, and IgE immunoglobulins (Fig. 3.2). These immunoglobulin-specific antisera are used routinely in even the most modest Clinical Immunology Service, frequently functioning in (forced) disguise as part of a Clinical Biochemistry Service, for the quantitative determination of the immunoglobulin classes in the circulation (radial immunodiffusion test) and for the assessment of the monoclonal or polyclonal nature of the immunoglobulins (immunoelectrophoresis) (see Chapter 7).

The reader will appreciate that differences in the amino acid

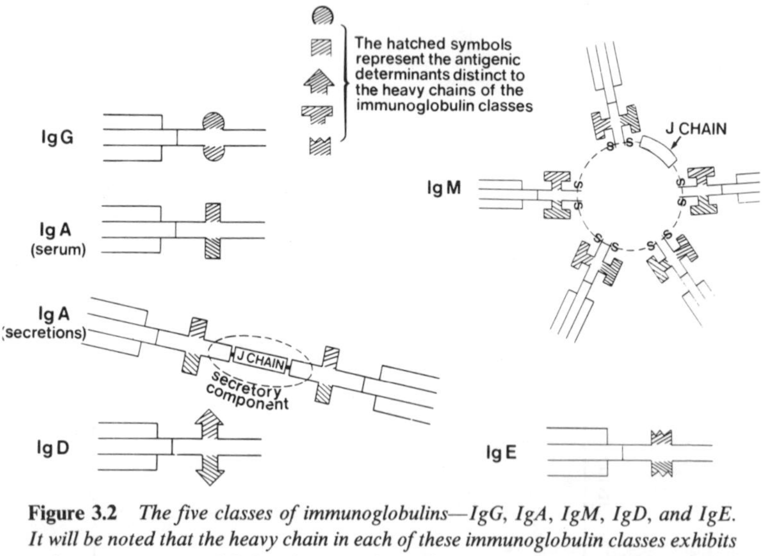

Figure 3.2 *The five classes of immunoglobulins—IgG, IgA, IgM, IgD, and IgE. It will be noted that the heavy chain in each of these immunoglobulin classes exhibits a distinctive immunoglobulin class-specific configuration (and probably amino acid sequence) toward the COOH-terminal region of the chain. These different configurations are recognized by the xenogeneic animal (i.e. the rabbit or goat) as distinct antigens, and the animal, therefore, produces antibodies specific for the heavy chains of each of these immunoglobulin classes.*

sequence and/or composition translate into differences in configuration. The amino acid sequence and composition impart to the antigen-binding region of the antibody molecule a unique configuration which permits it to bind to only one antigen to the exclusion of all other antigens. In other words, the antigen and antibody are configurationally complementary at their sites of interaction. The effect of a distinct amino acid sequence at the antigen-binding site of the antibody molecule is to impart to it a unique antigenicity. In fact, it has been demonstrated that the Fab regions of IgG antibody molecules directed toward different antigens, obtained from the same individual, exhibit antigenic specificity. This can be demonstrated in the following way. If human IgG antibodies to diphtheria toxoid (D.t.) are injected into a rabbit, the rabbit forms antibodies directed toward various antigenic determinant sites on the human IgG molecules, including the antigen-binding site designated as Ab (D.t.) (Fig. 3.3). If the rabbit anti-human IgG antiserum is absorbed with human IgG antibodies to tetanus toxoid, obtained from the same individual who supplied the IgG antibodies to diphtheria toxoid, all the rabbit anti-human IgG antibodies will be absorbed except for those rabbit antibodies directed specifically toward the antigen-binding sites on the human IgG antidiphtheria toxoid antibodies (Fig. 3.3). Thus, human antibodies of the same class (i.e. IgG) directed toward different antigens can be distinguished on the basis of the antigenic specificity of the antigen-binding site. This is referred to as the **idiotype** or **idiotypic specificity** of the immunoglobulin molecule, a characteristic which is not genetically transmitted. Thus, different antibody molecules of the same immunoglobulin class in the same individul are characterized by different idiotypic specificities. On the other hand, other markers (detected by their antigenicity in both humans and other animal species) referred to as **allotypes** or **allotypic markers** are genetically transmitted, with the result that all of the immunoglobulin molecules of the same individual will exhibit the same markers. Several of these allotypic markers are the INV and Gm markers, and they exist on the light and heavy chains of the immunoglobulin molecules.

PROPERTIES OF IMMUNOGLOBULIN CLASSES

Each of the immunoglobulin classes appears to have a distinct role to play—either by providing protective immunity or inducing pathology in the host.

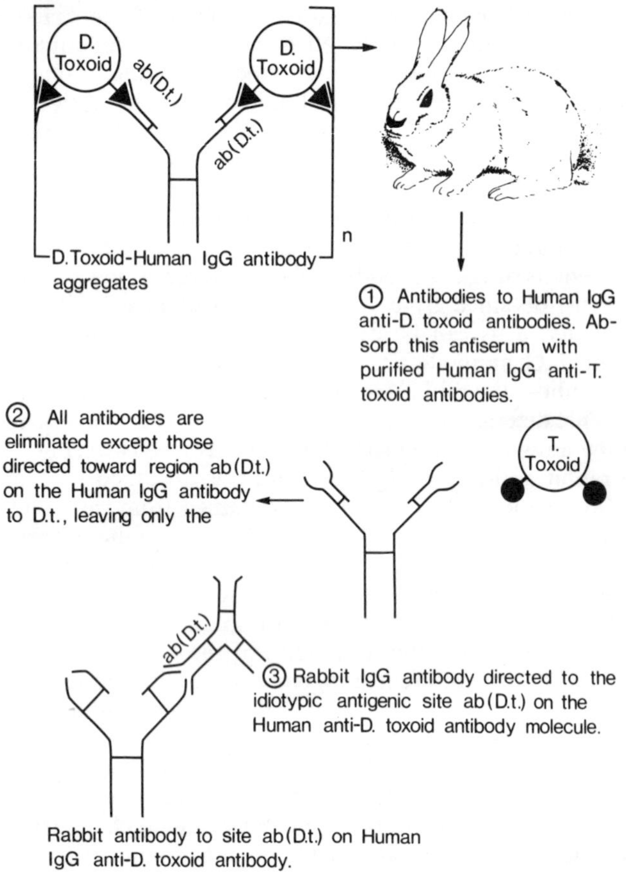

Figure 3.3 *The demonstration, via diagrammatic representation, of the antigenic specificity of the idiotypic sites of an antibody molecule.*

IgG

The IgG antibodies exist only as monomers (the basic four-chain units) (Fig. 3.2) and are found primarily in the circulation, where they normally constitute the bulk of antibody activity (Table 3.1). Some IgG antibodies may also be present in the interstitial fluid because these molecules, in view of their relatively small size (compared to IgM antibodies) can traverse, by emperipolesis, the stretched endothelial cells lining the postcapillary venules, especially at the stretched-out intercellular junctions. IgG antibodies are also found, albeit in low concentration, in secretions. The IgG antibodies are synthesized by the lymphocyte-plasma cell series of cells within the lymph nodes and the spleen. The IgG synthesizing cells appear to be limited to those lymph nodes directly accessible to or draining portals of entry in the peripheral parts of the body. They consist of the popliteal, inguinal, epitrochlear, axillary, and cervical lymph nodes rather than the deep thoracic and abdominal lymph nodes.

The IgG antibodies or IgG immunoglobulins can be segregated on the basis of genetically acquired surface configurations (which are distinct antigenic determinants when injected into a rabbit) into four subclasses—IgG-1, IgG-2, IgG-3, and IgG-4. The majority (75%) of induced antibodies are IgG-1 and IgG-3 immunoglobulins. They are also the primary complement-fixing antibodies. The IgG-2 and IgG-4 antibodies, on the other hand, fix complement poorly or not at all. Although placental transfer is restricted to the IgG immunoglobulins, the different subclasses of the IgG immunoglobulins differ in their capacity to cross the placenta; the IgG-1 immunoglobulins most easily cross the placental barrier while the IgG-2 immunoglobulins are the least endowed to do so.

Another property which distinguishes the immunoglobulins in the four IgG subclasses is their ability to bind to the macrophage receptor directed to the Fc of IgG. Thus, macrophages bind to the Fc of IgG-1 and IgG-3 but not to the Fc of IgG-2 and IgG-4 immunoglobulins.

Although these in vitro criteria which distinguish between the immunoglobulins in the four different IgG subclasses may appear to be trivial or subtle and their relevance from the immunochemical point of view rather obscure, their significance from a functional point of view becomes very apparent when considering the consequences should the individual synthesize antibodies incapable of facilitating complement fixation or phagocytosis. Such an individual will present with symptoms of immunodeficiency disease which may not be correctly diagnosed due to the presence of IgG immunoglobulins in the circulation in a significant concentration. The physician must be astute enough to recognize that circulating IgG and antibody-deficient immunodeficiency disease are not incompatible simultaneous findings if the IgG can be demonstrated to be primarily IgG-2 and IgG-4. Antibodies in these categories of IgG do not function well, if at all, as protective antibodies in the immunologic sense since they cannot fix complement and cannot enhance phagocytosis of the invading organism.

IgM

IgM antibodies are generally of the protective variety (Table 3.1) and exist as pentamers in the circulation (Fig. 3.2). The five basic four-chain units are held together by a high molecular weight peptide called the J (joining) chain (mol wt 15,000). Due to their large size, IgM antibodies are restricted to the circulation. On an equal mole basis, IgM antibodies are the most effective immunologically as each molecule possesses 10 antigen-binding sites. Due to the close proximity of the four-chain units, IgM antibodies are also more efficient at fixing complement than are the IgG antibody molecules, especially at threshold antibody concentration.

IgA

The IgA proteins are the predominant immunoglobulins in secretions bathing mucosal surfaces (Table 3.1). These tissues are frequently in direct continuity with and exposed to the external environment and, therefore, provide the portals of entry to and the first line of defense toward penetration and invasion by pathogenic microorganisms. The antibacterial and antiviral protection afforded by secretions is directly attributable to their content of specific IgA antibodies, although they also contain small quantities of IgG and traces of IgM antibodies. The ratio of IgA antibodies to IgG antibodies in secretions is usually the reverse of that which exists in the blood. The ratio of IgA:IgG in secretions is normally 4:1 to 6:1, whereas the ratio of IgA:IgG in serum is 1:3 to 1:6.

The secretions which exhibit IgA antibodies include saliva, tears, sputum, sweat, gastric juice, bronchial secretion, vaginal secretion, semen, and breast milk. In view of the fact that only IgG immunoglobulins can pass through the placenta, the newborn is normally deficient of IgA antibodies. Therefore, the only way for the neonate to acquire IgA antibodies is via the breast milk, which constitutes a good reason to encourage breastfeeding of infants. Furthermore, the IgA antibodies in breast milk are directed toward the pathogenic microorganisms most frequently encountered in the external environment by the mother and are those which would tend to parasitize and invade the gastrointestinal tract of the neonate.

The IgA antibodies are essentially protective antibodies capable of neutralizing antigens and pathogens at the portal of entry. They have not been directly implicated in the induction of pathology. In the gastrointestinal tract, IgA antibodies can be detected in intestinal contents following deliberate ingestion of live attenuated polio virus (Sabin vaccine) (oral immunization) or the unintentional ingestion of pathogenic bacteria such as *Vibrio cholerae* or *Salmonella typhi*. These intestinal (or copro) antibodies neutralize exotoxins and endotoxins and prevent the

Important

The antibodies formed following oral immunization with the Sabin polio vaccine are primarily IgA antibodies limited to the gastrointestinal tract. On the other hand, the antibodies synthesized following parenteral immunization with the killed polio virus (Salk vaccine) are primarily IgG antibodies localized to the circulation. Thus, parenteral immunization with the killed virus results in immunity to systemic infection with the polio virus but does not prevent the establishment of the carrier state. On the other hand, oral immunization with the live, attenuated virus results in long-term secretory IgA synthesis and prevention of the carrier state but no systemic immunity. It is obvious, therefore, that the ideal immunization to polio virus should consist of initial parenteral immunization with the killed virus followed by oral immunization with the attenuated virus. The decision by different public health bodies to recommend immunization with only one of the polio vaccines, the Salk or the Sabin, but not with both vaccines, defies logic and runs counter to our present appreciation of the roles of the different immunoglobulins in the provision of resistance.

adherence of the microorganisms to the intestinal mucosal cells and thereby their colonization and invasion into the body proper.

The IgA antibodies occur primarily as dimers in secretions and as monomers in the serum (Fig. 3.2). The IgA dimer is composed of two basic four-chain units held together by a polypeptide called the J chain (mol wt 15,000) and a larger protein molecule referred to as secretory component (mol. wt. 70,000). Secretory component appears to wrap itself around the Fc segments of the two juxtaposed four-chain monomer units. The greater rigidity and protection afforded to the IgA dimer by the J chain and secretory component probably impart to the molecule a greater stability in comparison to the other immunoglobulins, thus rendering it less susceptible to degradation by highly potent enzymes and acids especially present in the gastrointestinal tract. Presumably, the Fab sites are protected from denaturation by the gastric juice (pH 1 to 3) and enzymatic digestion in the stomach (by pepsin) or the intestine (by trypsin, chymotrypsin, etc.) by the presence of the J chain and the secretory component.

IgA is synthesized by cells of the lymphocyte-plasma cell series present in large numbers in the Peyer's patches and lamina propria of the gastrointestinal tract and in the connective tissues beneath the mucosa along the respiratory tract. A larger proportion of the plasma cells in these locations stain for IgA by immunofluorescence as compared to the plasma cells in the peripheral anatomically distinct lymphoid tissues (spleen, lymph nodes). The IgA monomers and dimers are both synthesized by the same plasma cell, the ratio of monomer to dimer depending upon the cell's capacity to synthesize the J chain. Thus, the monomeric IgA molecules which interact with the J chain are secreted as the IgA dimer. Both the IgA monomers and dimers diffuse through the submucosal connective tissue, diffuse through the mucosal basement membrane, and enter the intercellular spaces between the epithelial cells lining the basement membrane. However, only the IgA dimer is capable of interacting with the secretory component lining the epithelial cell membrane. This interaction is essential to facilitate the active transport of the IgA dimer through the epithelial cell and its secretion from the cell into the lumen. On the other hand, the IgA monomers secreted by the submucosal plasma cells (not complexed with the J chain) cannot traverse the mucosal basement membrane; these molecules diffuse toward and into the lymphatics and thence into the circulation, where they constitute the serum IgA.

Serum IgA consists of two subclasses—IgA-1 and IgA-2, identified serologically on the basis of antigenic differences (when injected into the xenogeneic animal) in the heavy chains. Ninety per cent of circulating IgA is composed of monomeric IgA-1 and approximately 10% is monomeric IgA-2. IgA-1 proteins are synthesized primarily in the extraintestinal, extramucosal lymphoid tissues, especially the spleen and bone marrow. On the other hand, the high percentage of IgA-2 immunoglobulins in mucosal secretions (35%) is reflected by the much higher percentage of IgA-2, compared to IgA-1, secreting plasma cells in gastrointestinal, bronchial, salivary, and mammary gland mucosae. Thus, the IgA-1 and IgA-2 proteins are, to certain degrees, synthesized in anatomically distinct organs, the IgA-1 by plasma cells in the lymph nodes, spleen, and bone marrow and the IgA-2 mainly by mucosally related plasma cells.

These findings explain the discordant, if not paradoxical, observations made in some patients in whom a deficiency of serum IgA is not reflected by a deficiency of secretory IgA. In other words, lack of serum IgA is frequently associated with an asymptomatic condition since the concentration of IgA in the secretions, where it constitutes the primary specific immunity, is normal or only slightly below normal. Serum IgA does not appear to be relevant in the provision of specific antibody-mediated immunity.

IgE

IgE immunoglobulins are present in the circulation in an exceedingly low, sometimes undetectable, concentration even utilizing the extremely sensitive radioimmunoassay for their detection (Table 3.1). Although IgE antibodies do not confer immunity of a classical (protective) nature to the host, they are responsible for some of the most serious life-threatening immunologically mediated conditions which one can encounter in the emergency ward—circulatory collapse and shock due to anaphylaxis, and respiratory failure secondary to bronchoconstriction due to or coincident with status asthmaticus (see Chapter 14).

IgE antibodies initiate the allergic reactions which are mediated by vasoactive amines released as a consequence of the basophil and/or mast cell-bound IgE antibody-allergen reaction. IgE antibodies adhere strongly to surface structures (receptors) on the mast cell and basophil. Interaction of these cell-bound IgE antibodies with the specific allergen results in the induction of lesions in the cell membrane and eventual degranulation and discharge of histamine, serotonin, eosinophil chemotactic factor, etc., all of which are normally stored in an inactive state within the metachromatically stained granules. The cells are not necessarily killed by the antibody-allergen reaction, as the damage inflicted as a consequence of this reaction is often reversible.

IgD

Thus far, with the exception of several investigations which purport to assign antibody activity to the IgD immunoglobulins, it is fair to conclude that antibodies have not been found to be associated with the IgD immunoglobulins. It has been shown that some of the circulating antibodies directed toward specific food allergens in patients allergic to these foods are IgD proteins. It has also been reported that some myeloma proteins of the IgD class can interact in vitro with certain selected antigens. Thus, the old axiom "seek well and thou shalt find" is alive and well in the field of immunoglobulins. However, to place things in proper perspective, the overwhelming majority of investigations aimed at demonstrating antibody activity associated with the IgD immunoglobulins have been unsuccessful in this regard. Therefore, the immunologic significance and role of this class of immunoglobulins can only be conjectured at the present time. During embryogenesis, IgD molecules appear on the surface of the B cell within 10 to 12 weeks of gestation, shortly after the appearance of IgM immunoglobulins on the B cell. This consistent finding suggests that IgD immunoglobulins were synthesized at one stage during the evolution of the species. The fact that IgD immunoglobulins do not appear to possess antibody activity postnatally in any of the species investigated would suggest that they had limited survival value, and Darwinian evolution dictated that IgD antibody synthesis stop, if in fact it ever occurred. IgD immunoglobulin may have been a primitive type of antibody synthesized during the early period of the phylogenetic development of the immune response. One reason for its demise may be its inability to fix complement, a property of great survival value if the antibody is to facilitate lysis of invading microorganisms (Table 3.1). IgG immunoglobulins, which fix complement, probably evolved subsequent to or concurrent with the appearance of complement and displaced IgD immunoglobulins in the further development of the immune response.

Important

It is important to note that only a minority of the molecules in any one of the immunoglobulin classes are, in fact, antibody molecules. By far the majority of the molecules are either redundant or are antibodies directed toward any or all of the myriad of antigens, many unidentified, to which we are exposed throughout our lives. Following accepted immunization procedures, it is rare for the antibody concentration in any of the immunoglobulin classes to exceed 10 to 20 mg%. Even after intense hyperimmunization in the experimental animal, the antibody concentration in the IgG class rarely exceeds 50 to 100 mg%, or less than 10% of the total IgG concentration.

CHAPTER 4

The Chemistry of Antigens (or *Anti*body *Gen*erating Factor)

Unlike antibody molecules, which are homogeneous within each class of immunoglobulins and which differ primarily in the amino acid composition at the N-terminal regions of the light and heavy chains of the Fab region (the antigen-binding sites), antigens come in all shapes, sizes, and composition. The term "antigen" is used to define a molecule which possesses antigenic determinants capable of inducing antibody formation. These antigenic determinants constitute only a very small percentage of the surface structure of the molecule. Antigenic sites have been shown to be composed of peptides consisting of 4 to 12 amino acids. Some general characteristics of antigens are as follows:

1. Antigens can be proteins, glycoproteins, lipoproteins, and nucleoproteins. The antigenic determinant sites are usually within the protein constituent of the antigen. The carbohydrate, lipid, and nucleic acid constituents are not in themselves antigenic or are weakly antigenic. A number of microbially derived carbohydrates, such as the pneumococcal polysaccharides and some synthetic derivatives of simple sugars such as dextran, are antigenic. These carbohydrate antigens are distinguished by their polymeric composition.

2. In general, the number of antigenic determinant sites on a molecule increases as the molecular weight of the molecule increases (Table 4.1).

3. In general, a protein is more antigenic if it is globular than if it is fibrillar in structure or if it possesses a rigid structure.

4. In general, a protein is more antigenic if it is catabolized in vivo than if it is not susceptible to enzymatic digestion.

5. In general, a protein is more antigenic if it has retention ability than if it is eliminated by one or two excursions through the kidney.

Table 4.1
The Relationship between Molecular Weight of the Antigen and the Number of Antigenic Determinant Sites

Antigen	Molecular Weight	Number of Antigenic Sites
Egg albumin	22,000	5
Human serum albumin	70,000	8–10
Human gamma globulin (IgG)	150,000	18–20
Human fibrinogen	400,000	30–40
Human red blood cell		>50,000

6. An antigen must be foreign to the circulation of the host.

A "hapten" is defined as a small molecular weight entity which, by itself, is incapable of inducing an immune response but which can interact with antibody directed against it. It becomes antigenic when coupled chemically to a large "schlepper" or carrier protein or if it autocouples spontaneously to autologous proteins following its administration. In this state, the hapten is transformed into an antigenic determinant on the carrier molecule and is capable of inducing the formation of antibodies directed to it and of interacting with the antibodies in vitro to give a precipitin reaction. Examples of haptens are drugs such as penicillin, sulphonamides, tranquilizers, anesthetics, and aspirin (acetylsalicylic acid).

By far the major, if not the paramount, contributions to our understanding of the composition of antigenic determinants must be credited to Karl Landsteiner. Between the years 1910 and 1940, Landsteiner conducted systematic investigations, along chemical lines, to define the specificity of the immune reaction. Landsteiner coined the term hapten for a low molecular weight, chemically defined compound which could only induce antibody formation when coupled to a larger carrier protein molecule. Landsteiner summarized the results of his investigations in his book entitled *The Specificity of the Serological Reaction*, which must be considered even today to be a classic, unsurpassed in its critical evaluation and elucidation of this area of immunology.

Landsteiner coupled phenylated acids, such as aminophenylarsonic (arsanilic), aminophenylbenzoic, and aminophenylsulfonic (sulfanilic) acids, to carrier proteins and observed that antibodies to the haptens formed in the rabbit were highly specific in their capacity to interact with the haptens. In this way Landsteiner demonstrated the extreme specificity of the antigen-antibody reaction. He also immunized rabbits with ortho-, meta-, and para-aminophenylarsonic acid-protein conjugates. These three arsonic acid derivatives are referred to as homologous haptens. Landsteiner showed that antibodies produced in the rabbit immunized with the ortho-aminophenylarsonic acid-protein carrier conjugate reacted primarily, if not only, with ortho-aminophenylarsonic acid, and to only a limited extent, if at all, with meta-aminophenylarsonic acid and para-aminophenylarsonic acid (Table 4.2). Similarly, the antibodies produced to the meta- and para-aminophenylarsonic acid haptens reacted only with the immunizing haptens. These results indicate that the immunogenicity of an antigenic determinant is relatively independent of its general chemical (elemental) composition but is dependent upon its overall configuration.

Findings of a similar nature with other unrelated compounds, such as dextran, bacterial polysaccharides, and synthetic polypeptides, have disclosed that the antigenic determinant need not be larger than a hexasaccharide (in the case of dextran) or a tetrapeptide (in the case of synthetic peptides). Furthermore, when the antigenic determinant is a terminal sequence on a synthetic polymer or a peptide linked covalently to a carrier protein, the terminal sugar or amino acid exerts the most dominant influence in terms of immunologic specificity. Thus, the antibody-binding site on the Fab region of the IgG antibody molecule must, at the very least, be of a dimension to accommodate six monosaccharide units or four amino acid residues. As discussed in Chapter 3, variations in the sequence and composi-

Table 4.2
The Relationship between the Structure of a Hapten Moiety and Its Capacity to Interact with Antihapten Antibodies Produced to a Homologous Hapten

Rabbit Immunized with Carrier Conjugated with	Reactivity of Antibodies with Respect to		
	Ortho-amino-phenylarsonic Acid	Meta-amino-phenylarsonic Acid	Para-amino-phenylarsonic Acid
Ortho-aminophenylarsonic acid	+++	±	±
Meta-aminophenylarsonic acid	−	+++	±
Para-aminophenylarsonic acid	−	−	+++

tion of the 8 to 10 N-terminal amino acids in the L and H chains of the Fab region of the antibody molecule could theoretically account for the necessary configurations and dimensions to accommodate all possible antigenic determinants.

It should be stressed that the antigenic determinants on a molecule need not be identical. There is no rule or formula which can be used to predict the proportion of identical and nonidentical antigen determinant sites on a molecule. Thus, some antigens possess large numbers of the identical antigenic determinant and other antigens display many serologically unrelated antigenic determinants in varying numbers. The former category consists of polymers composed of repeating identical subunits and includes dextran, the pneumococcal polysaccharides, Salmonella flagellin, polyvinylpyrrolidone, and synthetic polypeptide antigens. The majority of the naturally occurring antigens and those used for prophylactic immunization belong to the latter category, that is, antigens characterized by numerous, randomly distributed, unrelated antigen determinant sites.

ADJUVANTS

The immunogenicity, or the capacity to induce antibody formation, of an antigen or a hapten-carrier conjugate can be varied depending on the manner of administration of the antigen or hapten-carrier conjugate. Antibody synthesis to an antigen can be greatly augmented if it is administered together with or emulsified in any of a number of unrelated nonantigenic agents. These agents are referred to collectively as "adjuvants." The first adjuvant specifically utilized to enhance antibody synthesis was introduced by Freund in the late 1940s. It consists of three constituents—a mineral oil (Bayol), a detergent (Arlacel-A), and killed *Mycobacterium tuberculosis.* When a protein antigen is emulsified in this adjuvant prior to its initial (primary) administration into the animal via the subcutaneous or intramuscular route, it will be observed that the latent period of antibody synthesis is not significantly altered, but the concentration of circulating antibodies at the time of peak titer will be several magnitudes (10 to 100 times) higher and the duration of the immune response will be 3 to 5 times longer as compared to the immune response observed following primary immunization without the adjuvant. A nonantigen or a material normally displaying poor immunogenicity can be converted into a potent antigen if it is administered together with the adjuvant. Furthermore, the quantity of the antigen administered may be reduced by more than 90% without affecting the immune response if it is injected emulsified in the adjuvant.

The three-component adjuvant introduced by Freund is referred to as "complete Freund's adjuvant" (CFA) as compared to the two-component (Bayol and Arlacel-A) adjuvant referred to as "incomplete Fruend's adjuvant." The latter is not nearly as effective an adjuvant as is the complete adjuvant.

Although the complete Freund's adjuvant has been used extensively in animal investigations, its use in the human is limited due to the fact that it often induces the formation of very painful sterile abscesses which progress to ulcer formation and scarring. There have also been scattered reports that it is carcinogenic or that it promotes the induction of "spontaneous" tumors.

A number of other adjuvants which have been used experimentally are aluminum hydroxide, calcium alginate, and endotoxins of gram-negative bacteria.

The mechanism of action of the adjuvants is far from clear. The different actions may act in a synergistic fashion to facilitate what would otherwise be referred to as a hyperimmune response. Several adjuvant-induced actions are as follows:

1. Retention of the antigen at the site of injection for a long period of time and its slow release into the circulation. The effect is to provide an antigenic stimulus over a long period of time.
2. Stimulation of the reticuloendothelial (phagocytic) system. Not only are these cells increased in number, but their phagocytic activity is greatly enhanced.
3. Induction of cellular differentiation and proliferation in the draining lymph nodes and spleen, especially following the injection of the complete Freund's adjuvant. The spleen and particularly the draining lymph nodes are much enlarged and hyperplastic. The lymphoid follicles may be very much enlarged and may merge to the point that they obliterate the interfollicular spaces. Histologically, the picture may resemble one of giant follicular lymphoma with many blast cells and binucleate cells displaying minimal degrees of anaplasia and pleomorphism. Of course, there is no malignant transformation, and normal architecture and morphology are re-established within 2 to 4 weeks following the administration of the adjuvant.

The return to cytologic normalcy may be attributed to the action of suppressor cells induced by the Freund's adjuvant. As is discussed in Chapter 8, these cells function to inhibit the immune response. One action of suppressor cells is the abrogation of antigen-driven cellular (immunocyte) proliferation. It is not unreasonable to assume that suppressor cells are also capable of inhibiting adjuvant-stimulated cellular proliferation.

CHAPTER 5

The Cellular Basis of Antibody Formation (The Humoral Immune Response)

Knowledge of the antibody or humoral immune response stems primarily from analyses of the immune responses of mice and rabbits injected on one (primary immune response) or more (secondary or anamnestic immune response) occasions over a short period of time with very large doses of antigens. The knowledge of the immune response as it was accepted until the mid-1960s can be summarized in the following statements. These are restricted to events induced in the primary immune response so as not to confuse the reader with the secondary immune response, which is discussed later.

1. Antibodies can invariably be detected in the circulation by 2 to 4 days (mice) and 5 to 7 days (rabbits) following immunization. Antibody levels attain a peak 2 to 4 days later and antibodies persist in the circulation, in diminishing concentration, for 1 to 2 weeks (mice) and 4 to 6 weeks (rabbits).

2. The first antibodies to be detected are IgM antibodies. However, the IgM antibodies are almost totally displaced by IgG antibodies 2 to 4 days later.

3. During the latent (preantibody) phase of the immune response, mitotic figures can be observed at the corticomedullary junction in the lymph node and in the inner and outer marginal zones of the splenic follicles, giving rise to large numbers of pyroninophilic (blast) cells.

4. During the phase of active antibody synthesis, significant numbers of plasma cells can be seen along the medullary cords in the lymph node and the red pulp in the spleen.

5. By a combination of immunofluorescence and phase microscopy, some antibody-laden cells can be identified as plasma cells.

6. Antibody-containing cells at the peak of antibody synthesis transiently invade the circulation and infiltrate all the lymphoid

organs (including the thymus), the liver, the kidneys, and the bone marrow.

7. Antibodies are present in relatively low concentration in the circulation by 4 to 6 weeks postimmunization (rabbit), which coincides with the return to normal architecture of the spleen and lymph nodes.

8. Within 4 to 6 weeks postimmunization (rabbit), antibody-forming cells in an active phase of synthesis can no longer be detected in any of the lymphoid organs. However, cells capable of being rapidly reactivated can be detected in the spleen. These cells are referred to as **memory cells** and are morphologically identical to small, mature lymphocytes.

To facilitate a more in-depth appreciation of the humoral immune response, it is necessary to elaborate upon the statements presented above. It is not inappropriate to dissect the immune response into its noncellular and cellular components. Let us first discuss the noncellular aspects of the immune response. The characteristic features and the sequence of their appearance are:

1. A latent or eclipse period, which varies with the species of animal used and which refers to the interval of time between the injection of the antigen and the appearance of circulating antibody. The latent period may vary from 2 to 3 days in mice, rats, and guinea pigs; 5 to 7 days in rabbits; 8 to 10 days in dogs; and 10 to 20 days in humans.

2. The period of active synthesis and secretion of antibodies (antibody synthesis > antibody catabolism).

3. The period characterized by a static antibody level often referred to as the plateau phase of the antibody synthesis curve (antibody synthesis = antibody catabolism).

4. The period of antibody decay (antibody synthesis < antibody catabolism).

5. Absence of circulating antibody. The concentration of antibodies falls to a level where it is asymptotic with the horizontal axis. Antibodies can still be detected using highly sensitive radioimmunoassay techniques. This phase will not occur until weeks or months postimmunization. It, too, varies with the species of animal used. In humans, antibodies may still be detected in low concentration in the circulation 3 to 10 years postimmunization.

IMMUNE RESPONSE

A **primary response** is that which occurs following the initial contact with the antigen. A **secondary** or **anamnestic** (memory) **response** is that which occurs after a second exposure to this same antigen months or years after the initial exposure. An immune response following a third or fourth contact with the same antigen, even years after the primary immune response, will invariably exhibit the characterisics of the secondary, and not the primary, immune response. The primary and secondary immune responses in the rabbit are compared and contrasted in Table 5.1, and the comparison is valid for all animal species. The main features which distinguish the secondary immune response from the primary immune response are:

1. A much shorter latent period (1 day as compared to 2 to 4 days in the mouse; 2 to 3 days as compared to 5 to 7 days in the rabbit; 5 to 7 days as compared to 10 to 20 days in the adult human).

2. A much longer perior of active antibody synthesis. The period during which antibody synthesis takes place in the secondary response may be 3 to 5 times longer than that which characterizes the primary immune response.

3. A much higher concentration of antibodies at the peak of antibody synthesis. The concentration of circulating antibodies at the peak of the secondary response may be 10 to 100 times greater than the antibody concentration at the peak of the primary response.

4. The time interval between the appearance of IgM (early) antibodies and IgG (late) antibodies is blurred. In the secondary response, both can be detected in the circulation almost simultaneously in contrast to the situation in the primary response when the IgM antibodies precede the appearance of the IgG antibodies by 1 to 3 days. Furthermore, the concentration of the IgM antibodies relative to that of the IgG antibodies is much lower in the secondary response compared to the relative concentrations of the IgM and IgG antibodies in the primary response.

Table 5.1
Properties of the Primary and Secondary Precipitating Antibody Responses

	Primary Response	Secondary Response
Latent period (days)	4–6	1–2
Day of maximum antibody concentration postimmunization	10–14	4–8
Duration of immune response (weeks)	4–6	8–20
Antibodies detected in the circulation	IgM initially and IgG detected 2–3 days later	IgM and IgG detected at the same time
Ratio of IgG to IgM antibodies synthesized in immune response	2:1 to 4:1	10:1 to 50:1

Important

The above statements concerning the primary humoral immune response reflect the state of knowledge attained by the late 1940s. Unfortunately, the immunologic technique utilized at the time to detect and quantitate antibodies, the quantitative precipitin test, was rather primitive by today's standards and only reflected the presence of precipitating antibodies. The proposed mechanisms of antibody formation propounded in the 1940s and 1950s were based solely on the temporal aspects of the synthesis of precipitating antibodies. The introduction of the passive hemagglutination techniques in the mid-1950s made possible the detection of antibodies irrespective of their precipitating properties. Using both the quantitative precipitin test and the passive hemagglutination technique, Richter and Haurowitz observed that nonprecipitating antibodies can be detected in the circulation in high concentration for 1 to 2 years following the cessation of synthesis of precipitating antibodies without any further immunization. However, this finding of a long period of nonprecipitating antibody synthesis does not fit into the long-established framework of immunologic theory and has not been incorporated into the hypotheses concerning the mechanism of antibody synthesis. Nevertheless, it is not improbable that the seemingly contradictory findings of a short-term period of precipitating antibody synthesis (3 to 4 weeks) and a long-term period of immunologically mediated protection (3 to 5 years) following immunization with toxoids and viruses may be resolved by the fact that toxin and viral neutralizing antibodies need not be of a precipitating nature to be detected. They may, therefore, be nonprecipitating antibodies which continue to be synthesized for long periods of time following cessation of synthesis of precipitating antibodies.

SYNTHESIS OF ANTIBODIES

Where are the antibody molecules synthesized and what are the cells involved? Until the mid-1960s it was assumed that a single pluripotent immunocompetent lymphoid cell becomes activated to antibody formation following interaction with the antigen in the primary immune response and that it gives rise to the memory cells (Fig. 5.1). Numerous investigations carried out during the late 1940s and the 1950s—especially those by Coons, Dixon, Fagraeus, the Harrises, Nossal and Miller, and their associates—established the spleen and lymph nodes as the organs in which antibody formation takes place. It was established that antibody formation takes place primarily in the spleen following

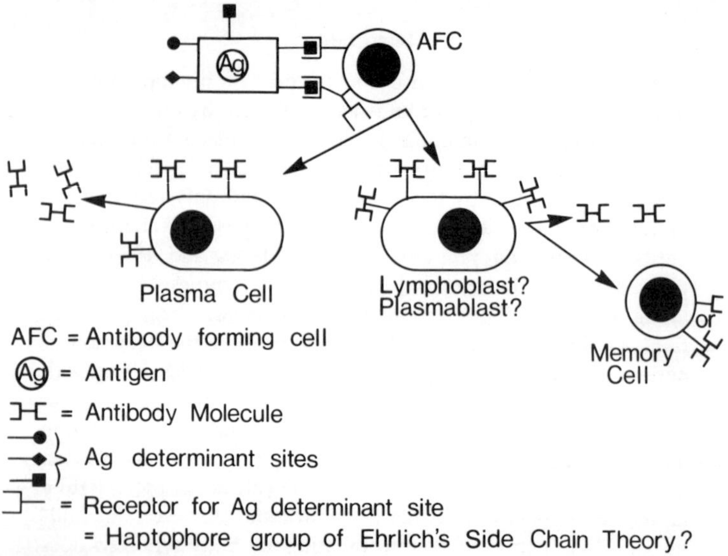

Figure 5.1 *Basic model to account for the induction of the immune response prior to the 1960s. A single pluripotent lymphoid cell was considered to be able to interact with, and be stimulated by, antigen. This cell, it was presumed, would transform following stimulation by the antigen into a lymphoblast and/or a plasmablast, during which stage it would present as an active, antibody-synthesizing and antibody-secreting cell. The memory cell, the progeny of the lymphoblast, is a small long-lived (up to 10 to 20 years) lymphocyte, present essentially in the spleen and capable of being almost instantaneously reactivated to antibody synthesis by subsequent exposure to antigen.*

intravenous injection of the antigen, and in the draining lymph nodes following intracutaneous or subcutaneous administration of the antigen. Within a short period of time, the antibody response was localized to the lymphocytic series of cells and their progeny—medium and large lymphocytes, lymphoblasts, plasmablasts, and plasma cells. On the basis of results of cell transfer experiments, different investigators attributed antibody formation to one or more of these cell types, and some investigators even attributed antibody synthesis to macrophages. Antibodies were consistently detected in high concentration in mature plasma cells by immunofluorescence, and this finding was interpreted as evidence in favor of very active antibody synthesis by the plasma cells. However, the application of tissue and single cell culture techniques did not support this interpretation. It was observed that the most active phase of antibody synthesis in vitro appeared to coincide with the generation of large lymphocytes and especially lymphoblasts and plasmablasts. Antibody synthesis was found to diminish or cease with the appearance of the mature plasma cells.

The paradox presented by antibody-laden plasma cells which do not appear to synthesize antibodies, and essentially antibody-free lymphoblasts and plasmablasts which appear to be primarily involved in antibody synthesis, can be explained in the following manner. The plasma cells contain antibodies due to the fact that, during the transformation of blast cells into mature plasma cells, the cells lose the capacity to actively secrete antibodies before they lose the capacity to synthesize antibodies, thus imparting the impression that plasma cells are actively engaged in antibody synthesis. The failure to detect significant quantities of antibodies in lymphoblasts and plasmablasts is attributed to the capacity of these cells to secrete the antibody molecules as soon as they are assembled within the cell.

Morphologic Changes in Antibody-forming Organs

Certain changes precede and accompany the synthesis and secretion of specific antibody molecules. Following subcutaneous, intracutaneous, or intramuscular immunization, the immune response is primarily localized to the regional draining lymph nodes. Within 24 to 48 hours of intracutaneous immunization, the most apparent histologic change in the draining lymph node is the unmistakable appearance of significant numbers of pyroninophilic blast cells or plasmablasts (also referred to as immunoblasts), first in the interfollicular areas and then in the paracortical and deep cortical areas as well. Blast cells continue to increase in numbers in these locations during the following 24 to 48 hours. At this time, plasmablasts can be detected in much greater numbers in the outer marginal zones of the primary follicles. These cells traverse the paracortex and enter the medulla. Within an additional 24 to 48 hours, the medullary cords and sinuses appear to be filled with mature plasma cells, while plasmablasts can still be detected in the deep cortical regions. By this time, immunoblasts will have disappeared from the outer cortex and are replaced by small, mature-looking lymphocytes. Germinal centers begin to evolve in the primary follicles with the appearance of large numbers of blast cells which undergo numerous mitotic divisions. Within another 48 to 72 hours, the cellular reaction begins to subside and there is restoration of normal architecture and morphology. The follicle centers begin to take on the appearance of normal germinal centers characterized by moderate numbers of blast cells, larger numbers of medium-sized lymphocytes, and the typical macrophages with "tingible bodies" representing nuclear debris ingested by these macrophages. By the 10th to 14th day following immunization, only a few plasma cells can be seen in the medulla.

By the application of the immunofluorescence technique, it can be shown that the plasmablasts and plasma cells detected in the deep cortex and the medullary cords by the 4th to 6th day following immunization possess specific antibodies to the immunizing antigen, thus relating these cells directly with the immune response. However, antibodies are not detected in the plasmablasts observed in the outer cortex during the initial phase (days 1 to 3) of the immune response. These cells are, therefore, not the precursors of antibody-forming cells detected 2 to 3 days later. The early cortical immunoblast response may represent the proliferation of T cells or antigen-recognizing cells (ARC) (see below); it may also constitute the initial phase of a cell-mediated immune response to the antigen which is either aborted in favor of the antibody response or is masked by the more aggressive antibody response. The exact relationship of the germinal center proliferative response to the immune response is not understood at the present time. (Could these cells be the precursors of the suppressor cells?)

The changes in the spleen following intravenous immunization are similar to those in the lymph node following intracutaneous immunization. The first blasts following immunization can be detected among the lymphocytes constituting the T cell-dependent periarteriolar lymphocyte sheath surrounding the follicular arteriole. This blast reaction is followed within several days by the appearance of large numbers of plasmablasts among the cells in the outer marginal zones of the follicles in the white pulp. The plasmablasts then appear to migrate into the red pulp, where they appear to transform to plasma cells. Within 10 to 12 days following immunization, only a few plasma cells can be detected. Normal architecture is restored within an additional 5 to 10 days.

Only a minority of the antibody-forming blast cells revert to small, mature, long-lived lymphocytes—referred to as **memory cells**—which reside primarily in the spleen. When the host is reimmunized with the original antigen months or years following the primary immune response, it is these memory cells which now respond with antibody formation in the characteristic secondary immune response.

Immunization of animals with "physiologic" quantities of antigen—that is, quantities of the antigen which would normally be provided by a bacterial infection—does not result in greater than normal numbers of plasmablasts and plasma cells, nor does it result in any obvious alterations in the gross or microscopic morphology of the cortex or medulla of the lymph nodes or the white or red pulp of the spleen. What is observed is enlargement of primary follicles, with both the germinal center and mantle zone cells participating in the hyperplastic reaction. In the rabbit, blast cells are detected in the outer mantle zones of the lymphoid follicles by 4 to 6 days postimmunization, following which they, along with small numbers of plasmablasts and plasma cells, can be detected in close proximity to the medullary cords. Antibodies are detected in the circulation very shortly thereafter.

Plasma cells are abundant in the spleen and lymph nodes following repeated or hyperimmunization with large amounts of the antigen, especially if the antigen is combined with an adjuvant, a situation which is only encountered in laboratory-contrived experiments. This plasma cell response may be considered to constitute a pathologic response of the immune system confronted with an excessively large number of antigen molecules. A large number of antibody-synthesizing blast cells are generated in the immune response, but a majority of the antibody-forming cells give rise, through either transformation or proliferation, to antibody-secreting plasmablasts which, in turn, give rise to moribund plasma cells (life-span 2 to 4 days). This mechanism, the transformation of antibody-forming blast cells to short-lived plasma cells, may be considered to constitute a safety valve provided by nature for the elimination of unneeded immunocompetent cells once the immune response is terminated, thus preventing excessive or prolonged antibody synthesis beyond that necessary to ensure protection to the host. Amyloidosis subsequent to continuous or oft-repeated immunization may very well represent a breakdown in this mechanism.

A relationship between the amount of antigen administered and the lymphoid cell response was suggested by Sterzl and his colleagues more than two decades ago, but it was not spelled out in specific terms and is rarely referred to in contemporary textbooks. It was proposed that an inverse relationship exists between the extent of the immune response and the percentage of the antibody-forming cells which revert to the status of memory cells. In other words, the total number of antibody-forming cells would be greater but the percentage of these cells which revert to memory cells would be smaller in the case of an aggressive immune response as compared to a threshold immune response. Animals immunized with very small (threshold immunogenic or subimmunogenic) quantities of an antigen may fail to exhibit detectable antibodies in the circulation. However, such animals have indeed been immunized since they can mount a secondary, not a primary, immune response following reinjection of the original antigen. Thus, it is possible for an immunocompetent cell to pass through the various proliferative and/or transformational and/or maturational stages of the antibody-forming cell cycle followed by de-differentiation into a memory (small lymphocyte) cell in the apparent absence of any antibody-secretory phase. It is also possible, however, if not probable, that antibody formation may take place in the "nonresponsive" animals referred to above but may not be detected due to the relatively insensitive serologic assays used to detect antibodies. Therefore, it cannot be stated with any degree of certainty that the induction of immunologic memory can bypass the antibody-synthetic phase of the immune response.

Functions of T Cells and B Cells

Current knowledge of the cellular interactions in the immune response, especially the distinct roles played by the thymus-derived (T) cells and the bone marrow-derived (B) cells, dates from investigations carried out by Claman, Chaperon, and Triplett at the University of Colorado, the results of which were reported in 1966. These investigators utilized inbred mice and the plaque-forming cell (PFC) response as the means to detect the formation of antibodies by the spleen cells toward the sheep red blood cell (SRBC) antigen. Mice subjected to 600 rads whole body irradiation temporarily lose the ability to give a PFC response upon immunization with SRBC. These investigators observed that the immunocompetent state could not be reconstituted by the administration of either syngeneic bone marrow or thymus cells alone. However, most unexpectedly, the administration of a mixture of syngeneic bone marrow and thymus cells reestablished immune responsiveness to the SRBC antigen in these otherwise immunoincompetent mice. This finding constitutes a milestone in contemporary immunology, as it provided the first evidence for the participation of a least two distinct lymphocytes in the humoral immune response.

It was subsequently demonstrated that the virgin immunocompetent cell provided by the thymus (the T cell), and not the cell provided by the bone marrow (the B cell), interacts initially with the antigen and undergoes blastogenesis and mitosis following interaction with the antigen. However, this T cell does not synthesize antibodies. The virgin immunocompetent cell provided by the bone marrow (the B cell) does not appear to interact initially in a detectable manner with the antigen, but it does transform into or generate the cells which synthesize the antibodies. These findings imply that the T cell but not the B cell possesses a receptor on its surface, the structure of which is configurationally complementary to that of the antigen determinant site, thus facilitating interaction with the antigen. The concept of a receptor is now widely accepted, although it was a novel and highly controversial concept as recently as the mid-1960s. The T cell is, therefore, referred to as the antigen-recognizing cell or antigen-reactive cell (ARC) and the B cell as the antibody-forming cell (AFC). Results of numerous investigations in the mouse and the rabbit have disclosed that the virgin ARC cell is a unipotent cell, precommitted to interact with a single antigen or antigen constellation, whereas the virgin AFC cell, or at least its precursor, does not appear to be subject to this restriction. The virgin precommitted AFC cell is potentially a pluripotent cell but becomes a unipotent cell only after it is stimulated into antibody synthesis. In other words, a committed antibody-forming cell is only capable of synthesizing antibodies to a single antigen.

One postulated role of the T cell is to present the antigen to the antibody-forming B cell in such a way as to facilitate the interaction between the antigen and the B cell, by lining up the antigenic determinants along the surface of the B cell. The T cell or ARC is, therefore, also referred to as the **helper cell** in the antibody response to denote its functional role.

Important

1. It has become common practice to refer to the lymphocytes participating in the humoral immune response as the immunocompetent T and B cells. The reader should realize, however, that the immunocompetent T and B cells represent only minor populations of cells in the thymus and bone marrow, respectively. The vast majority of the cells in the thymus and bone marrow have functions other than immunologic ones.

2. It must be pointed out that the bases for the identification of an immunologic role for these cells were investigations conducted solely in selected strains of inbred mice. It has since been shown that the cellular interactions in other species, such as the outbred rabbit, may not be identical to those in the mouse, even in the ontogenic sense. It may, therefore, be preferable to refer to the participating cells in terms of their functional roles rather than their ontogenic origins. Thus, the T immunocompetent cell (and its progeny) is referred to as the "antigen-reactive" or "antigen-responsive" or "antigen-recognizing cell" (ARC) or "helper cell."

The B immunocompetent cell (and its progeny) is referred to as the "antibody-forming cell" (AFC).

3. The reader will have concluded by now that the terms "virgin" and "recognizing" (or reactive or responding) in referring to the "virgin immunocompetent antigen-recognizing cell" (the ARC) are incompatible. The term recognition implies previous exposure to or interaction with the antigen. A more appropriate term to define the virgin immunocompetent ARC would be the "antigen-cognizing cell," or ACC. However, the term ARC is now comfortably incorporated into the lexicon of immunologic terminology and it would take a great effort to dislodge it and replace it with another term.

The demonstration of the obligatory T cell-B cell interaction in the primary immune response to numerous antigens, especially the ubiquitous sheep red blood cell (SRBC) antigen, contrasts sharply with the nonparticipation of T cells in the secondary or anamnestic immune response to all antigens investigated. These observations constituted the basis for the investigations which provided a rational, scientifically based response to the frequently posed question: "Why is the primary immune response so much more sensitive to irradiation, steroids, and immunosuppressive drugs than is the secondary immune response?" The answer is that the primary immune response involves virgin ARC T cells which are highly sensitive to irradiation, steroids, and immunosuppressive drugs, whereas the secondary immune response involves only the memory B cells which are far less sensitive to each of these agents. The relative insensitivity to immunosuppressive drugs of the primary immune response to antigens which do not appear to require mediation by T cells (T-independent antigens, see below) is attributed to the fact that virgin AFC B cells, like memory B cells, are also relatively insensitive to immunosuppressive agents.

Functions of the Macrophage

There is general agreement that the macrophage plays an important role in the induction of antibody formation. More precisely, there exists an acute awareness of the need to incorporate a cell with the demostrated capacities of the macrophage into the scheme of cellular interactions leading to antibody formation. It has been speculated that the macrophage initiates the events which culminate in antibody synthesis by interacting with the antigen, breaking it down, and liberating the antigenic determinants capable of interacting with and activating the immunocompetent cells. Results of in vitro experiments strongly indicate such a role. It has been demonstrated that macrophage-processed antigen is more antigenic on an equal weight basis than is the native antigen, suggesting that the antigen is normally partially metabolized or altered by interaction with the macrophage. However, it has not been unequivocally established whether this finding in vitro should be considered as coincidental to, or a major contribution in, the induction of antibody synthesis in vivo. The precise role of the macrophage and the point of its intervention in the immune response in vivo have still not been elucidated. It should be pointed out that investigations which implicated the phagocytic cell in the immune response utilized particulate antigens such as bacteria and erythrocytes, which must be degraded in order to facilitate liberation of the antigenic determinants. Recent investigations have utilized more refined, soluble, low molecular weight antigens which need not be broken down in order to liberate antigenic determinants and, therefore, may not require the mediation of the phagocytic cell.

Important

It is instructive to note that large molecular weight proteins such as "native" human gamma globulin (HGG) are highly antigenic when injected into xenogeneic animals and they induce copious amounts of antibodies. This is not surprising since it appears to be the norm. It is the anticipated response based on previous experiences extending back three to four decades. Serum proteins have been used as antigens because they are homogeneous, nontoxic, nonreplicating, and nonparticulate; in short, they constitute "clean antigens" as opposed to bacterial antigens which are usually described as "dirty antigens."

What is surprising, however, is that HGG is antigenic in the xenogeneic animal like the rabbit only when it is injected in the "native" aggregated or polymeric state. HGG is **not** antigenic when it is injected into the rabbit in the deaggregated or monomeric state. It is a fact that HGG and other serum proteins, which have been utilized as typical antigens for years and have furnished the investigative results which constitute the basis of our understanding of immune mechanisms, aggregate spontaneously from the moment that the blood is drawn into the syringe. What is usually referred to as "pure HGG" or "pure albumin" is actually a purified aggregate of the protein. Thus, if the aggregated serum proteins are removed by ultracentrifugation, the nonaggregated serum proteins (which are probably the true native proteins) do not induce an immune response following their injection into the rabbit, irrespective of the amount injected. In fact, the deaggregated protein induces a state of immunologic tolerance to the aggregated serum protein. On the other hand, the aggregated serum protein is a highly potent antigen in the rabbit, and it induces a greater immune response than does the untreated "native" serum protein. The explanation for these observations is that only the aggregated proteins following interaction with the ARC cells interact with the macrophages during the induction phase of the antibody response. The macrophages normally process the antigen and liberate the antigenic determinants in an immunogenic state. On the other hand, the deaggregated serum proteins, following interaction with the ARC cells, do **not** interact with the macrophages. They are, therefore, not degraded, the antigenic determinants are not liberated in a form which imparts immunogenicity to them, and the immune response is abrogated if in fact it was ever initiated.

It is, therefore, fortuitous that the use of artificially aggregated purified serum proteins as antigens has enabled investigators to elucidate the cellular interactions which appear to characterize the normal immune response. This is ironic since the serum proteins in the aggregated form would probably not be used today as model antigens in view of our current appreciation of the fact that they are really not antigenic in the nonaggregated, monomeric state which defines their normal composition in the circulation in vivo.

On the assumption that the macrophage plays a definitive role in the sequence of intercellular reactions which culminate in antibody formation by the AFC cells, where might we consider that it participates? Obviously, it must interact with the antigen either before or after the ARC cell enters the picture. As stated above, the original premise that the macrophage-antigen interaction is the initial reaction in the sequence leading to antibody formation was based on the assumption that the ARC cell could not possibly interact with a cellular antigen, such as an erythrocyte or bacterium, due to steric hindrance. However, this is not a valid assumption, as Richter and Abdou demonstrated that "virgin" ARC cells of an unimmunized normal rabbit are quite capable of instantaneously interacting with red blood cell membrane (stromal) antigens in the absence of prior macrophage interaction. Thus, it is more plausible to assume that the macrophage reacts with the antigen following its interaction with the ARC cell. It is postulated that the receptor for the antigen determinant site is liberated by the ARC cell following interaction with the antigen (Fig. 5.2) and that this receptor will adhere to the determinant site and protect it from being degraded following phagocytosis of the antigen by the macrophage (Fig. 5.3). It is proposed that the macrophage degrades and catabolizes the entire antigen molecule except for those sites which are protected by their coating of autologous receptor molecules, the antigenic determinant sites (Fig. 5.3). The latter are then either expelled from the macrophage directly into the circulation and eventually encounter the virgin AFC cells in the spleen and/or lymph node; or they may be directly transmitted to the virgin AFC cell following contact between the macrophage and the virgin AFC cell (Fig. 5.4); or they may reassemble on the surface of the ARC cell which originally provided the receptors (and which is now denuded of receptors) and be transmitted to the virgin AFC cell following contact of the latter cell with the ARC-antigen determinant complex (Fig. 5.5).

This proposed scheme of cell-cell interactions leading to antibody synthesis is favored by the author. It is consistent with current experimental findings and imparts rational roles to the three cells involved in antibody synthesis—the macrophage, the lymphoid ARC, and the lymphoid AFC. Furthermore, it incorporates the ARC helper cell at two different points in the sequence of cell-cell interactions—initially to provide the protective "coat" to the antigen determinant in the form of a receptor, and later to provide the "scaffolding" for the identical receptor-antigen determinant complexes to line up and be "presented" to the virgin AFC. The signal to activate the AFC to antibody synthesis is amplified many times since all the antigenic determinants

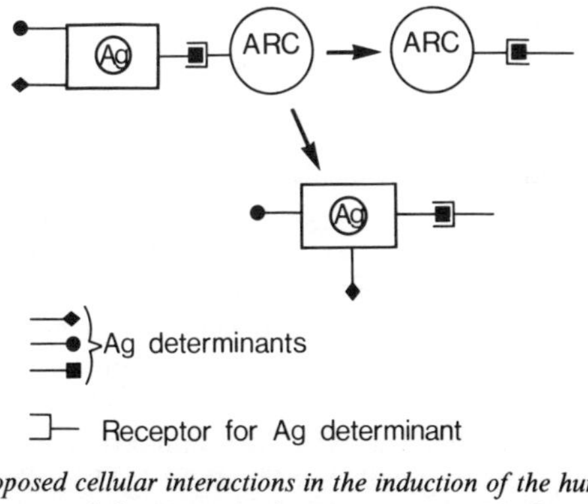

Figure 5.2 *Proposed cellular interactions in the induction of the humoral immune response. Interaction of the antigenic determinant site with the receptor on the antigen-reactive cell (ARC) results in the formation of either ARC-antigen determinant complexes or antigen-receptor complexes.*

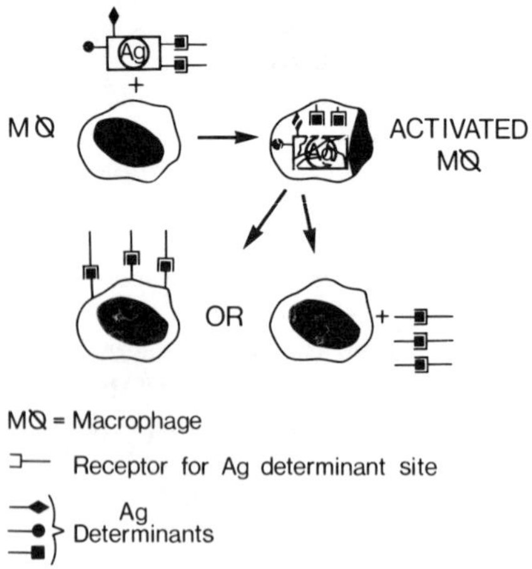

Figure 5.3 *Proposed cellular interactions in the induction of the humoral immune response. The antigen, consisting of the carrier portion of the molecule with its attached determinant sites and those determinant sites now protected with a coating of autologous protein provided by the ARC receptor sites, is phagocytized by the macrophage. The entire antigen molecule, except for the protected antigen determinant sites, is degraded and catabolized. Only the undegraded protected antigen determinants escape unscathed, and they become attached to surface structures on the macrophage or are secreted into the microenvironment of the cell.*

complexed to the attached ARC cell would be identical. The latter role(s) proposed for the ARC is in keeping with that postulated for the helper cell, and the scheme presented in Figures 5.2 to 5.5 provides the mechanism whereby the ARC helper cell carries out its function following immunization with a multideterminant heterogeneous antigen. The proposed scheme allows for the generation of memory cells from immune lymphoblasts (or immunoblasts) and the "siphoning off" or elimination of excessive numbers of lymphoblasts by their transformation to plasmablasts and moribund plasma cells (Fig. 5.6).

The AFC precursor or progenitor cell is pluripotent, that is, it is endowed with the potential to synthesize antibodies of different specificities. However, once it is stimulated to synthesize antibodies, it becomes unipotent and synthesizes and secretes antibodies of only one specificity and most probably of only one class. There is still some confusion about the latter point, as some evidence suggests that the AFC can convert from an IgM to an IgG antibody-forming cell. Synthesis of IgM antibodies appears to proceed without any significant proliferation of the antibody-forming cells, whereas synthesis of IgG antibodies appears to

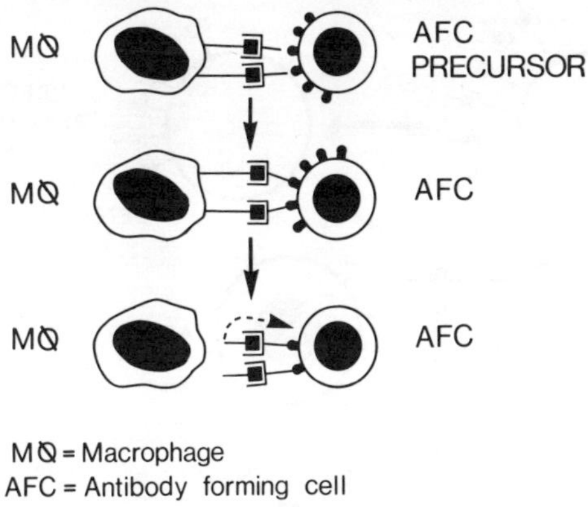

Figure 5.4 *Proposed cellular interactions in the induction of the humoral immune response. The macrophage-antigen determinant-receptor site complex interacts with the precursor of the AFC. The antigen determinant-receptor complex is transferred from the macrophage to the AFC precursor and it is then internalized into the cell, which transforms to an overt antibody-forming cell.*

coincide with proliferation of these cells. Thus, antimitotic agents are much more effective in inhibiting the synthesis of IgG antibodies than they are in inhibiting the synthesis of IgM antibodies.

Important

1. The bicellular nature of the immune response (the T-B cell interaction) is not the rule. The majority of antigens investigated require involvement of both the T and B cells in the antibody response, and these are referred to as "thymic-dependent antigens." Other antigens do not (apparently) require the participation of the T cells, and these are referred to as "thymic-independent antigens." These antigens tend to be composed of linear polymers of repeating identical antigenic determinants which would naturally "line up" along the B cell surface following their interaction, presumably via receptors, with the B cell. The existence of these antigens serves to make us aware of the alternate mechanisms with which the animal is endowed to facilitate the formation of antibodies. Undoubtedly, there are other mechanisms which we have not yet identified.

2. It is important to stress that the antigens utilized in immunologic investigations tend to be chemically "purified" antigens, synthetic antigens, or naturally occurring polymeric-type antigens such as POL (polymerized flagellin of Salmonella). Many microbiologists and those immunologists concerned with microbial im-

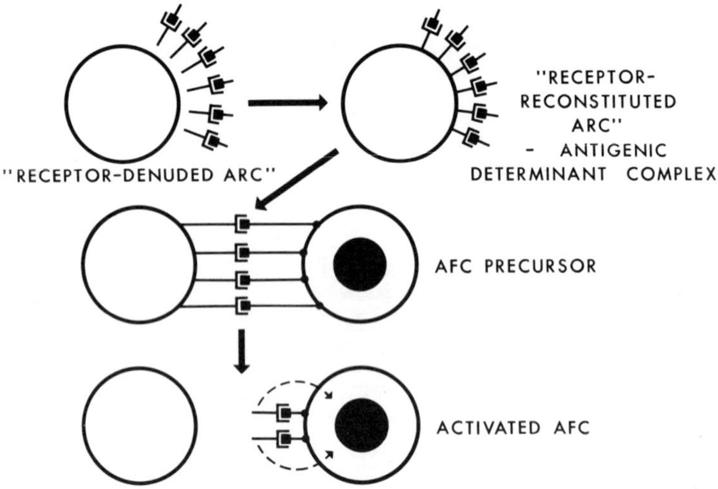

Figure 5.5 *Proposed cellular interactions in the induction of the humoral immune response. The receptor-antigenic determinant complexes encounter a "receptor-denuded" ARC cell which originally provided the receptors for these determinants and interacts with this cell. As a result of configurational complementariness between cell surface structures on the "receptor-denuded" ARC cell and the free receptors bound to the antigenic determinants, the cell will accommodate only the identical receptors originally shed. Thus, all the receptor-antigen determinant complexes on any one reconstituted ARC will be identical. The antigenic determinants will be "presented" to the immediate precursor of the AFC and will be incorporated into the AFC, activating it and initiating antibody synthesis.*

munity have persistently questioned whether results obtained with relatively low molecular weight noncellular, purified, degraded, and chemically altered antigens necessarily reflect the true picture of the immune response as it relates to immunity to infectious microorganisms. Unquestionably, it is much easier to work with chemically purified and defined "clean" antigens, especially if they are commercially available, than it is to work with undefined microbial preparations containing a heterogeneous population of antigens. The latter is not in fashion. Nevertheless, it may be that the neat packaging of the immune responses as either T-dependent or T-independent does not reflect the realities of protective immune mechanisms and is only valid within the context of investigations dealing with laboratory-purified antigens. It has, in fact, been demonstrated on more than one occasion that the simultaneous administration into a thymectomized T cell-deprived animal of a T-independent antigen along with a normally T-dependent antigen will result in antibody formation toward both antigens.

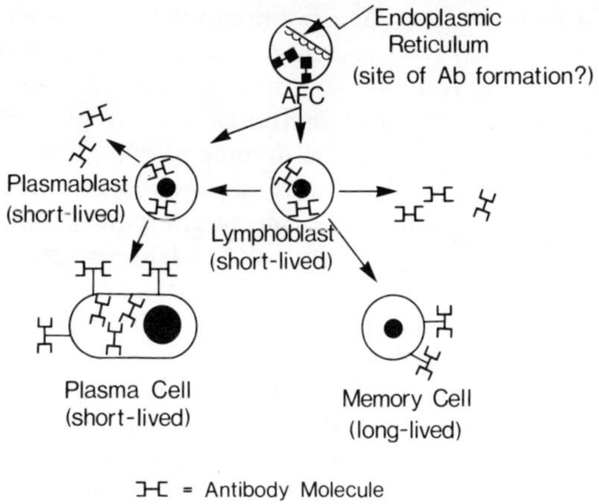

Figure 5.6 *Proposed cellular interactions in the induction of the humoral immune response. The AFC transforms into a lymphoblast or a plasmablast, and mitotic divisions then occur. The plasmablasts differentiate to plasma cells which are end stage, short-lived cells. The lymphocyte progeny of the immune lymphoblasts constitute the memory cells.*

Thus, the strict T dependency of an antigen can be subverted simply by resorting to the institution of conditions which govern an immune response under natural physiologic conditions—the simultaneous exposure of the immune system to a large number of antigens.

EFFECT OF THYMECTOMY ON IMMUNE RESPONSE

In view of the fact that thymus- and bone marrow-derived cells have been implicated as the major participants in the humoral immune response and the thymus-derived cells as the major participants in the cell-mediated immune response (see Chapter 6), the reader may wonder as to the consequences for the host following extirpation or ablation of these organs. Experiments carried out in the mouse have disclosed that neonatal extirpation of the thymus results in the almost total abolition of the capacity to give a cell-mediated immune response several weeks later when the mouse would normally have attained immunologic maturity. It was, therefore, concluded that the thymus possesses the effector cells which participate in the cell-mediated immune response and that these cells continue to remain in the thymus as the animal matures.

The humoral immune response is not as markedly affected by neonatal thymectomy as is the cell-mediated immune response.

In point of fact, the immune response to some antigens (thymus-dependent antigens) is significantly affected by neonatal thymectomy, whereas the response to other antigens (thymus-independent antigens) is only marginally, or not at all, affected by neonatal thymectomy. Since the thymus provides the helper cells which participate in the humoral immune response with respect to thymus-dependent antigens, one might expect that antibody formation with respect to thymus-dependent antigens would be totally abolished following neonatal thymectomy. However, as stated above, the immune response to thymus-dependent antigens is diminished to a significant degree but is not totally abrogated. Reconciliation of these two seemingly irreconcilable positions was achieved by the demonstration that the helper T cells are liberated from the thymus and are seeded into the peripheral lymphoid organs in the prenatal and/or immediate postnatal period. Therefore, neonatal extirpation of the thymus abrogates the cell-mediated immune response but not the humoral or antibody immune response, even with respect to thymus-dependent antigens.

Immune Response in Bursectomized Chickens

Investigations carried out by Glick about 20 years ago implicated the bursa of Fabricius as the source of the antibody-forming cells or their precursors in the bird. The bursa of Fabricius is a small lymphoid organ located at the junction of the rectum and the cloaca and consists of masses of mainly small mature lymphocytes. It has a well defined cortex and medulla and histologically resembles the Peyer's patches. The tissue extends as folds into the lumen of the rectum.

Glick observed that adult chickens which had been neonatally bursectomized could not synthesize antibodies. He concluded that the bursa of Fabricius provides the progenitor or precursor cells of the antibody-forming cells. However, such was the state of the discipline at that time that Glick was only able to publish these extremely important and relevant results in the *Journal of Poultry Science.* Glick's findings have had a major impact in furthering our knowledge of the cellular basis of the immune response. It is now accepted that the thymus and bursa of Fabricius (or its equivalent in nonavian species) constitute the "central lymphoid organs" and that the spleen, tonsils, lymph nodes, and infiltrations of lymphoid cells, such as the lamina propria of the gut, constitute the "peripheral lymphoid tissues." There is controversy as to which category the appendix and Peyer's patches should be placed in. Those investigators who consider that these two lymphoid organs constitute the mammalian homologue of the avian bursa of Fabricius place them in the category of central lymphoid organs, while others group them with the spleen and lymph nodes as peripheral lymphoid organs. The distinction between the central and peripheral lymphoid tissues is based on the following considerations:

1. Proliferation of thymic and bursal cells occurs in the absence of external stimulation, antigenic or otherwise. On the other hand, proliferation of cells in the lymph nodes and spleen appears to be a response to external stimulation.

2. Extirpation of the thymus or bursa of Fabricius (in the bird) at the neonatal stage results in marked depression of the ability of the animal to subsequently render a cell-mediated immune response or a humoral immune response, respectively. However, extirpation of the spleen and/or lymph nodes does not have this effect.

3. The spleen, lymph nodes, and most recently the appendix have been shown to possess morphologically distinct and identifiable "thymic-dependent areas" and "bursal-dependent areas." In the lymph node (Fig. 5.7), the former constitute the interfollicular, parafollicular, and deep cortical areas, whereas the latter constitute the primary follicles themselves. In the spleen (Fig.

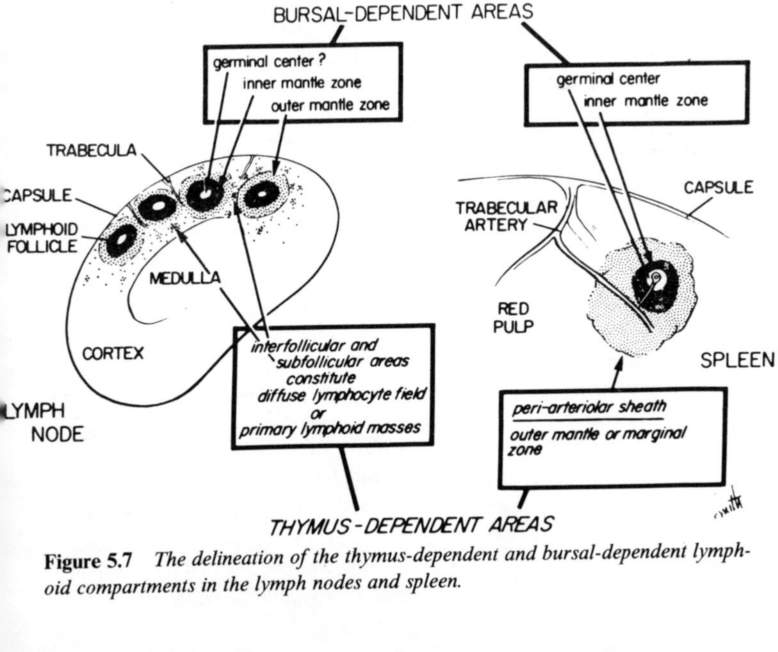

Figure 5.7 *The delineation of the thymus-dependent and bursal-dependent lymphoid compartments in the lymph nodes and spleen.*

5.7), the thymic-dependent areas are the perivascular infiltrates of cells located at one pole of the elliptically shaped follicle. Examination will reveal a small blood vessel (a branch of the follicular artery) in the middle of the cell infiltrate, referred to as the periarteriolar sheath. The bursal-dependent areas in the spleen consist of the lymphoid follicles.

4. Following neonatal thymectomy, the thymus-dependent areas in the lymph nodes and spleen remain unpopulated with cells for the duration of the life of the animal. There is usually a compensatory hyperplasia of the cells adjacent to the thymus-dependent areas. On the other hand, neonatal bursectomy in the chicken results in a permanent depletion of cells in the bursal-dependent areas of the lymph nodes and spleen.

5. A majority of the thymus and bone marrow cells have been shown to possess distinct "organ-specific" antigens. These cells infiltrate the peripheral lymphoid organs as thymus-derived and bone marrow-derived cells, respectively. Other than the thymus and bone marrow, only the appendix of the remaining lymphoid organs has been found to possess cells with an "organ-specific" antigen(s) which identifies these cells as appendix cells. These cells, like the bone marrow and thymus cells, infiltrate the peripheral lymphoid tissues as appendix-derived cells. Thus, on the basis of cell surface "organ-specific" antigens, the appendix should be classified as a central lymphoid organ along with the thymus and bone marrow, although it also exhibits properties of a peripheral lymphoid organ in that it possesses thymus-derived and bone marrow-derived lymphocytes.

Important

1. The dramatic immunologic consequences of thymectomy (in the mouse, rat, or chicken) and bursectomy (in the chicken) can only be obtained if the organs are extirpated in utero or in the very early postnatal period. If one waits until the animal is 1 to 2 weeks of age before surgical extirpation of the appropriate organ, sufficient seeding of thymic or bursal cells to the peripheral organs will have taken place. The effect of this dissemination of cells is to distort or minimize the sequelae of thymic or bursal extirpation.

2. Mammals do not possess a bursa or Fabricius. However, all indications point to a "bursal equivalent" in these animals, including humans, but we do not yet know the identity of the bursal equivalent. Some evidence, as yet unconvicing, points to the gut-associated lymphoid tissues (appendix and/or Peyer's patches) as the homologue of the avian bursa. It would appear, though, that

the immunocompetent B cells or their precursors, in both birds and humans, migrate prenatally to the bone marrow where they mature and from which they subsequently migrate to the peripheral lymphoid organs (spleen, lymph nodes). It is only their ontogenic source, embryologically speaking, which remains to be resolved.

Direct implantation of syngeneic thymus tissue into the rectus abdominus muscle following extirpation of the thymus results in repopulation of the thymus-dependent compartments of the lymph nodes and spleen with T cells and the reestablishment of normal architecture. However, if the syngeneic thymus tissue is implanted in a semipermeable chamber (permeable to protein molecules but not to cells), the thymus-dependent compartments of the lymph nodes and spleen are not fully repopulated. These findings imply that the cells which inhabit the thymus-dependent areas of the lymph nodes and spleen need not be derived from the thymus but require the presence of a soluble factor released from the thymus in order to respond with blastogenesis and proliferation. A large number of investigators have, over the past 10 years, presented evidence in favor of not one but several thymic hormones (i.e. thymosin, thymopoietin) secreted by the thymic epithelial cells capable of transforming non-T cells into cells with T cell characteristics. The next decade will surely be witness to great refinements in the isolation procedures, the characterization of these hormones and their utilization in the treatment of diseases characterized by thymic failure or absence.

It may also be predicted that a similar hormone(s) will be isolated from bone marrow cells to which will be attributed the function of maintaining the cells in the B or bursal-dependent compartments in the lymph nodes and spleen.

THEORIES OF ANTIBODY FORMATION

Over the years, a large number of theories have been proposed, considered, and rejected in the attempt to explain the mechanism of antibody formation. Those investigators who accepted the principle that a theory must conform to and satisfy rational considerations and must adhere to the restrictions of mathematical models and statistical analyses tended to accept the **instructional theory** of antibody formation, originally propounded by Breinl and Haurowitz in the 1930s and subsequently elaborated upon by Alexander, Mudd, and Pauling. This theory was certainly a plausible one, as it incorporated the contemporary and then novel role of DNA as the master planner and executor of protein synthesis within the cell. The DNA molecules, it was assumed, constitute the templates onto which the various amino acids line up, interact, and then peel off as long peptide chains which undergo interaction with other peptide chains to form the more complex proteins. Pauling and Haurowitz both proposed that antigen penetrates the antibody-forming cell and interacts with the DNA template for gamma globulin synthesis, altering its structure sufficiently so as to change the sequence of amino acids adhering to this template at this site. They proposed that the specificity is not necessarily conferred at the stage of polypeptide synthesis, but at a later stage when the folding of the chains takes place. Thus, the configuration of the peptide formed at the site of antigen-DNA interaction would be configurationally complementary to the antigen. This theory allows for the unlimited formation of different antibodies or antibodies of different specificities.

It withstood the test of time until the mid-1950s, when Jerne proposed the **natural selection theory** which was followed by Burnet's **clonal selection theory** to explain antibody formation. Jerne postulated that the normal circulating gamma globulins consist of distinct populations of molecules carrying reactive sites capable of interacting with all potential antigenic determinants other than those already existing in accessible areas of the body with which they would not be able to interact as these are "autologous" antigens. The function of the antigen is to interact with the naturally occurring gamma globulin (antibody) directed toward it and bring it to the cell which synthesized it initially. The antibody and/or antigen would somehow be taken into the cell and stimulate it to synthesize more replicas of this naturally occurring antibody.

Burnet incorporated Jerne's concepts into his clonal selection theory. Burnet originally proposed that preprogrammed or precommitted pluripotent immunocompetent cells are produced in the fetus capable of interacting with all antigens (endogenous and exogenous) with which the host may come into contact postnatally. However, in this initial form, the theory failed to resolve a number of questions which, from a philosophic point of view, initially deterred acceptance of this theory and any other theory based on the principle of precommittment. Several of these questions were as follows:

1. How does the theory take into account the fact that autoimmune disease occurs very infrequently in the normal immunologically mature population? Since the theory proposed that prepro-

grammed cells capable of interacting with all exogenous and endogenous antigens are generated in the fetus, then all the immunocompetent cells could theoretically be stimulated to autoantibody synthesis postnatally. Such is fortunately not the case, and autoimmune disease is not a prevalent illness in the immunologically mature adult population. But if the theory were to be accepted as valid, why do we not experience autoimmune diseases with the high frequency the theory would dictate?

2. How does the theory take into account the fact that an individual may be incapable of producing antibodies to a particular antigen but be capable of synthesizing normal levels of antibodies to all other antigens? Such a situation should not occur if all immunocompetent cells are pluripotent prior to activation.

To resolve these questions, Burnet proposed that specifically precommitted unipotent clones of immunocompetent cells, each capable of responding to only one major antigenic determinant, are generated in the fetus rather than precommitted pluripotent non-clonally selected immunocompetent cells capable of reacting with all exogenous and endogenous antigens. Burnet further stipulated that any precommitted immunocompetent cells which would encounter the specific antigen(s) in utero would be destroyed, and thus entire clones would be eliminated. Since endogenous autoantigens but not exogenous antigens normally penetrate the fetal circulation, only those clones of cells precommitted to respond to autoantigens would be obliterated. In this manner, only those clones of cells directed toward exogenous antigens would be expected to survive fetal life, and these cells, upon encountering exogenous antigens postnatally, respond with antibody formation. To take autoimmune disease into account, Burnet allowed for the emergence of "forbidden clones" of cells postnatally, capable of interacting with autoantigens and synthesizing autoantibodies, thus facilitating the "spontaneous" emergence of autoimmune disease (this matter is further elaborated upon in Chapter 12). The interaction with the antigen is facilitated by the existence of an antigen-binding site on the surface of the appropriate cell, presumably a lymphocyte, configurationally complementary to the potential antigen determinant. Each binding site, or receptor, would be characteristic of a particular clone of cells. Following the interaction between the antigen and the cell surface receptor, the cell will be stimulated to produce gamma globulin molecules of a type characteristic of the clone.

Both of these theories borrowed heavily from the **side chain theory** originally proposed by Paul Ehrlich in 1898. Ehrlich considered that virgin or potential antibody-forming cells possess specific surface receptors, which he referred to as side chains or haptophores, which could interact with configurations (antigenic determinant sites in our modern terminology) on the appropriate antigen (Fig. 5.1). Interaction of these receptors with the antigen would trigger the cell to produce and secrete more of these side chains, which actually constitute the antibodies in our modern terminology. It is indeed remarkable that Ehrlich was able to conceptualize a mechansism for antibody formation which is, in fact, an acceptable explanation today for the immune response to so-called "T-independent" antigens in spite of the fact that the composition of antigens and antibodies was totally speculative and the lymphocyte was considered a totally redundant and/or irrelevant cell in his time.

The essential feature of both the Jerne and Burnet theories is the assumption that antibodies can be synthesized in the total absence of antigenic stimulation. The Jerne-Burnet hypothesis was, therefore, challenged for many years from a philosophic point of view because it did not make provision for and was not precise as to how the immune system could conceivably be endowed with the foresight needed to anticipate all possible antigens on pathogenic microorganisms while still in the prenatal state. They did not consider whether there could be sufficient clones of cells to permit responses to the hundreds, if not thousands, of antigens present in the environment.

Nevertheless, contemporary research has confirmed the basic validity of this theory. Richter and Abdou showed that the normal, unimmunized rabbit and Wigzell and his associates showed that the normal, unimmunized mouse possess virgin immunocompetent cells capable of interacting with randomly selected antigens. Investigations of these cells in the late 1960s disclosed that they were the antigen-reactive or -recognizing ARC cells and not the antibody-forming AFC cells or their precursors and that they were normally confined to the thymus in the mouse and the bone marrow in the rabbit. Abdou and Richter confirmed that these cells are clonally selected. They isolated individual clones by passage of the ARC-containing cell suspensions through antigen-sensitized glass bead columns followed by elution of the adherent cells from the beads, a technique first introduced by Wigzell. These isolated clones of cells, upon transfer to irradiated, immunoincompetent hosts whose own ARC cell population had been destroyed by total body irradiation, could only confer immune responsiveness to the antigen originally used in the glass bead column for the isolation of these cells. Conversely, the ARC cells which did not adhere to the antigen-sensitized glass beads could confer immune responsiveness to all antigens with which the host was challenged except to the antigen originally used on the glass bead column.

It must be stressed that this work was conducted with normal, immunologically mature adult rabbits which had not been previously immunized to any of the antigens used in the study of ARC cells and which did not possess either plaque-forming cells in any of the lymphoid organs or circulating antibodies directed toward these antigens. This is in contradistinction to similar work done with the mouse which could be suspect on the basis that the unimmunized mouse invariably possesses both plaque-forming cells in the spleen and usually low levels of circulating antibodies directed toward a broad range of antigens. Thus, one could consider that the "normal, unimmunized" mouse is not really unimmunized and that the virgin antibody-forming cells are really immune cells. What remains to be seen is whether the clonal selection theory, with all its ramifications, applies to the normal human. This matter is further discussed in the chapters concerned with autoimmune diseases (Chapter 12), immunologic tolerance (Chapter 11), and immunodeficiency diseases (Chapter 10).

Important

The flow of knowledge concerning the interacting virgin immunocompetent cells in the primary response, and memory cells in the secondary immune response, has not kept pace with the flow of questions which have surfaced as a consequence of results obtained from the utilization of new, more sensitive assays for the detection of immunoresponsive cells, especially those in the circulation. The investigations which gave rise to our knowledge of the immunocompetent B and T cells were conducted essentially in vitro with the spleen, bone marrow, and thymus cells, but not the circulating cells, of one or two highly inbred strains of mice. The results obtained to date from all this work carried out in the mouse do not, however, provide answers to several questions which clinical immunologists pose today:

1. If, as appears to be the case in the rodent, the spleen in humans is the primary depository of the antigen-induced memory cells, one might anticipate that extirpation of the spleen following a primary immune response would result in deprivation of antibody-forming memory cells to the original immunizing antigen and failure of the individual to respond immunologically to that antigen. If that were the case, then why do not splenectomized adults succumb to infections with pathogenic organisms to which

they undoubtedly responded with an antibody response at some time prior to splenectomy? Since they no longer possess antigen-specific memory cells, they should be unable to mount any antibody immune response to previously encountered antigens.

The reader must avoid becoming confused with the roles attributed to the spleen in the primary and subsequent (secondary) immune responses to the identical antigen. In the primary immune response, both the spleen and the draining lymph nodes participate in the immune response, the spleen following intravenous immunization and the lymph nodes following intradermal or intramuscular immunization. Thus, the precursors of the AFC cells may reside in both the spleen and lymph nodes. However, the memory cells generated in the primary response appear to home in to the spleen; they do not appear to reside in the lymph nodes. Thus, a secondary immune response is primarily a function of the spleen, irrespective of the mode of immunization.

2. Since neither the virgin immunocompetent (ARC and pre-AFC) cells nor memory cells appear to exist in the circulation except during the height of the immune response when the AFC cells may infiltrate the circulation, what precisely are the circulating cells which are detected in the postimmunization state capable of responding with blastogenesis and mitosis when confronted with the original immunizing antigen in vitro? Furthermore, these cells can be detected in the circulation for long periods of time (years, not months) following immunization. If they are not conventional memory cells, then what is the functional identity of these circulating cells which undergo blastogenesis in the presence of the specific antigens. If they are conventional memory cells, then the long-held view that memory cells are restricted to the spleen is not valid.

3. The results of in vitro investigations of the "primary" immune response to sheep erythrocytes (SRBC) of both mouse spleen cells and human circulating cells have implicated T cells in the in vitro response. However, these in vitro responses are clearly secondary and not primary responses since both the unimmunized mouse and human possess antibodies to SRBC in high titer in the circulation, suggesting that immunization with SRBC or cross-reactive antigens must have taken place previously, unknown to the investigator. Since secondary responses in vivo are considered not to involve T cells, are the results obtained in the in vitro assays artifacts or might they indicate the existence of bypass or secondary mechanisms not normally activated in vivo?

Until answers to these highly relevant questions are forthcoming, attempts at regulating or manipulating the humoral immune response in humans will have to carried out in a partial vacuum of knowledge. The present state of knowledge does not ensure a very high success rate in our collective efforts to intervene immunologically in diseases with a proven immunologic etiology and pathogenesis to the assured benefit of the affected individual.

CHAPTER 6

Cell-mediated Immunity

The term "cell-mediated immunity" (CMI) implies that cells, rather than antibodies, are concerned with the provision of resistance to infectious agents. It is an umbrella term which includes all immune reactions where the terminal event(s) and/or most apparent manifestation(s) of the immune response or reaction is mediated by cell-cell interactions and/or cell-derived mediators other than antibodies.

The immune responses, reactions, and/or diseases which today are defined as cell-mediated include: (a) the allograft (transplant) rejection reaction; (b) a large number of autoimmune diseases, especially those affecting the parenchyma of the anatomically distinct organs; (c) cancer immunity; (d) immunity induced in response to a number of bacteria (Mycobacterium, Brucella, Treponema), viruses, fungi, and parasites; (e) a number of skin diseases resulting from sensitivity to otherwise innocuous chemical and biologic agents (**contact sensitivity**); and (f) **delayed hypersensitivity skin reactions**, the reactions following intradermal challenge with synthetic chemicals (i.e. (DNCB)) and extracts derived from certain bacteria (old tuberculin, lepromin), fungi, parasites, viruses, and plants (poison ivy, poison oak). For many years, these skin reactions were referred to as **tuberculin-like reactions** since they strongly resemble the tuberculin reaction described in detail by investigators concerned with understanding the relationship between resistance (or susceptibility) to tuberculosis following immunization with *Mycobacterium tuberculosis* and the prognostic significance of the skin reaction elicited following challenge of the immunized individual with tuberculin, a soluble constituent of the tubercle bacillus. This skin reaction elicited to tuberculoproteins in the individual or animal infected or immunized with the tubercle bacillus was originally referred to as bacterial allergy or infectious allergy and defined as a delayed reaction by Zinnser in 1921 on the basis of its slow evolution following intradermal challenge with the antigen.

The delayed hypersensitivity skin reaction (DHSR) served as a prototype of a cell-mediated immune reaction from the 1920s to the 1960s. The DHSR is clearly immunologic in character since (a) previous exposure to the antigen is mandatory; (b) a minimum time (latent period) must elapse between exposure to the antigen and challenge with the antigen for the reaction to occur (the sensitization period); (c) an anamnestic, or memory, response may be induced; in instances where sensitivity has disappeared following first exposure to the antigen, the latent period for the reestablishment of sensitivity is much shorter; and (d) specific tolerance (or desensitization) can be instituted to the sensitizing antigen.

TUBERCULOSIS AND THE DELAYED HYPERSENSITIVITY SKIN REACTION

The histories of tuberculosis and delayed hypersensitivity are so interwined and interdependent that it would appear appropriate to discuss some of the early experiences. It was Robert Koch, in the 1880s, who isolated and identified many of the disease-causing microorganisms, including *Mycobacterium tuberculosis* which causes tuberculosis. His indefatigable and systematic investigations demonstrating the cause-effect relationship of bacteria with specific disease states resulted in his enunciation of a systematized methodological approach toward the identification and isolation of disease-causing bacteria, now referred to as the Koch principles. In his work with tuberculous animals, Koch noted that infected and normal animals respond in distinct fashions to challenge with tuberculin and in their response to inoculation with the live tubercle bacilli. Intradermal challenge with tuberculin results in the delayed skin reaction in tuberculous, but not in normal, guinea pigs. Following the intradermal injection of live tubercle bacilli into a normal guinea pig, a localized nodule appears within 10 to 14 days at the site of inoculation. The nodule increases in size and undergoes necrosis and ulceration while the bacilli are disseminated throughout the body and eventually kill the guinea pig. However, when the tubercle bacilli are injected intradermally into tuberculous guinea pigs, the response is quite different (the Koch phenomenon): The inflammation in the skin lasts only a few days and is followed in rapid succession by necrosis, ulceration, and healing by fibrosis (scarring), and the infection does not spread beyond the point of inoculation. It became apparent to Koch that prior infection with the tubercle bacillus leads to resistance to infection with this organism.

By the mid-1920s, Calmette and Guerin had succeeded in culturing an attenuated strain of mycobacteria called BCG or bacillus of Calmette and Guerin. In a number of controlled studies in the 1950s and 1960s using large numbers of adults and children, immunization with BCG was shown to impart resistance toward infection with tuberculosis. Both the primary and post-primary (or reactivation) types of tuberculosis were consistently reduced by 75 to 90%; furthermore, the vaccinated individuals incurred a very low incidence of miliary tuberculosis, tuberculous bronchopneumonia, or tuberculous meningitis as compared to far greater incidence of these three conditions in the control groups. Nevertheless, it must be admitted that a great deal of controversy still surrounds the efficacy of BCG in the induction of resistance to tuberculosis. Results of a number of recent studies, especially several carried out in India, failed to confirm the previous conclusions that immunization with BCG increases the resistance to infection with tuberculosis. A factor which was not considered in these latter studies is the varying nature of BCG, in terms of its content of the appropriate antigens from one batch to another, especially when the organism is grown in a number of unrelated laboratories. Therefore, the failure to induce resistance to tuberculosis in a BCG-immunized population may be attributed to a faulty or inadequate BCG vaccine.

As was pointed out by Rich and by succeeding investigators, the immunized individual displays a true sensitivity to the live *M. tuberculosis* and to a relatively innocuous soluble extract, old tuberculin (OT) or the purified protein derivative of old tuberculin (PPD), as compared to the normal individual. In fact, OT or PPD behave as toxins when injected into the immunized individual. The reaction following intradermal challenge with OT usually takes the form of a localized inflammation which may progress to dermonecrosis, ulceration, and scar formation, a lesion not unlike that produced by diptheria toxin in the Schick test. Fever, nausea, vomiting, lymphadenopathy, and sometimes death may result when OT is administered systemically.

Furthermore, the extensive caseation and cavitation in the lungs of tuberculous individuals who had previously been immunized to the tubercle bacillus suggests that the cellular immunity to the infectious organism is responsible, in an almost perfidious manner, for the heightened clinical symptoms and pulmonary pathology. That is probably true, but it is not the fault of the cell-mediated immune system. Unfortunately, the portal of entry for the tubercle bacillus is most frequently the respiratory tract. The tubercle bacilli, upon penetrating the respiratory mucosa and encountering the sensitized cells, elicit the same severe inflammatory reaction in the lungs (which leads to caseation, fibrosis, and cavitation) as occurs in the skin subsequent to the intradermal penetration of the organism (dermonecrosis, fibrosis, and scarring). Depending on one's point of view, it may be concluded that immunity is not always beneficial to the host; this matter is discussed fully within the context of immunopathology in Chapter 14.

The term **delayed hypersensitivity** is a misnomer, as it suggests an exaggerated sensitivity or allergy which is delayed in onset in response to the inducing stimulus. In fact, delayed hypersensitivity is neither a hypersensitivity or allergy nor is it significantly delayed in onset.

It is true that the capacity of the individual to give a skin reaction to tuberculin following vaccination with BCG (a cell-mediated immune response) develops a bit more slowly (3 to 4 weeks) in contrast to the more rapid induction of the capacity to give an Arthus skin reaction (2 to 3 weeks) following immunization with an antibody-inducing antigen (a humoral immune response). However, as stated above, delayed hypersensitivity refers not to the slow onset of sensitivity but to the slow evolution of the skin reaction following intradermal antigen challenge in contrast to the two other immunologically specific skin reactions commonly used in clinical immunology which occur much more rapidly following intradermal antigenic challenge—the immediate and the Arthus reactions characteristic to Types I and III immune reactions, respectively (see Chapters 7 and 14).

Delayed hypersensitivity is also not an exaggerated sensitivity or allergy to the inciting agent. Allergies like hay fever or asthma are exhibited by only a small minority of individuals (5 to 10%), all of whom are equally exposed to the antigen (or allergen). The allergic response is, therefore, not the usual or expected response to the allergen; rather, it is generally accepted that the allergic individual has a genetically determined predisposition to respond in this abnormal manner to otherwise innocuous substances. On the other hand, cell-mediated immunity is the immune mechanism universally selected by nature to be activated in response to an antigen like the tubercle bacillus. All individuals suitably exposed to this antigen will invariably develop the capacity to give delayed skin reactions if challenged intradermally with the antigen. Therefore, it would be more appropriate, and scientifically more valid, to refer to this reaction as a delayed skin reaction (DSR) or cell-mediated immune skin reaction rather than as a delayed hypersensitivity skin reaction.

CHARACTERISTICS OF THE DELAYED SKIN REACTION

The delayed skin reaction is a visible manifestation in the skin of a cell-mediated immune response. The reaction becomes obvious 12 to 24 hours after challenge and reaches maximum intensity after an additional 24 to 48 hours. This reaction should be contrasted with the histamine-mediated erythema-wheal-flare reaction characteristic of the allergen-induced skin reaction (discernible in minutes, maximum intensity in 10 to 20 minutes) and the Arthus reaction initiated by the deposition of immune complexes along the basement membrane of small blood vessels (evident by 4 hours, maximum intensity by 6 to 12 hours). The delayed skin reaction at its zenith is characterized by a nonpitting edema and induration, attributable to massive infiltration of mononuclear cells—small, medium, and large lymphocytes, macrophages, histiocytes, foam cells—and multinucleated giant cells resulting from the fusion of two or more macrophages. There is destruction and necrosis of adjacent muscle bundles and collagen fibers and swelling of the ground sustance. Perivascular "cuffs" of these cells are a common observation, with the cells actually adhering to the inner walls of the small blood vessels (postcapillary venules) or forming a frank thrombus. In a severe reaction, small vessel occlusion by thrombus results in localized areas of tissue breakdown and necrosis, followed by healing by fibrosis and scar formation. The usual reaction is much milder and does not normally culminate with ulceration and scar formation. Reversion to normal results by absorption of the exudate and subepithelial healing.

INFILTRATION OF MONONUCLEAR CELLS

What initiates and sustains the massive infiltration of mononuclear cells in the challenged skin site? Following the transfer to a normal animal of ^{3}H-thymidine-labeled lymphoid cells obtained from a syngeneic sensitized animal and intradermal challenge of this normal recipient with the specific antigen, it can be shown by radioautographic analysis of a biopsy specimen of the challenged skin site that only 1 to 5% of the infiltrating mononuclear cells are donor cells, that is, actively sensitized cells. The vast majority of the infiltrating cells, more than 95% of the cells, are nonsensitized cells of host origin. It is, therefore, necessary to explain how and why normal, nonsensitized mononuclear cells can be recruited by the antigen to infiltrate the challenge site.

Upon initial sensitization of the host with an antigen which characteristically induces a cell-mediated immune response, inherently precommitted T cells of a particular subclass armed with surface membrane receptors for this antigen react with the antigen. This reaction triggers a series of intracellular events which culminate with cells becoming "sensitized" or endowed with the capacity to liberate invader-repelling mediators following subsequent interaction of these cells with the original sensitizing antigen (Fig. 6.1).

LYMPHOKINES

The mediators are referred to collectively as **lymphokines**. They include transfer factor (TF), mononuclear cell chemotactic factor (MCF), mitogenic factor (MF), migration inhibitory factor (MIF), cytotoxic factor or lymphotoxin (LT), macrophage-activating factor (MAF), osteoclast-activating factor, and interferon. To date, more than 20 mediators have been identified as originating from sensitized lymphocytes and from monocytes, and undoubtedly other factors remain to be discovered. It must be kept in mind, however, that the lymphokines have been isolated from and tested in cell cultures maintained under artificially controlled conditions which can charitably be described at best as highly unphysiologic. Undoubtedly, a few of these lymphokines are real in that they are probably also synthesized in vivo. However, it is highly probable that a majority of the lymphokines are artifacts, synthesized by the cells in response to abnormal, unphysiologic signals or stimuli or released from the cells during their degenerative phases in vitro. Since the normal in vivo detoxifying mechanisms are not operative in vitro, these factors will accumulate. Those which have effects on the cells in agreement with contemporary concepts concerning the mechanism of the cell-mediated immune reaction are referred to as lymphokines. Nevertheless, several of the lymphokines enumerated above have withstood the test of time and have been shown to be distinct entities. Furthermore, they are sufficient to explain the evolution of the delayed skin reaction in a sensitized individual following intradermal challenge with the antigen.

Circulating sensitized cells passing through the challenge site interact with the antigen, resulting in the release of lymphokines into the microenvironment. The MCF attracts unsensitized "innocent bystander" cells into the challenge site, and MIF prevents these cells from emigrating. TF acts on these normal cells and converts them into responder cells. These newly recruited, passively sensitized cells cannot be functionally distinguished from

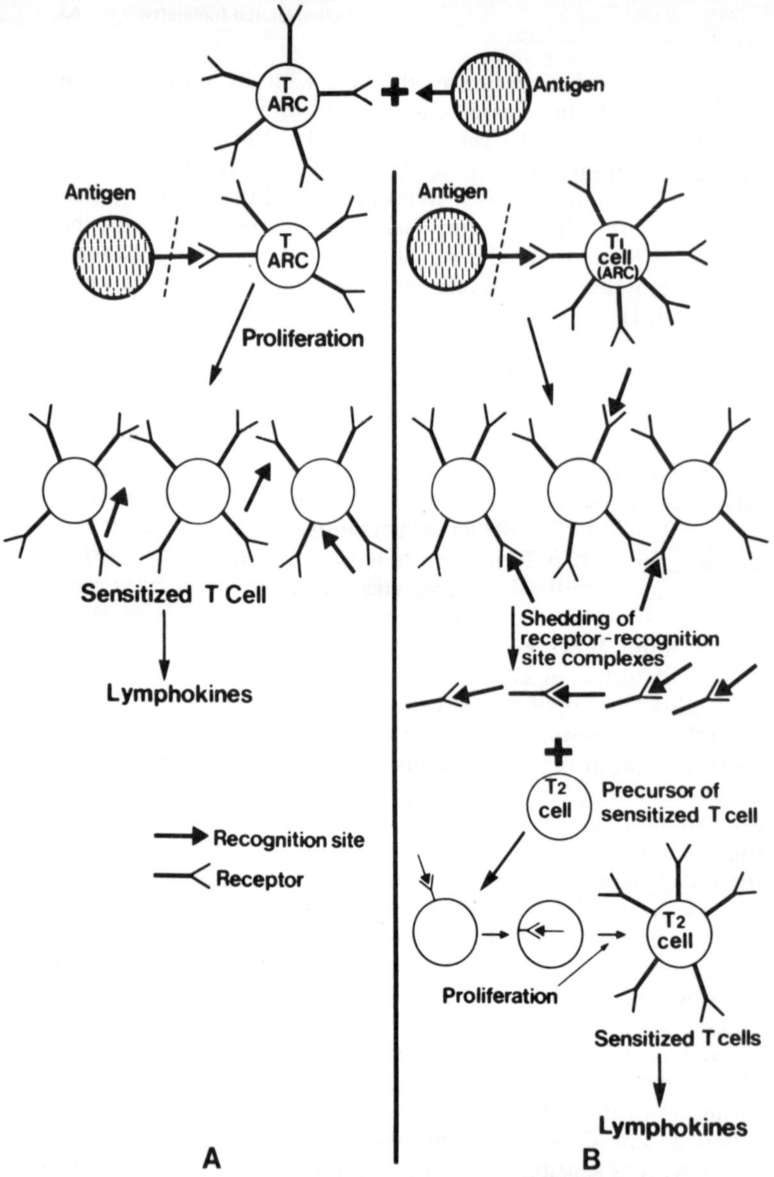

Figure 6.1 *The cellular interactions in the induction of sensitized lymphocytes in the cell-mediated immune response. (A) pre-1970s scheme involved only one T cell which could be activated by the sensitizing antigen and which would transform into and/or generate the sensitized T cell. (B) post-1970s scheme involves at least two T cells, one analogous to the T ARC helper cells in the antibody response and the other a precursor T cell which transforms into and/or generates the sensitized T cells.*

actively sensitized cells. Thus, TF serves as an amplification factor, as the TF secreted from a single sensitized lymphocyte can probably recruit 10 to 100 normal cells. MF acts on the actively sensitized cells and on the recruited passively sensitized cells, inducing blast transformation and proliferation of these cells. The progeny revert to small and medium-size lymphocytes. MAF acts on the infiltrating monocytes and the macrophages by "activating" or "arming" them so that they are much more actively phagocytic. These activated phagocytes attack any "sick" bystander autologous cells and foreign cells (i.e. the invading microorganisms) but not normal autologous cells. LT acts on all foreign cells and kills them by an as yet undefined mechanism. Like MAF-transformed macrophages, it does not act on normal syngeneic cells. The demonstration that an osteoclast-activating factor is also secreted by the sensitized lymphocytes upon contact with the antigen facilitates the elucidation of the pathology of the inflamed joint in rheumatoid arthritis.

Important

The reader may still be somewhat confused as to the disctinctness of the effector mechanisms in humoral and cell-mediated immunity—antibodies and lymphokines, respectively. The properties which distinguish antibodies from lymphokines are presented in Table 6.1. It is imperative to note that antibodies secreted by B cells can interact only with the specific antigen (the same antigenic determinant, to be more precise), whereas lymphokines are secreted primarily by the sensitized T cells upon confrontation with the specific sensitizing antigen and they act nonspecifically and indiscriminately on bystander or infiltrating lymphocytes, macrophages, fibrocytes, and muscle cells. The lymphokines do not interact with the sensitizing antigen.

Table 6.1
Properties Which Distinguish Antibodies from Lymphokines

Property or Activity	Antibodies	Lymphokines
Synthesized by B cells	Yes	No
Synthesized by T cells	No	Yes
Interact with specific immunizing antigen	Yes	No
Act on cells in nonspecific fashion	No	Yes
Are protein in nature	Yes	Yes
Constitute a homogeneous family of compounds	No	No
Reactive sites have a similar configuration and structure	Yes	No

ANTIGEN-SPECIFIC RECEPTORS

Although antibodies are not directly involved in the induction and maintenance of the delayed skin reaction, the reaction is mediated by sensitized cells which express a specificity toward the antigen comparable to that displayed by antibody molecules. The specificity of the cell-mediated immune reaction dictates that the antigen must interact with surface configurations or receptors on the surface of the sensitized cell configurationally complementary to the antigen. However, the nature and composition of the receptors have not been determined. It has been proposed that antibodies with a high affinity for lymphoid cells, referred to as cytophilic antibodies, become irreversibly bound to the cell surface and constitute the "receptors" for the antigen. Accordingly, the sensitized lymphocyte is actually a complex of antibody with a previously innocent, bystander lymphocyte, the lymphocyte acting in a passive capacity as the carrier of the antibody molecules. However, such passively sensitized lymphocytes cannot passively transfer the capacity to elicit a delayed skin reaction, a property characteristic and definitive for actively sensitized lymphocytes. Therefore, although antibodies with a high affinity for normal lymphocytes exist in the circulation following immunization, this proposed mechanism to account for cell-mediated immunity has not won wide support.

If conventional and cytophilic antibodies are eliminated as the providers of the antigen-specific receptors on the sensitized lymphocyte, it must be assumed that the receptors are synthesized by the appropriately stimulated lymphocytes during the sensitization period of the immune response and that the receptors constitute essential components of the cell surface. Whether the receptors are similar to the Fab segment of the antibody molecule may only be speculated upon at the present time.

ORIGIN OF SENSITIZED CELLS

The sensitized cells, or more specifically their precursors, seem to arise from among the lymphocytes which compose the T cell-dependent areas of the lymph nodes and spleen. The most striking morphologic changes during the induction of cell-mediated immunity to a locally applied antigen occur in the draining lymph nodes, especially when the antigen consists of a skin allograft or an epicutaneously applied chemical sensitizer such as DNCB.

The lymph nodes hypertrophy to 2 to 3 times their original size and weight during the first 4 to 6 days postsensitization. Microscopically there is marked proliferation of cells in the T-dependent areas of the draining lymph nodes (the interfollicular, paracortical, and deep cortical areas) with resultant compression of the lymphoid follicles by the 2nd to 3rd day. Large numbers of pyroninophilic blast cells can be detected by the 4th day within the T-dependent areas, and they appear to migrate to the inner margins of the cortex where it interfaces with the medulla. These cells then appear to invade the medullary cords, penetrate the venous sinuses, and thence the circulation, where they may be detected in small numbers by days 4 to 6. Within the lymph node, the bursts of cell division result in the generation not of more blast cells but of small lymphocytes by days 6 to 8. The onset of the capacity to elicit a cell-mediated delayed skin reaction appears to coincide with the appearance of these newly generated small lymphocytes in the circulation. These are the effector sensitized T cells which infiltrate the allograft or the skin site challenged with DNCB.

A percentage of these sensitized cells are long-lived recirculating cells; they can, therefore, be detected in the circulation for months or years postsensitization (in contrast to the absence of antibody-forming cells in the circulation during an antibody response except at the peak of the immune response when they may temporarily invade the circulation). The precursors of these immunologically committed sensitized lymphocytes remain in the lymph node where they were initially generated, and they constitute the pool of cells which can be rapidly reactivated following reimmunization with the same antigen.

Important

It is important to stress the difference between the cell-mediated immune response and the humoral or antibody immune response on a purely morphologic level, as other distinguishing criteria are listed in Table 6.1 and have been discussed above. The humoral immune response, following aggressive immunization with an antigen capable of inducing a humoral immune response, is characterized by an initial mild immunoblast response in the T cell-dependent areas (which can be attributed to proliferation of T ARC cells) which is quickly overtaken by a much more marked blast response in the B cell-dependent lymphoid follicles. The primary follicles may become greatly enlarged and be identified by the appearance of germinal centers which may also hypertrophy markedly before finally contracting to normal dimensions. This is followed by the generation of plasmablasts and plasma cells which can be detected in large numbers first in the deep cortex and then in the medulla. On the other hand, the most dramatic change in the lymph node during the induction of a cell-mediated response is a blast cell response in the T cell-dependent areas with no detectable changes in the B cell-dependent lymphoid follicles. The pyroninophilic blast cells undergo several mitotic divisions, and the progeny of the terminal mitotic division transform to small lymphocytes which constitute the specifically sensitized cells.

The reader may, at this point, conclude that the experimental animal or human immunized with an antigen can respond with either a humoral or cell-mediated immune response, but not with both. In fact, it has been demonstrated that, with many antigens to which the anticipated and verified response is a humoral one, the initial response appears to mimic, morphologically, a cell-mediated immune response. Animals injected with subthreshold (for the antibody response) quantities of conventional protein antigens emulsified in Freund's adjuvant, or subjected to a dose of total body irradiation sufficient to inhibit the antibody response but not the cell-mediated immune response, can be shown to respond with a cell-mediated immune response within the first 7 to 14 days postimmunization. However, this immune response is largely masked in the immunized normal animal due to the almost simultaneous or intercurrent synthesis of antibodies. Since the antibodies and the sensitized cells exhibit the identical antigenic specificity, that is, they react with the identical or adjacent antigen determinant sites on the antigen molecule, the circulating antibodies can more easily interact with and neutralize the antigen determinants (due to the absence of steric hindrance as encountered with the sensitized cells). Therefore, the delayed skin reaction cannot be induced following intradermal challenge with the antigen, and the cell-mediated immune response is not considered to have occurred.

The converse is also true. It has been demonstrated that individuals immunized with BCG or old tuberculin to give the anticipated cell-mediated immune response do in fact synthesize antibodies toward at least eight constituents of the antigen. These antibodies can be detected by conventional immunoassays (i.e. precipitation in gel). However, these antibodies do not appear to play a role in the induction of the delayed skin reaction, probably because the antibodies in this instance are not directed toward the determinant sites with which the sensitized cells interact and, therefore, do not impede interaction of the antigen with infiltrating sensitized cells.

A question which is invariably asked by those individuals who constantly seek to equate and contrast the variety of participating cells in the humoral and cell-mediated immune responses is whether more than one type of T cell is involved in the induction of cell-mediated immunity. Until the 1970s, it was assumed that a single T cell could subserve the functions of both antigenic recognition and specific commitment or sensitization (Fig. 6.1). However, results of investigations in the 1970s strongly implicate at least two distinct T cell lines in the induction of the sensitized T cells. One of these T cells appears to act in the capacity of a helper cell (analogous to the helper T ARC cell in the antibody response) as it facilitates the generation of sensitized T cells from precursors of the sensitized cells (Fig. 6.1).

Thus, the cell-mediated immune response appears to mirror the humoral immune response insofar as both responses are characterized by the existence of virgin, precommitted antigen-recognizing "helper" cells (ARC cells) which interact with the antigenic determinant sites via specific surface membrance receptors. On the other hand, the properties which distinguish between the humoral and cell-mediated immune responses support the generally held view that they are distinct immune responses. These are (a) the essential participation of B cells in the humoral immune response and the absence of B cell participation in the cell-mediated immune response; (b) the differing morphologic features in the affected lymphoid tissues; and (c) the roles of antigen-specific antibody molecules as opposed to non-antigen-specific lymphokines as the effector agents in the humoral and cell-mediated immune responses, respectively.

CHAPTER 7

Immune Reactions Used to Assess the Immunocompetent State

IN VITRO IMMUNE REACTIONS

An immune reaction, whether its consequences are protective or pathologic, is defined strictly in terms of its specificity. All the other criteria which define the immune reaction may be considered as commentary. In the absence of the criterion of specificity, the reaction is not an immune reaction, although it could be so defined on the basis of a half-dozen ancillary properties. The basis of the immune reaction is the interaction of the antigenic determinant on the antigen molecule with the specific antigen-binding site on the F(ab) segment of the antibody molecule. In order to appreciate the antibody-antigen reaction, which forms the basis for an understanding of immunology, one must first become aware of the conditions governing this reaction.

In nature, the antibody molecule, whether it be an IgG, circulating IgA, IgD, or IgE, has two, only two, and always two antigen-binding sites. These sites are located at the amino-terminal end of F(ab) regions (Fig. 3.1). IgM, being a pentamer of the four-chain unit, has 10 sites, and secretory IgA, being a dimer, has four such sites. The point is that the smallest naturally occurring protein exhibiting antibody activity is the basic four-chain structure, and it possesses two antigen-binding sites.

Naturally occurring antigens, on the other hand, may have any number of identical and/or different antigenic determinant sites in their structure, with as few as two or as many as 50,000.

Each antigen-binding site is referred to as a valence. Thus, the IgG antibody molecule always has a valence of two, whereas the antigen may have a valence of two to 50,000.

A characteristic of the antigen-antibody reactions is the marked difference in their sensitivity to detect antibody (Table 7.1). This point will be elaborated upon in the subsequent discussion. Appreciation and understanding of the factors which limit or

Table 7.1
Relative Sensitivity of Antibody-Antigen Reactions

Serologic Procedure	Relative Sensitivity
A. In vitro	
1. Precipitation in fluid or gel	1
2. Immunofluorescence	2–5
3. Complement fixation	10–100
4. Bacterial agglutination	100–1,000
5. Hemagglutination (active or passive)	100–1,000
6. Nephelometry	1,000–10,000
7. Radioimmunoassay	10,000–100,000
8. Enzyme-linked immunosorbent assay (ELISA)	10,000–100,000
B. In vivo	
1. Toxin neutralization	10–100
2. Anaphylaxis	1–5
3. Skin reaction	1
Arthus reaction	

enhance the sensitivity of the immune reactions permit their rational utilization in diagnostic immunology.

To facilitate an understanding of the antigen-antibody reaction, we will assume that the soluble protein antigen has two identical antigenic determinant sites (not normally the case) and that the IgG antibody has two antigen-binding sites (normally always the case) (Fig. 7.1).

Immune Precipitation in Liquid Medium (the Precipitin Test)

Let us assume that an antiserum (usually used undiluted) containing IgG antibodies (Ab) directed to a divalent antigen (Ag) is deposited into the bottom of a capillary tube and the antigen solution (usually a 0.1 to 0.5% solution in saline) is layered on top of the antiserum (Fig. 7.2). The antiserum, being the more dense reactant, should always be added first to the tube, followed by the antigen solution. A white precipitate will form at the interface within minutes, and the precipitation band will widen and may actually fall to the bottom of the tube, to be replaced by a second precipitation band. This test is referred to as the **interfacial precipitin ring test** and is the most primitive yet the most specific and appropriate screening test for the detection of antibodies. What causes the precipitation of the antibody by the antigen?

Let us assume that we have incubated equal numbers of

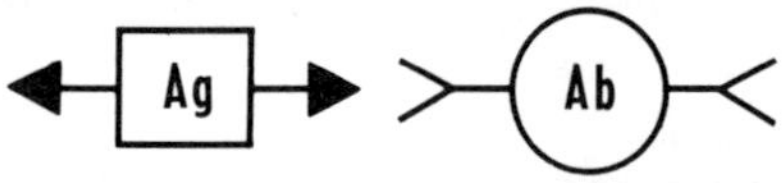

Figure 7.1 *A diagrammatic representation of a divalent antigen and divalent antibody. As per definition, each reactant possesses two combining sites.*

divalent antibody and antigen molecules (Fig. 7.1). The antigen and antibody molecules are normally in solution and are, therefore, hydrophilic. At physiologic pH, there is a positive (+) and negative (−) charge at the amino and carboxyl terminals of the molecule, respectively. Additionally, there are negative (−) charges due to the free carboxyl groups of aspartic and glutamic acid and positive (+) charges due to the free epsilon amino groups of lysine. The sites on the antigen and the antibody molecules where interactions occur are usually positively or negatively charged, respectively, and, therefore, there is a great deal of water of solvation helping to maintain the hydrophilic properties of the antibody and antigen molecules. Following interaction of the antibody with the antigen, there is a loss of net charge at the sites of interaction since the antigenic determinants and the antigen-binding sites are oppositely charged. Water molecules are expelled, and the Ag-Ab chain begins to take on the characteristics of a long uncharged aliphatic fatty acid chain, which is hydrophobic. Once the Ab-Ag chain is sufficiently long, the hydrophobicity will dictate that it become water-insoluble and precipitate out of solution (Fig. 7.3). Under conditions of antigen excess or antibody excess, the Ab-Ag complexes cannot become long enough to become sufficiently hydrophobic; therefore, they do not precipitate out of solution (Fig. 7.3).

The limitations of the precipitin test, carried out in the liquid or gel phase, are that (a) the antibody concentration must be relatively high (greater than 20 mg %) and (b) the antibody must be a precipitating type of antibody. The advantages are (a) the simplicity of the technique and (b) the specificity of the reaction, which is partly a reflection of its lack of sensitivity.

Important

1. As the different techniques used to detect and quantitate antibodies are described, the reader will not fail to note that they become increasingly more sensitive. Paradoxically, as the sensitivity of a technique increases, the less specific the reaction becomes. This is due to the fact that, as the technique becomes exceedingly sensitive, it will permit the detection of the ever present small number of antibody molecules which are directed toward contaminating or cross-reacting antigens. These antibodies are normally not detected by the precipitin reaction.

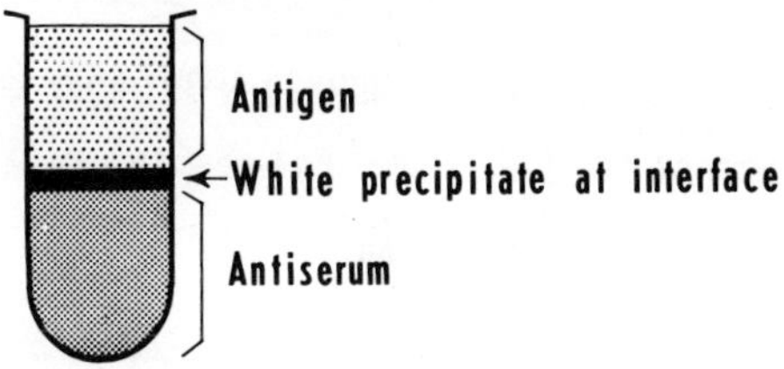

Figure 7.2 *The interfacial ring or precipitin test.*

2. The reader will easily understand that in the example given above, where both the antibody and antigen molecules are divalent, 50% of the immune precipitate is composed of antigen and 50% of antibody since equal numbers of antigen and antibody molecules are incorporated into the Ab-Ag chain under optimal conditions for Ab-Ag precipitation (see below). However, as discussed previously, a naturally occurring antigen tends to possess many more antigenic determinant sites on its surface than there are antigen-binding sites on the surface on an antibody molecules (10 to 100 as compared to two, respectively). It can be demonstrated that the ratio of antibody molecules to antigen molecules in the immune precipitate obtained under optimal conditions is directly proportional to the ratio of the valences of the antigen and the antibody molecules:

$$\frac{\text{No. of antibody molecules in precipitate}}{\text{No. of antigen molecules in precipitate}} \cdot \alpha \frac{\text{Valence of antigen molecule}}{\text{Valence of antibody molecule}}$$

If the valence of the antigen molecule is 10 to 20 (which is not unusual with naturally occurring antigens), then it can be easily calculated that 80 to 90% of the immune precipitate is composed of antibody molecules. Thus, the limiting factor in the facilitation of immune precipitation is the concentration of antibody molecules, not antigen molecules.

Once an antibody-antigen reaction has been detected by the interfacial ring test, the amount of antibody in the serum can be precisely determined by the use of the **quantitative precipitin test**, first introduced by Heidelberger and Kendall in 1935 (Fig. 7.4). In this test, the antigen is usually dissolved in 1 ml of saline and doubling dilutions are made in 1-ml volumes. One milliliter of the antiserum, usually diluted 1:5 or 1:10, is then added to each of the tubes, the contents are shaken, and the tubes are incubated

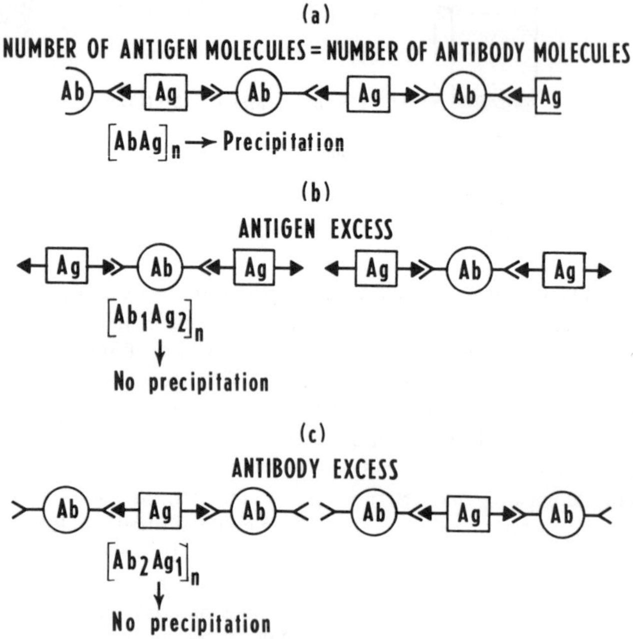

Figure 7.3 *The precipitation of divalent antibody by divalent antigen.*

in a water bath for 60 minutes at 37°C. They are examined every 5 to 10 minutes. As can be seen in Figure 7.4, tube 4 displays the first signs of a visible Ab-Ag reaction, which is opalescence. This is followed by turbidity, flocculation, and precipitation. These reactions also take place, to varying degrees, in the tubes on each side of tube 4. Tube 4 also will be found to contain the most precipitate. By definition, tube 4 contains the antibody and antigen in optimal proportions, that is, the ratio of antigen to antibody which facilitates maximum co-precipitation of antigen and antibody. This relationship is referred to as the "Dean-Webb antibody constant antigen variable optimal proportions ratio." The precipitate can be dissolved in a dilute acetic acid solution and the protein content determined spectrophotometrically. Since normally greater than 90% of the immune precipitate is composed of antibody molecules, the protein content of the immune precipitate can be considered to represent the antibody content of 1 ml of the antiserum.

The limitations and advantages of this technique are similar to those described above for the interfacial ring test.

This technique was used extensively in the 1930s and 1940s to quantitate the concentration of antibodies (i.e. antipneumococcal

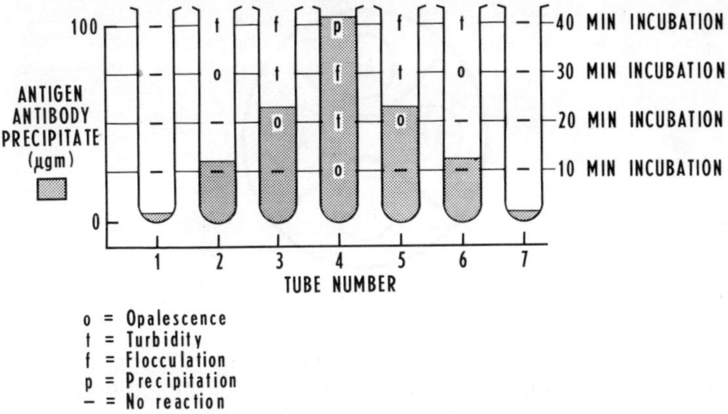

Figure 7.4 *The quantitative precipitation reaction. Antigen is added in a 2-fold dilution sequence to tubes 1 to 7. The antiserum, in a constant concentration, is added to all the tubes. Therefore, the system is in relative antigen excess in tubes 1 to 3 and in relative antibody excess in tube 5 to 7. Note: The absence of precipitation in tube 7 may also be attributed to insufficient antigen to facilitate immune precipitation.*

polysaccharide antibodies) in the antisera prepared in animals for chemotherapeutic use in patients with suspected infectious disease (i.e. diplococcus pneumonia). Its use today is almost totally limited to that of a laboratory exercise in the immunology laboratory course.

Precipitation in Agarose Gel (Semisolid Medium)

By the early 1950s agar gel medium had replaced the liquid phase for the demonstration of immune precipitation. An example is the Ouchterlony technique, whereby the flat bottom surface of a Petri dish is covered with the agarose solution (0.5%) to a depth of 3 to 4 mm. The agarose is permitted to solidify at room temperature. Four wells of equal dimensions placed equidistant to each other are then dug out of the agar by the use of templates, and these are then filled with saline solutions of either the antigen or the antiserum (Fig. 7.5). The antigen and antibody molecules will diffuse toward each other in the agarose phase, and they will co-precipitate when they meet at or near optimal proportions. The precipitin band may appear to migrate toward either the antigen or the antibody well. However, this is an illusion. What does happen is that the precipitate initially formed between the antigen and antibody molecules will usually dissolve, either because of antigen excess or antibody excess conditions, and the precipitate band will reform in the direction of the reactant

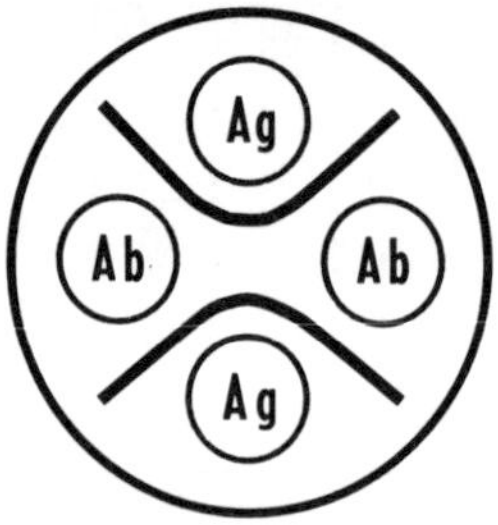

Figure 7.5 *Antibody-antigen precipitation in a gel.*

present in the lesser concentration. The greater the concentration of the antigen relative to the concentration of the antibodies, the closer to the antiserum well will the final stationary precipitin band be formed, and vice versa. Thus, one can simultaneously determine the relative concentrations of the same antigen in a number of unknown specimens or the relative concentrations of the same antibodies in different antisera.

Here again, the use of this technique is limited by the need to have relatively high concentrations of antibodies and the need of the antibodies to be a precipitating type.

Immunoelectrophoresis—Immune Precipitation in Gel following Electrophoresis of Antigen(s) in Gel

By this technique, the antigen(s) is first subjected to electrophoresis in the gel medium followed by diffusion of the antibody and antigen molecules toward each other in the gel resulting in lines of precipitation (Fig. 7.6). The advantage of this method, as compared to the straightforward diffusion in gel discussed above, is that separation of the antigens in the antigen solution can be effected first by electrophoresis, following which each individual antigen can be identified by precipitation in the gel with the respective antibodies.

This technique permits the investigator to determine the degree of (antigenic) heterogeneity of the different serum protein families, bacterial culture filtrates, vaccines, and purified antigens such as the "purified protein derivative" (PPD) of tuberculin. The latter can be shown by immunoelectrophoresis to consist of at least 8 to 10 distinct antigenic constituents, so that reference to it as a "purified" antigen would seem to be inappropriate.

The greatest use of immunoelectrophoresis in the clinical immunology laboratory lies in its ability to permit the simultaneous detection of the IgG, IgM, and IgA immunoglobulin classes of proteins (not their quantitation) and their monoclonal or polyclonal nature as defined by the shape of the precipitin arcs

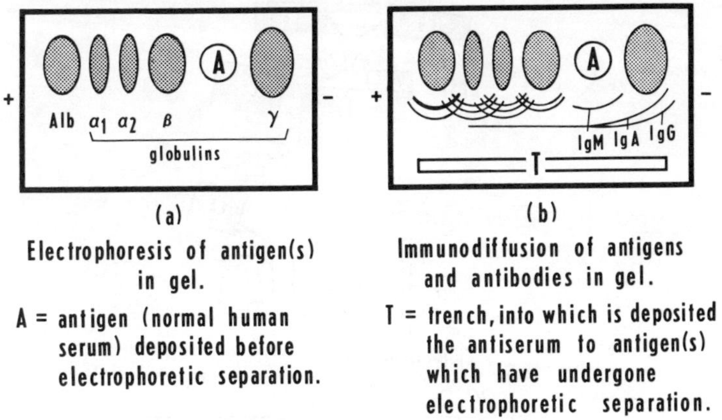

+
Alb α1 α2 β γ
globulins
A
-
+
A
IgM IgA IgG
T
-
(a)
Electrophoresis of antigen(s) in gel.
A = antigen (normal human serum) deposited before electrophoretic separation.
(b)
Immunodiffusion of antigens and antibodies in gel.
T = trench, into which is deposited the antiserum to antigen(s) which have undergone electrophoretic separation.

Figure 7.6 *Immunoelectrophoretic analysis of serum proteins.*

formed subsequently in the gel between the immunoglobulins and the xenogeneic antiserum.

Important

The limitations of this method are that (a) an antigen can only be identified if antibodies have been formed toward it, (b) the antibodies to each individual antigen must be present in a concentration exceeding 10 mg%, and (c) the antibodies must be of the precipitating type.

Complement and Complement Fixation

Complement (C′) consists of at least nine normally circulating innocuous protein complexes. These are designated C′1 to C′9 (Fig. 7.7). Following interaction of the antigen (Ag) with the antibody (Ab) (IgG or IgM), C′1 interacts with the Ab-Ag complex, resulting in its activation and initiation of a cascade reaction resulting in activation of each of the components of the C′ system, beginning with C′1 and ending with C′9. As the different complement components are activated, they release highly active mediators into the microenvironment. Several of these are neutrophil chemotactic factor, anaphylatoxin (histamine-releasing agent), proteolytic enzymes, etc. If the antigen happens to be a bacterium or red blood cell, cytolysis will occur almost immediately following activation of C′7, C′8, and C′9, which appear to be activated simultaneously. The lysis is due to enzymatically induced focal destruction of the cell membrane with reversal of the sodium-potassium pump followed by osmotic lysis. The term complement fixation is a misnomer, based on the original belief that the complement components actually adhere

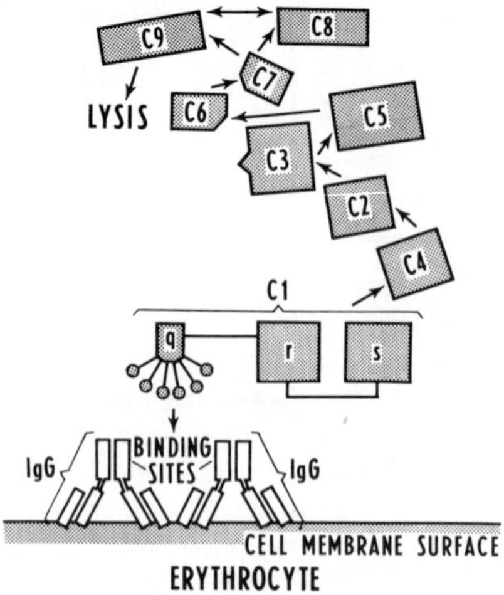

Figure 7.7 *The classical complement fixation reaction. The antigen is the red blood cell, and the antibody is IgG antibody directed toward the red cell. (The author would like to thank the UpJohn Pharmaceutical Company for permission to use this illustration.)*

to the antigen-antibody aggregate. This is not so, and, in fact, only several of the nine major constituents of the complement system, primarily C′1 and C′3, adhere to the antigen-antibody complex.

The complement system can be activated by the **classical and alternate pathways** (Fig. 7.8). In the classical pathway, the components are activated in sequence beginning with C′1 and ending with C′9 (actually C′8 and C′9 are activated simultaneously). In the alternate pathway, the complement system becomes activated as a result of interaction of the complement-fixing reactants with C′3, bypassing C′1, C′2, and C′4. The remaining constituents of the complement system are activated in the same way as in the classical pathway. Each component must be present in a concentration sufficient to permit the activation of the factor following it or the reaction stops.

From the historical point of view, complement fixation was originally defined in terms of activation of the first four components—C′1, C′4, C′2, and C′3 in that order, with lysis following activation of C′3. In the absence of activation of the first three complement constituents, C′1, C′4, and C′2, the reaction was not considered to be one of complement fixation, irrespective of the manifestations of the reaction.

Recently, however, it has been unequivocally demonstrated

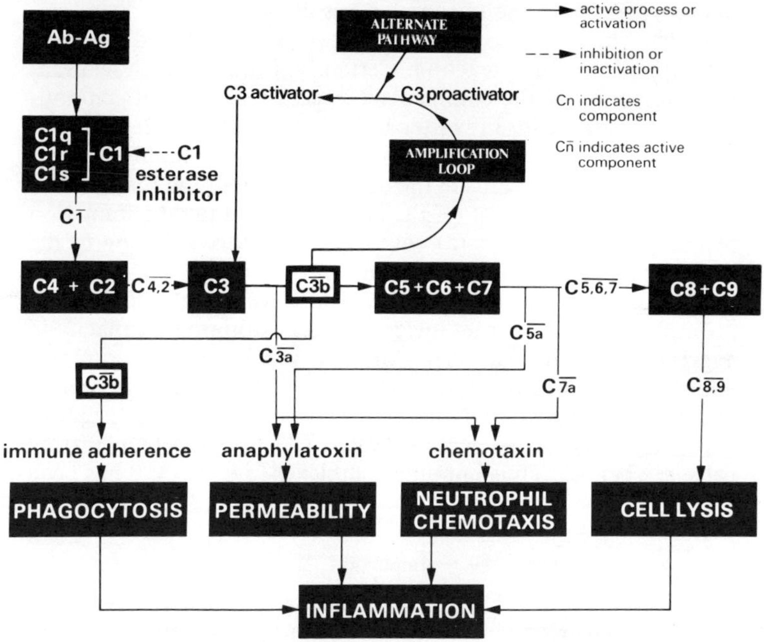

Figure 7.8 *Complement fixation. The classical pathway of complement fixation is initiated at the C′1 level by the antigen-antibody complex. The alternate pathway is initiated at the C′3 stage. The complement fixation reaction serves as a mechanism for the activation of pharmacologically active mediators. (The author would like to thank Behring Diagnostics, Hoeschst Pharmaceuticals, Canadian Hoechst, Ltd., for permission to use this illustration.)*

that the complement system can be activated by certain materials *without* participation of C′1, C′2, or C′4. These materials constitute a group of seemingly unrelated substances, i.e. inulin, dextran, bacterial endotoxins, polyvinylpyrrolidone, casein. The reactions induced in vivo as a result of their administration are indistinguishable from antigen-antibody-induced anaphylactic shock, and they are, therefore, referred to as anaphylactoid reactions. It has been demonstrated that the agents causing anaphylactoid reactions do, in fact, fix complement by reacting directly with C′3 and bypassing C′1, C′2, and C′4 (the alternate pathway of complement fixation). The activation of C′3 is dependent upon prior interaction of the foreign substance with a number of normally circulating proteins known collectively as the "properdin system."

If the complement system existed only to interact with the

microorganism-antibody complex, resulting in lysis of the microorganism, the host would rarely if ever suffer from deleterious consequences of this reaction. Certainly, it has been shown that the interaction of the complement system with the antigen-antibody complex results in swifter and greatly enhanced degradation and elimination of the antigen. If the antigen is a highly virulent pathogenic microorganism, the complement fixation reaction has great survival value as it results in the lysis and rapid elimination of the pathogen due to (a) complement factors adhering to the immune complex, thus increasing the size of the complex and facilitating phagocytosis by the macrophages and neutrophils; (b) "complement-fixed" immune complexes exhibiting a capacity to aggregate (conglutination?), forming much larger complexes which are more easily eliminated by the phogocytic cells; and (c) macrophages, neutrophils, and lymphocytes possessing receptors, capable of interacting with activated C′3 (C′3 receptor-bearing cells, see below). Thus immune complexes to which C′3 has been "fixed" can be eliminated by interaction with C′3 receptor-bearing cells.

Important

Antibodies by themselves are not cytotoxic. In fact, they may even stimulate proliferation of the organism. It is the antibody-complement system which is cytotoxic.

A number of pharmacologically very active factors (or mediators) are formed and/or activated and/or released during the immune complement-fixation reaction (Fig. 7.8). The majority of these factors function to provide more protection to the host by amplifying the inflammatory response. However, at least two of the factors, anaphylatoxin(s) and neutrophil chemotactic factor(s), may provoke a life-threatening situation in the host if they are not neutralized or if they are generated in excessive amounts during the C′ fixation reaction. The anaphylatoxin is capable of inducing degranulation of platelets, mast cells, and basophils, resulting in the release into the circulation of a number of very potent pharmacologically active agents, such as histamine, serotonin, and blood-clotting factors. The former two are capable of inducing vascular collapse and shock. This type of noncardiogenic shock should be contrasted with cardiogenic shock, anaphylactic shock as a consequence of the release of histamine and serotonin from mast cells following the interaction of the allergen or the antigen with IgE antibodies fixed onto these cells (see Type I reaction, Chapter 14), and endotoxin-induced shock attributed to the activation of anaphylatoxin(s) from circulating serum protein precursors following activation of the complement system via the alternate pathway (Table 7.2). The clotting factors re-

Table 7.2
Properties Which Distinguish between Immunologically Mediated and Nonimmunologically Induced Shock

Condition	Conditions or Reactants Involved				
	Preimmunization with Antigen or Allergen	Type of Antibodies Involved	Primary Reactants Involved	Secondary Reactants Involved	Circulating Mediators Inducing Shock
Cardiogenic shock	No	None	None	None	None
Anaphylactic shock	Yes	IgE antibodies	Immune complexes on mast cells	None	Histamine, serotonin
Endotoxin shock	No	None	None	Anaphylatoxins, following C′ fixation by alternate pathway	Histamine, serotonin, proteolytic enzymes
"Immune" C′ fixation shock	Yes	IgG	Immune complexes in the circulation in high concentration	Anaphylatoxins following C′ fixation by classical pathway	Histamine, serotonin, proteolytic enzymes

leased from the platelets initiate intravascular coagulation, especially within the small blood vessels where the blood flow is sluggish. The neutrophil chemotactic factor is primarily responsible for the massive infiltration of polymorphonuclear leukocytes at the site of the reaction. These cells release very potent proteolytic enzymes into their microenvironment capable of causing local tissue necrosis and the clotting of blood by activation of the coagulation system.

Endotoxic shock, following infection with any of a number of gram-negative microorganisms, is due to the release of endotoxins from the organism which activate complement via the alternate pathway, resulting in the activation of anaphylatoxins and neutrophil chemotactic factors. The Schwartzman reaction, induced by the intravenous injection of an endotoxin 24 to 48 hours following a sensitizing injection of the same or even a different endotoxin, is also considered to be the result of a similar sequence of reactions. Disseminated intravascular coagulation (DIC) is a characteristic feature of this reaction.

Although complement is required for the effective eradication of invasive microorganisms, it can only become involved after antibodies have reacted with the antigen. The Fc region on the reacted, but not the native, circulating IgG antibody molecule is capable of activating C′1 by converting it into an esterase. Autoconversion of inactive C′1 into C′1 esterase is normally kept in check by the presence of a C′1 esterase inhibitor. The absence of this inhibitor in the circulation, as occurs in the clinical condition referred to as hereditary angioneurotic edema, results in indiscriminate activation of the complement system with pathologic consequences, such as recurrent urticaria or subcutaneous edema. Laryngeal edema is perhaps the most dramatic and life-threatening consequence of uncontrolled activation of the complement system and must be tended to immediately to prevent death from asphyxiation (respiratory failure).

Complement is quantitated in terms of the hemolytic titer of the serum in question when it is reacted with antibody-sensitized erythrocytes. The hemolytic titer is the inverse of the maximum dilution of the serum which can facilitate lysis of the antibody-erythrocyte complex. The hemolytic titer of normal serum is about 200 to 400. A serum with a hemolytic titer of 400 would be considered to contain 400 hemolytic units of complement. A hemolytic unit is, therefore, the minimum quantity of complement which can induce lysis of antibody-sensitized erythrocytes under optimal conditions.

Fresh guinea pig serum is the preferred source of C′ in view of its uniformly high hemolytic titer (800 to 3,200). Should fresh guinea pig serum not be available, fresh rabbit serum or human serum may be used as sources of C′, although their hemolytic titers are much lower. One or more of the components of C′ is heat-labile. Heating the fresh guinea pig serum (or any other serum used as a source of C′) for 30 to 60 minutes at 56°C results in total loss of C′ hemolytic activity. Since such treatment of antisera does not result in any deleterious effects on the antibody molecules, heating antisera at 56°C for 30 to 60 minutes is a routine procedure for the selective elimination of C′.

The guinea pig serum may be frozen and kept at −20°C for many months, if not years, without losing any significant hemolytic activity. However, storing the guinea pig serum for only a week at 4°C will invariably result in a significant loss of C′ hemolytic activity. A common way to store guinea pig serum is in the form of a lyophilized powder in which state the C′ is stable and the powder can be stored at 4°C for an indefinite period of time. It is only necessary to reconstitute the powder with water prior to its utilization in C′ fixation tests.

Certain clinical conditions are characterized by a marked decrease in the circulating hemolytic complement titer. The hemolytic complement titer in hereditary angioneurotic edema (HANE) or certain forms of immunodeficiency disease (hypocomplementemia) may be zero or as low as 10 or 20. The hemolytic complement titers in patients with immune complex disease (i.e. systemic lupus erythematosus), immunologically induced (poststreptococcal) glomerulonephritis, or collagen disease (i.e. polyarteritis nodosa) will also be decreased from the normal by 50 to 75%. The hemolytic complement titer will also be low in cases of liver dysfunction (cirrhosis, hepatitis, hepatoma), uremia, protein-losing enteropathies, and malignant diseases of the lymphoid system due to diminished synthesis of one or more of the complement components. Thus, the semiquantitation of hemolytically active complement in the serum is important in the differential diagnosis of a number of clinical conditions.

The utilization of the complement system is also very useful in the diagnosis of an infection. More precisely, the complement fixation reaction is used to indicate whether the patient has formed antibodies to the suspected infectious agent. Wasserman, at the turn of this century, was the first to utilize the complement fixation reaction in the diagnosis of an infection, in this case syphilis. This is known as the Wasserman test. Let us, therefore, use syphilis as an example to demonstrate how the complement fixation reaction is utilized in the diagnosis of an immune response to an infectious agent.

If the antigen (in this case *Treponema pallidum* organisms, which cause syphilis) is incubated with the serum of a patient containing antibodies to the organism (the serum is heated at 56°C for 30 minutes to inactivate its endogenous complement) and a known quantity of complement in the form of fresh guinea pig serum (the amount of complement usually used is 3 to 5 hemolytic units), the complement will be consumed secondary to the interaction between the *T. pallidum* and the specific antibodies (Fig. 7.9*a*, step 1). If one now adds antibody-sensitized indicator erythrocytes (Fig. 7.9*a*, step 2), the erythrocytes will not be lyzed since all of the complement added initially will have been con-

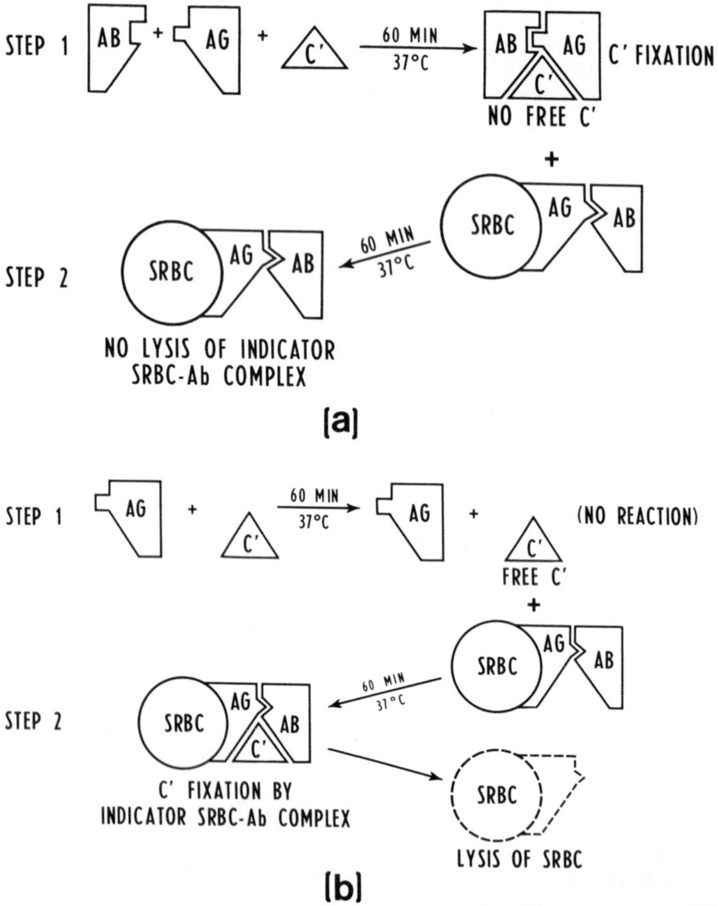

Figure 7.9 *The complement fixation reaction in (a) the presence and (b) the absence of specific antibodies to the suspected antigen.*

sumed in the interaction with the antibody-*T. pallidum* complexes and none is available to lyse the antibody-sensitized erythrocytes. Thus, failure to observe lysis of the indicator antibody-sensitized erythrocytes indicates a positive complement fixation by the suspected serum and, therefore, the presence of specific antibodies directed toward *T. pallidum*. On the other hand, lysis of the indicator antibody-sensitized erythrocytes in step 2 indicates no complement fixation by the suspected serum in step 1 and, therefore, no or undetectable quantities of specific antibodies to *T. pallidum* (Fig. 7.9*b*).

In practice, the Wasserman test utilizes an extract of beef heart in place of the *T. pallidum* organisms, as the beef heart extract is fortuitously just as effective in interacting with the anti-*T. pallidum* antibodies as is the *T. pallidum* itself. It is, therefore, ironic that the classical example of the complement fixation reaction utilizes a substitute for the true antigen.

Important

The limitations of this method are (a) the antibodies must be present in a sufficiently high concentration, (b) the antibodies must be of a complement-fixing type, and (c) one must not add an excessive amount of complement to the system or it will not all be consumed in step 1 of the reaction. The reaction would then be falsely interpreted as a negative complement fixation reaction.

Agglutination Reaction

The agglutination reaction is much more sensitive than the precipitin reaction for the detection of antibodies. This reaction is about 10 to 100 times more sensitive than the complement fixation reaction and 100 to 1,000 times more sensitive than the precipitin reaction. The reason for the increased sensitivity lies in the fact that only a minute, almost insignificant fraction of the agglutinated cell mass is composed of antibody molecules, in marked contrast to the precipitate formed by soluble antigens and antibodies which is composed primarily (80 to 95%) of antibody molecules. The factors which determine the ratio of antigen to antibody in the antigen-antibody complex formed under optimal conditions are their valencies and their relative sizes. The antibody molecule has a valence of only two and is a protein molecule with a molecular weight which is of the same magnitude as most soluble antigens. In the case of the agglutination reaction, the antigen is normally a cell, either a bacterium or an erythrocyte. Not only does the antigen, therefore, possess an overwhelming number of determinant sites relative to the antibody molecule (the valency is often greater than 1,000), but it is at least 10^8 to 10^9 times its size. The role of the antibody is only to bring the antigenic cells together in sufficiently close apposition so as to impart visible clumping or agglutination of the cells (Fig. 7.10).

Important

1. The antibody molecule must be a divalent molecule in order to effect agglutination.
2. The reaction is *not* dependent on the complement-fixing capacity of the antibody molecule.
3. The reaction is *not* governed by the precipitating properties of the antibody. Agglutination can be induced equally by precipitating and nonprecipitating antibodies.

The agglutination reaction involving erythrocytes can also be utilized to detect antibodies to protein antigens. The protein antigen is coupled irreversibly to the erythrocyte carier through the use of the chemical coupling agent bis-diazotized-benzidine (BDB). The BDB molecule is unstable because it has two highly reactive diazonium groups which react with phenylalanine and tyrosine residues on both the antigen and the erythrocyte surface, forming stable diazo bonds. The protein antigen is attached to the erythrocyte as a protein-BDB-erythrocyte conjugate. In the presence of antibodies to the protein antigen, the protein-erythrocyte complexes are agglutinated in the same way as are erythrocytes in the presence of antierythrocyte antibodies. This reaction is referred to as the passive hemagglutination reaction.

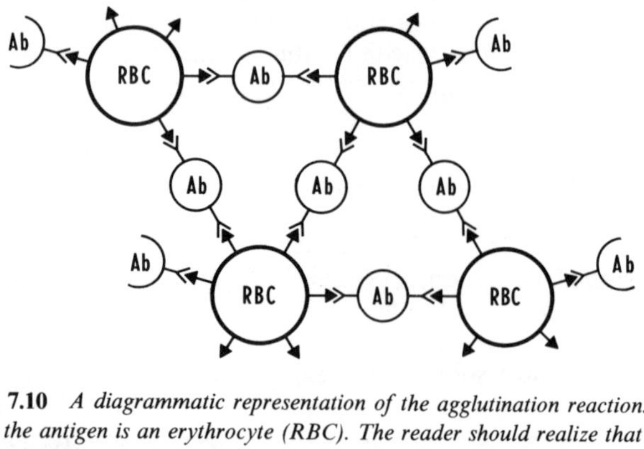

Figure 7.10 *A diagrammatic representation of the agglutination reaction. In this figure, the antigen is an erythrocyte (RBC). The reader should realize that the size of the antibody molecule (Ab) is really many magnitudes smaller than the RBC.*

Certain protein antigens and nonprotein (carbohydrate) antigens cannot be coupled to the erythrocyte surface with BDB. However, they can be strongly absorbed onto the erythrocyte surface following treatment of the erythrocytes with a dilute solution of tannic acid. In this case, the antigen is not irreversibly bound to the carrier erythrocyte and is continually eluted off when the antigen-erythrocyte conjugates are suspended in aqeous medium. However, sufficient antigen remains adherent to the erythrocyte surface to allow for the antigen-erythrocyte complexes to be agglutinated by antibodies directed toward the antigen. This, too, is an example of a passive hemagglutination reaction.

The primary advantage of using the passive hemagglutination reaction rather than the precipitation or complement fixation reactions to detect antibodies is the far greater sensitivity provided by the passive hemagglutination reaction (Table 7.1). Antibodies in too low a concentration to facilitate the precipitation and complement fixation reactions can still strongly agglutinate antigen-erythrocyte complexes up to titers of 1,000 to 10,000. Furthermore, the antibodies need not be of the precipitating or complement-fixing types to be detected. Thus, antibodies which cannot be detected by the conventional immunoassays can be easily detected and semiquantitated by the passive hemagglutination reaction.

Immunofluorescence

This technique, first described by Coons at Harvard University in the 1940s, enables one to visualize microscopically antigens or deposits of antibodies and/or complement on tissues or cells without disturbing the morphologic integrity or architecture of the tissue. Thus, one can detect (a) cell surface and intracellular antigenic constituents and determine their location within the tissue; (b) the location and type of autoantibody and complement deposited in the tissue; (c) virus particles within the tissue, i.e. hepatitis virus; and (d) circulating antibodies to pathogenic bacteria, viruses, fungi, and protozoa.

The basis for this technique lies in the fact that ultraviolet irradiation is converted to visible light after it strikes a fluorescent compound. The latter extracts energy from the invisible short wavelength ultraviolet (U-V) irradiation transforming it to visible light of longer wavelength and lesser energy. Fluorescent compounds used most frequently are fluorescein and rhodamine and the colors of the light emitted are yellow-green and orange-red, respectively. Thus, if visible light emanating from the U-V source is blocked and only U-V irradiation is permitted to strike the tissue-fixed fluorescein-conjugated compound, visible light will be emitted from the tissue specimen wherever the fluoresceinated compound has localized (Fig. 7.11*a*).

As an example of the use of this technique, let us consider how we would visualize the presence of IgG immunoglobulin (designated "antigen" in Fig. 7.11*b*) on the surface of a lymph node cell. One may use either frozen sections (5 μ thick cryostat-cut sections) or sections made following fixation of the tissue with alcohol at 4°C. The tissue specimen is incubated with rabbit (or goat or horse) antibodies to human IgG (designated "antibody" in Fig. 7.11*b*) coupled with fluorescein isothiocyanate. Upon examination by fluorescence microscopy, the generally black or darkened background will be sprinkled or interspersed with discrete points or areas of yellow-green light, thus disclosing the presence of the antigen, IgG immunoglobulin (Fig. 7.11*b*). By comparing a photograph of the immunofluorescent pattern with that taken in dark field or phase contrast, one may determine the percentage of IgG-bearing cells as well as ascertain the morphologic integrity of all the cells in the microscopic field.

A variation of this technique is the indirect or "sandwich" technique. This is a two-step, rather than a one-step, technique but is the one mainly used in practice. In this case (Fig. 7.11*c*) the initial antiserum, rabbit antihuman IgG, is not conjugated to the fluorescent compound. Instead, a second antiserum, horse antirabbit IgG, is conjugated to the fluorescent compound.

The sandwich technique allows for a greater degree of flexibility and, therefore, utilization than does the direct technique. A single fluorescein-conjugated antiserum, i.e. horse antihuman IgG, can be used following the screening of any number of human sera for circulating antibodies or autoantibodies directed toward various extrinsic and autologous antigens, respectively, in fixed tissue specimens. The nature of the antigens is not a factor here.

Examples of immunofluorescent patterns that one may see in practice are depicted in Figure 7.12. The sera of three patients with suspected systemic lupus erythematosus (SLE) were investigated for the presence of antinuclear antibodies by the immunofluorescence "sandwich" technique. Cells were first incubated with the patients' sera for 30 minutes at room temperature, washed, and then incubated with fluorescein-conjugated goat antihuman gamma globulin antibodies. Antinuclear antibodies present in the patients' sera adhere to the nuclei and are visualized

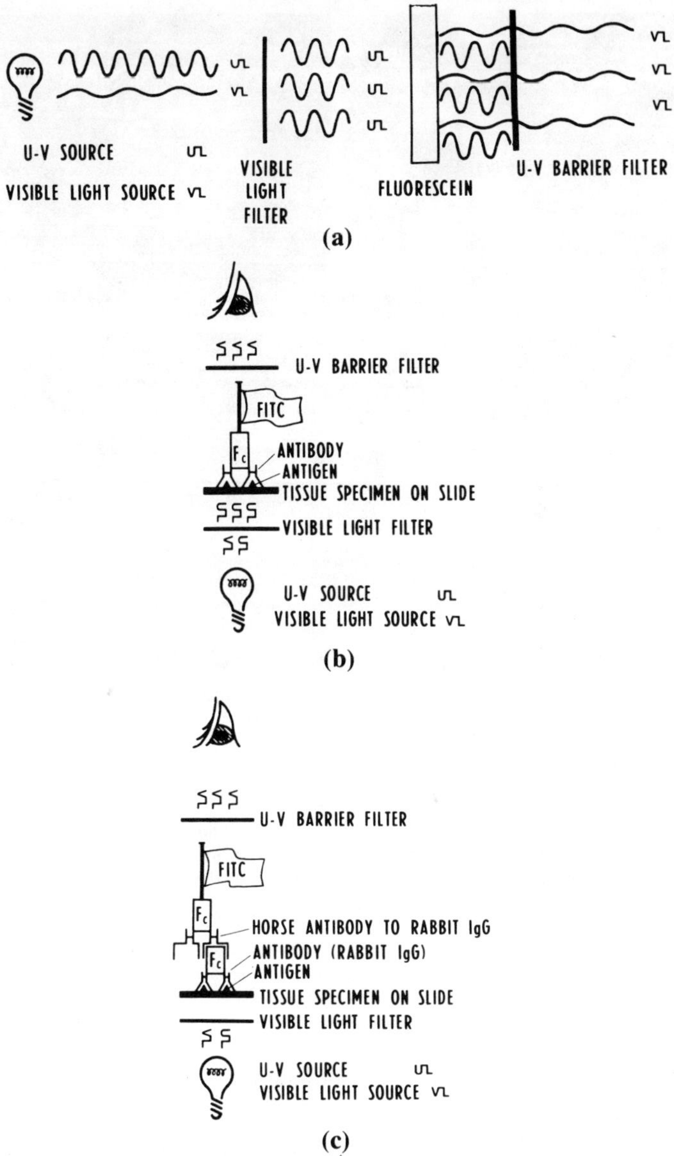

Figure 7.11 *The immunofluorescence technique. (a) A diagrammatic representation. (b) The direct immunofluorescence assay. (c) The indirect immunofluorescence assay or "sandwich" technique.*

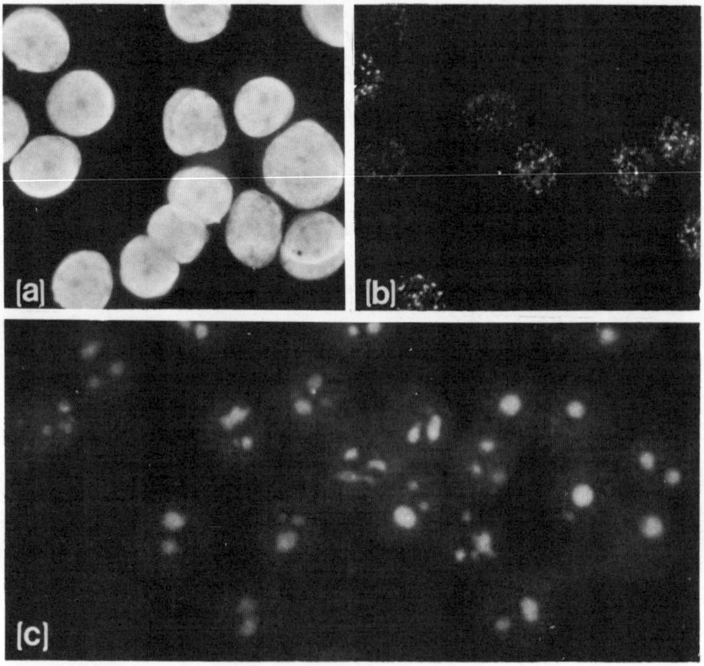

Figure 7.12 *An example of immunofluorescence staining (indirect or sandwich technique). The reader should keep in mind that all the white objects in the black and white photomicrographs actually look green-yellow to the eye on microscopic analysis, as the fluorescent dye used is FITC. (a) Serum of a patient with systemic lupus erythematosus (SLE). Homogeneous staining of the nuclei of buccal mucosa cells. (Original magnification ×400.) (b) Serum of a patient with SLE. Speckled staining of the nuclei of buccal mucosa cells. (Original magnification ×400.) (c) Serum of a patient with SLE. Nucleolar staining of the nuclei of buccal mucosa cells. (Original magnification ×400.)*

with the fluorescein-conjugated goat antiserum to human gamma globulin.

Radioimmunoassay

This is by far the most sensitive method for the detection and quantitation of antigens and antibodies discussed thus far and is equaled in terms of sensitivity only by the ELISA technique (see below). The application of the technique necessitates having one of the reactants coupled to a radioactive tracer, i.e. ^{131}I, ^{125}I, ^{3}H. The labeled reactant should be the one the binding to which by the control or known preparation is to be competitively inhibited by the serum of the patient. The assay for the concentration of circulating insulin serves to illustrate the mechanics of the radioimmunoassay procedure. The insulin molecule constitutes the antigen, and the known antibodies are provided by the serum of a specifically immunized rabbit (or goat or guinea pig), i.e. rabbit antihuman insulin antiserum (referred to as the xenogeneic antiserum). The three constituents required to carry out the assay are: (a) a calibrated quantity of ^{131}I-labeled insulin (Ag*), (b) the calibrated xenogeneic antiserum (Ab), and (c) the patient's serum containing insulin in an unknown concentration (Ag).

The patient's serum containing an unknown quantity of insulin or Ag is mixed with the xenogeneic anti-insulin antiserum, which has antibodies or Ab directed toward insulin, and a known quantity of radiolabeled insulin or Ag* is added. The Ag* is used in an amount which normally would interact with all the antibodies (Ab) in the aliquot of xenogeneic antiserum used. Any unlabeled insulin (Ag) present in the patient's serum will competitively interfere with the binding of some of the radiolabeled insulin (Ag*) with the xenogeneic antibodies (Ab). The decrease in the binding of radiolabeled insulin (Ag*) to the xenogeneic antibodies is, therefore, a reflection of the competitive binding of the radiolabeled (Ag*) and unlabeled (Ag) insulin for the same insulin-binding sites on the antibody molecules. The greater the concentration of insulin (Ag) in the circulation of the patient, the more effectively will the serum inhibit the binding of radiolabeled insulin (Ag*) to the xenogeneic antibodies.

Various means are used to measure the binding of the radiolabeled constituent to the specific antibodies. One method depends upon the differential precipitation of the antigen, antibodies, and immune complexes by ammonium sulphate (the Farr technique). The immune complexes as well as unreacted antibodies are precipitated by 40% saturated ammonium sulphate, whereas many antigens are not precipitated under this condition. Thus, the unreacted antigen is retained in the supernatant. Essentially all of the Ag* will be taken down in the immune precipitate if the only reactants are the radiolabeled antigen (Ag*) and the specific antiserum (Ab). However, in the presence of unlabeled Ag present in the patient's serum, the concentration of total antigen (Ag + Ag*) in the assay is increased relative to only Ag*. The result is that: (a) some Ag bind to Ab, resulting in (b) insufficient free Ab to bind all of the Ag*. Consequently, (c) Ag* can be detected in the supernatant.

Another system commonly used, as it is commercially available and very reliable, is based upon the irreversible binding of one of the reactants to an insoluble polystyrene surface (Fig. 7.13). The

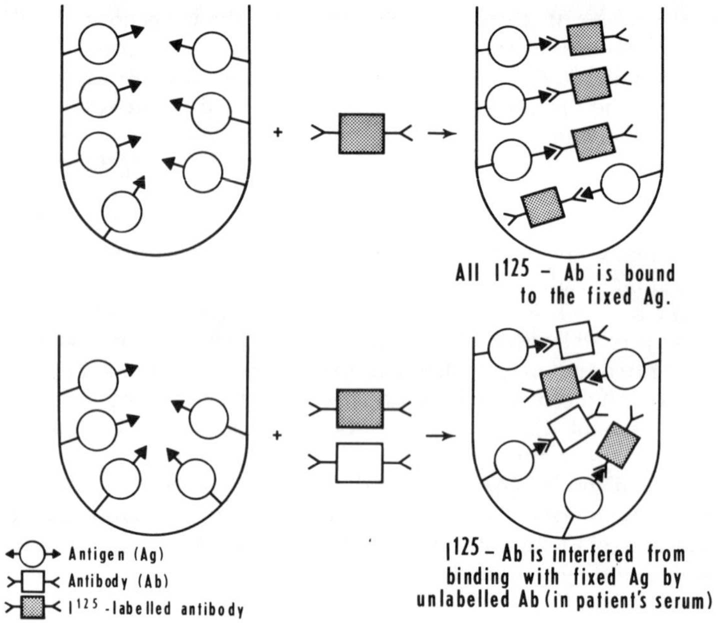

Figure 7.13 *A radioimmunoassay procedure, depicting the competitive binding of radiolabeled and unlabeled antibody for the same insolubilized antigen. In the presence of unlabeled antibodies, a proportion of the labeled antibody molecules will be prevented from interacting with the antigen molecules or will be displaced from the antigen. They can be detected in the supernatant fluid. The greater the number of unbound radiolabeled antibody molecules, the greater the number of antibody molecules in the serum under investigation.*

insolubilized matrix consists of antibodies (if the reactant to be investigated is the antigen) or of antigen (if the reactant to be investigated is the antibody). In the example cited in the figure, the antigen (i.e insulin) is fixed to the matrix in order to facilitate the determination of the concentration of the specific (anti-insulin) antibodies in the circulation of the patient under investigation.

Antibodies (i.e rabbit anti-insulin) labeled with ^{125}I are added in just sufficient numbers to totally saturate the fixed antigen molecules. If a serum is added which contains no antibodies directed toward the antigen, there will be no interference with the binding of all the ^{125}I-labeled antibodies to the fixed antigen. On the other hand, if the serum added contains antibodies directed toward the antigen, then the nonlabeled antibodies will compete with the I^{125}-labeled antibodies for the identical antigenic sites on the fixed antigen and some of the ^{125}I-labeled antibodies will remain in the supernatant. The percentage of ^{125}I-labeled antibodies in the supernatant, not bound to the fixed antigens, bears a stoichiometric relationship with the quantity of nonlabeled antibody molecules added. By comparing the non-bound ^{125}I-labeled antibody molecules in the presence of a patient's serum with that nonbound in the presence of graded known quantities of unlabeled antibody molecules, one can calculate the μg% of the (anti-insulin) antibodies in the circulation of the patient (Fig. 7.14).

The radioimmunoassay technique can be used to determine the concentration in the circulation of hormones, enzymes, drugs, immunoglobulins and other serum proteins, organ-specific oncogenically related protein constituents (i.e. alpha fetoprotein, carcinoembryonic antigen), etc. All that is required is that they be able to act as antigens in the xenogeneic hosts and induce the formation of specific antibodies. The antibodies can be irreversibly fixed to the surface of the polystyrene tube and the known calibrated indicator reagent is the radioactively labeled antigen, i.e. hormone, enzyme, immunoglobulin, or organ-specific protein. Its concentration in the circulation of the patient can be determined as described above.

Nephelometry

The use of optical techniques for the demonstration of antigen-antibody reactions dates back to the 1920s and 1930s. In the late 1930s, Levoisoleur claimed that rabbits injected with simple sugars or amino acids responded immunologically to these substances. Levoisoleur demonstrated, using homemade light-scattering equipment, that a beam of light directed at a glass tube containing the "immune" rabbit serum and the sugar (or amino

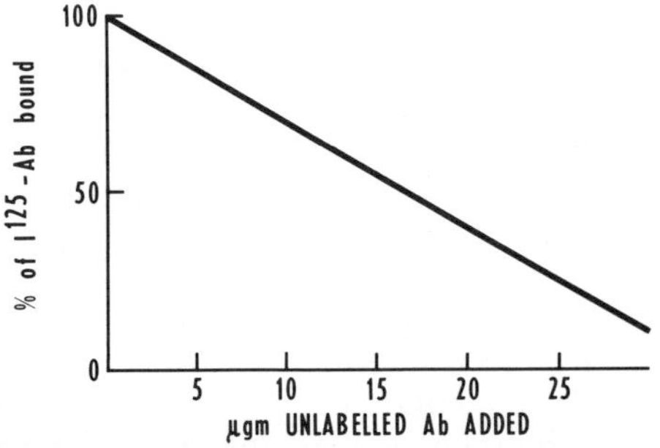

Figure 7.14 *The percentage of radioactively labeled antibodies (Ab) bound to the insolubilized antigen as a function of the quantity of unlabeled antibodies present in the assay mixture.*

acid) "antigen" deflected the transmitted light differently from that observed in the control tubes containing only one of these reactants. Levoisoleur concluded that the difference in the scattering of the light by the experimental tube compared to the control tubes could be attributed to formation of complexes between the "antigen" and factors in the rabbit serum which he considered to be antibodies formed in very low concentration to the injected simple sugars (or amino acids). The factors in the rabbit "immune" sera could not be identified as specific antibodies by the use of the conventional crude and insensitive techniques of that era. However, optical techniques were not taken seriously until the 1970s with the advent of automated instrumentation which allowed the quantitative analysis of antigens and antibodies by these techniques.

When incidence light at a particular angle is directed at a "narrow window" through a tube containing antigen and antiserum, the transmitted light is refracted as it goes through the tube and is scattered in variable angles to a degree markedly different from that observed in the presence of only antigen or antiserum. The precise measurement of this scattered light forms the basis of the analytic methods. Nephelometry is the technique whereby the light scattered from the antigen-antibody solution in a tube at a specific angle is precisely measured. It should be contrasted with turbidimetry, which is the measurement of the reduction in transmitted light due to light scattering.

The intensity of the scattered light is dependent upon a number of factors, the major ones being the molecular weight of the solute and its concentration. Since the immune complex formed between conventional soluble antigens, i.e. human serum albumin, and antibodies, i.e. rabbit antibodies, is anywhere from 4 to 10 times the mass or molecular weight of the individual constituents, the intensity of the scattered light (or Ls), especially the change of intensity with time (or dLs/dt), from a tube containing these reactants will be much greater than the intensity of the scattered light from a tube containing only the antigen or the antiserum. This change in intensity of scattered light is directly related to the concentration of the reactants—the antigen and the antibody. One can, therefore, set up the assay to provide a plot for the concentration of either of these two reactants, providing one of them is used as a reference standard.

Nephelometry has been utilized extensively during the latter half of the 1970s to quantitate the concentration of the serum protein, especially the immunoglobulins, the components of the complement system, transferrin, C′1-esterase inhibitor, myoglobin, etc. As little as 100 ng per ml of a protein antigen can be detected by nephelometric analysis.

Enzyme-linked Immunosorbent Assay (ELISA)

The enzyme-linked immunoassay is the most recent of the three reagent-labeled immunoassays, the other two being immunofluorescence (IF) and radioimmunoassay (RIA). The IF technique is the only immunoassay which lends itself to the determination of the intracellular localization of the agent under investigation, but it is a laborious procedure and is very subjective because the degree of fluorescence emanating from any one area on the microscope slide cannot be quantified. The RIA is an extremely objective, sensitive technique for the detection of either antigen or antibody. However, it has at least one serious limitation—a dependency on unstable radioactive isotopes with finite, in some cases rather short, half-lives. The ELISA technique is objective and can be quantified using currently available automated instrumentation. Since it is independent of radioactive isotopes, the enzyme-linked reagent has a long shelf life.

The basis for the ELISA technique is the use of a highly active enzyme which, when linked to either the antigen or the antibody, does not lose enzymatic activity and does not affect the immunologic properties of the carrier molecule. The substrate for the enzyme should be stable and soluble under all conditions. Ideally, the substrate should be colorless before and be strongly colored after it is acted upon by the linked enzyme. The color change is determined by spectrophotometric analysis. The intensity of the color is directly proportional to the amount of enzyme in the test system, which is a function of the degree of binding of the enzyme-linked antibody or antigen to its immunologic substrate. (Fig. 7.15). Therefore, with the appropriate controls, one can establish the exact concentration of the immunologic substrate (antigen or antibody) for the enzyme-linked conjugate (enzyme-antibody or enzyme-antigen conjugate, respectively).

In practice, the ELISA technique may be used to determine the concentration of an antigen or an antibody in solution, or it can be used to detect cells capable of synthesizing and storing either the antigen or the antibody components of the immune system under investigation in sections of even formaldehyde-fixed tissues.

In the former instance, one of the immunologic substrates is covalently linked to an inert insoluble matrix, such as cellulose, or it is adsorbed onto polystyrene or polypropylene beads, discs, or tubes. Let us assume that the objective of the exercise is to determine the level of IgG in human serum. Anti-IgG antibodies (prepared in an animal such as the rabbit) are coupled to the insoluble matrix, i.e. polypropylene tubes or discs (Fig. 7.15). The human serum is then added, in graded amounts, to the insolubilized rabbit anti-IgG antibodies, and this is followed by incubation for 15 to 30 minutes. Unattached human serum constituents are then washed off, and the enzyme-carrier conjugate (the carrier in this case is rabbit antihuman IgG) is added, followed by incubation for another 15 to 30 minutes. Free enzyme-carrier conjugate is washed off, the enzyme substrate (the chromogen) is added, and the tubes are incubated for a period of time characteristic of the particular enzyme-substrate combination used. The colored supernatant obtained from the test tubes is then analyzed in a spectrophotometer along with the supernatants of control tubes to which were originally added known (standard) amounts

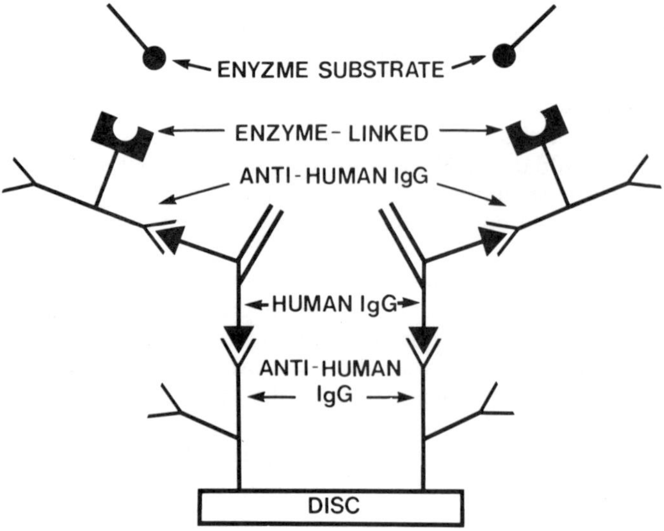

Figure 7.15 *A diagrammatic representation of the enzyme-linked immunosorbent assay (ELISA). In this example, the (rabbit) antihuman IgG antibody molecules have been linked to an insoluble matrix. The serum constituent to be detected and quantified, human serum IgG, is then incubated (as whole serum) with the matrix-(rabbit) antihuman IgG complex. The nonadherent human IgG molecules are washed off and the matrix-(rabbit) antihuman IgG-human IgG complexes are interacted with enzyme-linked (rabbit) antihuman IgG antibody molecules. The nonadherent enzyme-linked molecules are washed off, and the chromogen is added.*

of human IgG instead of serum. By plotting the results of the spectrophotometric analysis against the known concentrations of IgG used in the controls, a straight-line relationship is observed. Thus, the concentration of IgG in the test sample can be determined very precisely. The sensitivity of the ELISA assay approaches that of the RIA assay.

If it is intended to use the ELISA assay to determine, by light microscopy, the percentage of IgG-synthesizing cells in a tissue specimen, the enzyme-carrier conjugate (the carrier is rabbit antihuman IgG) is incubated with the tissue for 15 to 30 minutes, and the excess enzyme-carrier conjugate is washed off. The chromogenic substrate for the enzyme is now added, and incubation is carried out for the appropriate interval of time. For this assay, the substrate must be a chromogen which does not only change color when acted upon by the enzyme but also precipitates following interaction with the enzyme. Cells which contain droplets of the precipitated chromogen may be considered to have synthesized IgG immunoglobulins.

In this manner, the ELISA assay may be used to determine the number of IgG, IgM, IgA, IgD, and IgE-synthesizing cells in any of the lymphoid tissues.

In view of the great sensitivity of this assay, extreme care need not be taken to avoid denaturation of the protein constituents in the tissue specimen; therefore, tissues which have been fixed in formaldehyde rather than in liquid nitrogen may be analyzed successfully. This is not true for the immunofluorescence (IF) assay. Due to the much lower sensitivity of the IF assay relative to the ELISA assay, it is necessary to ensure minimum denaturation of the native proteins in the cells. Therefore, the tissue must be fixed by the least denaturing technique, that is quick-freezing in liquid nitrogen. Formaldehyde-fixed sections will have too little of the undenatured protein (i.e. human IgG) to be detected by the immunofluorescence assay.

The Hemolytic Plaque-forming Cell Response

This technique allows one to determine the actual number of antibody-forming cells at the stage of active synthesis and secretion of antibodies.

The animal, for example the rabbit, is injected intravenously with the antigen, i.e. sheep red blood cells (SRBC). Within 7 to 10 days, antibodies can be detected in the circulation. If one sacrifices the animal on day 7 and prepares a suspension of spleen cells, one may detect antibody-secreting cells by their ability to lyse SRBC in the presence of complement. If the cells (spleen cells and SRBC) are suspended in a semisolid gel and complement is added, a perfectly rounded, well-defined hemolytic translucent plaque (0.5 to 2 mm in diameter) will be formed around each antibody-secreting cell. This is referred to as the "direct hemolytic plaque assay" (Fig. 7.16).

The reaction is carried out as follows. The SRBC (antigen) and splenic (lymphoid) cells (antibody-forming cells) are mixed in varying ratios, agarose (kept at 48°C) is added, and the mixture of SRBC, spleen cells, and agarose is shaken at 48°C and pipetted onto the surface of a Petri dish at room temperature. Within 1 to 2 minutes, the mass solidifies or gels, and the SRBC and lymphoid cells are maintained immobile in the semisolid matrix of the agarose. The thickness of the gel should not exceed 3 to 5 mm. The Petri dish is covered and incubated at 37°C for 1 to 2 hours. During this time, the splenic lymphocytes secrete antibodies into the surrounding microenvironment where they encounter the SRBC (the antigen) and interact with them. If one now overlays the agarose with complement (fresh guinea pig serum), the sensitized SRBC will undergo rapid lysis (see complement fixation reaction described above). The areas of hemolyzed SRBC, the hemolytic plaques, can be easily identified on examination of the Petri dish surface, since the lysed areas will be red and translucent whereas the nonlysed areas will be opaque. A hemolytic plaque should have a lymphoid cell at its center. The number of hemolytic plaques represents the minimum number of antibody-secreting cells. Since one knows the number of lymphoid cells in the original cell suspension and the number of cells plated, one can easily calculate the number of antibody-secreting plaque-forming cells per 10^6 splenic lymphoid cells.

Important

1. The antigens that can be used are limited to erythrocytes or those antigens which can be coupled to erythrocytes, i.e. proteins, certain carbohydrate antigens.

2. The antibodies which react with the SRBC to lyse them in the presence of complement to form the hemolytic plaques are mainly IgM antibodies because they fix complement much more avidly and effectively than do the IgG antibodies, which are also usually secreted simultaneously by the antibody-forming cell. Therefore, one measures primarily the IgM antibody-secreting cells by this method. One can also detect IgG antibody-secreting cells by a variation of the hemolytic plaque assay referred to as the "indirect hemolytic plaque assay." Antiserum directed toward

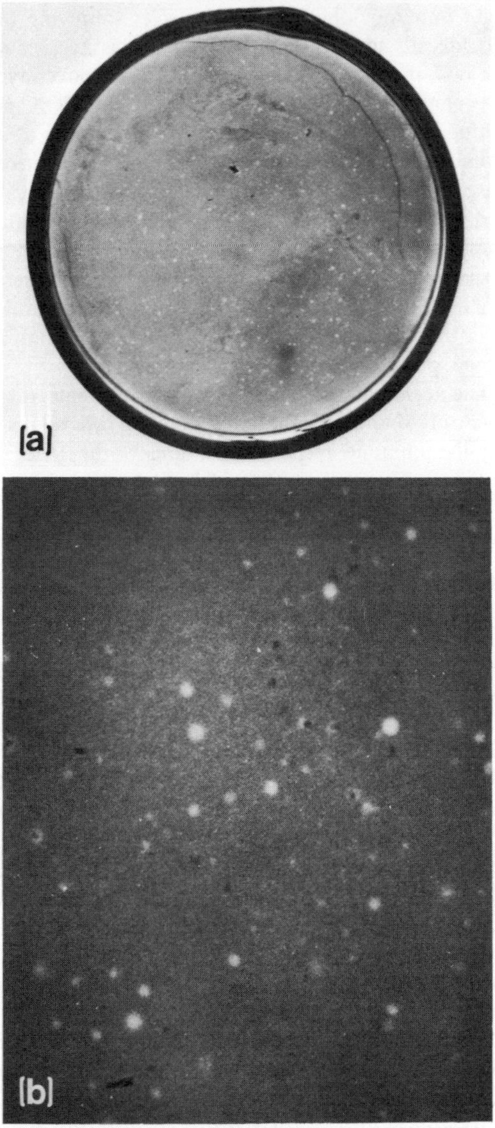

Figure 7.16 *The hemolytic plaque-forming cell assay in agarose gel medium. (a) Hemolytic plaques as viewed in the entire Petri dish under low magnification. (Original magnification ×4.) (b) Hemolytic plaques under higher magnification. (Original magnification ×40.)*

the IgG immunoglobulins of the species supplying the immune lymphoid cells for the hemolytic plaque assay (i.e. rabbit anti-mouse IgG, if mouse spleen cells are plated) is overlayed onto the agarose containing the lymphoid cells and the SRBC either at the beginning of the incubation period or at the time of addition of the complement. The effect of these anti-IgG antibodies is to increase the sensitivity of the IgG antibody-SRBC complexes formed during the incubation of the erythrocytes and immune lymphoid cells to hemolysis by complement, by adding a second tier of antibody molecules to the immune complexes. The effect is similar to the increased sensitivity of the immunofluorescence assay in the two-stage (sandwich technique), as compared to the one-stage, procedure.

3. The technique only allows one to estimate the minimum number of IgM and IgG antibody-secreting cells at a point in time during the immune response. Obviously, the total number of antibody-secreting cells generated over the entire period of antibody formation will be much greater.

The Blastogenic Response of Lymphocytes to Stimulation with Specific Antigens

Circulating lymphocytes of immunized individuals, upon incubation in vitro with the specific immunizing antigen (i.e. diphtheria toxoid, tetanus toxoid) in the appropriate culture medium, undergo blastogenesis and mitosis. The peak of the blastogenic response occurs by day 5 to 7 of culture. The extent of the blastogenic and proliferative response can be quantitated by determining the incorporation of ^{3}H-thymidine into the newly synthesized DNA of the dividing cells. The ^{3}H-thymidine is added on day 5 or 6, and the cultured cells are processed for determination of isotope content 24 hours later.

Since the circulating cells of unimmunized normal individuals do not undergo blastogenesis and mitosis in response to stimulation with specific antigens, the blastogenic response of circulating cells of immunized individuals must be considered as indicative of specific immune responsiveness or immunocompetence.

It should be noted that circulating cells capable of responding with blastogenesis and mitosis upon stimulation with a specific antigen can be detected in the circulation of the immunized individual for years following exposure to the antigen. The responding cells would, therefore, appear to be long-lived recirculating lymphocytes. Whether these lymphocytes are conventional memory cells remains to be determined.

IN VITRO REACTIONS WHICH INDICATE IMMUNOCOMPETENCE

The Blastogenic Response of Lymphocytes to Stimulation with the Plant Mitogens Phytohemagglutinin (PHA), Concanavalin-A (Con-A), and Pokeweed (PWM)

A number of plant constituents are capable of inducing transformation and proliferation of lymphocytes in vitro. These substances are referred to as mitogens. The cells are cultured in the presence of the mitogen for a period of 3 days, and ^{3}H-thymidine is added 2 to 18 hours prior to the termination of the culture. The extent of blastogenesis can be quantitated by measuring the incorporation of ^{3}H-thymidine into the newly synthesized DNA of the dividing cells. The uptake of ^{3}H by the cells is recorded as counts per minute (cpm). Furthermore, the percentage of radioactively labeled cells can be determined by autoradiographic analysis of the cells.

PHA and Con-A induce mitosis of T cells. Results of initial investigations suggested that PWM is a B cell mitogen. Subsequent investigations, using purified cell suspensions, disclosed that PWM could induce mitosis of B cells but only in the presence of T "helper" cells. In point of fact, T cells undergo even more extensive proliferation in response to PWM stimulation than do the B cells. Furthermore, the monocyte plays a major role in the reaction since cells depleted of phagocytic monocytes respond poorly to all three mitogens. Failure of the circulating lymphocytes, in the presence of normal monocytes, to respond to these nonspecific mitogens is indicative of a potential or actual immunoincompetent state.

Rosette Formation

Subpopulations of circulating mononuclear cells (lymphocytes and monocytes) can be isolated and analyzed for receptors and immunologic activity following their interaction with untreated and specifically treated xenogeneic erythrocytes (indicator cells) to form rosettes. A rosette is usually defined as a mononuclear cell surrounded by more than four indicator red blood cells which are tightly adherent to the mononuclear cell. Some rosettes are characterized by a single layer of indicator erythrocytes compressed tightly against the central mononuclear cell, while others may appear to be composed of several layers of indicator erythrocytes adherent to the central mononuclear cell (Fig. 7.17). The rosetted cells are more dense than the nonrosetted cells and can be separated from the latter by centrifugation in a Ficoll-Hypaque

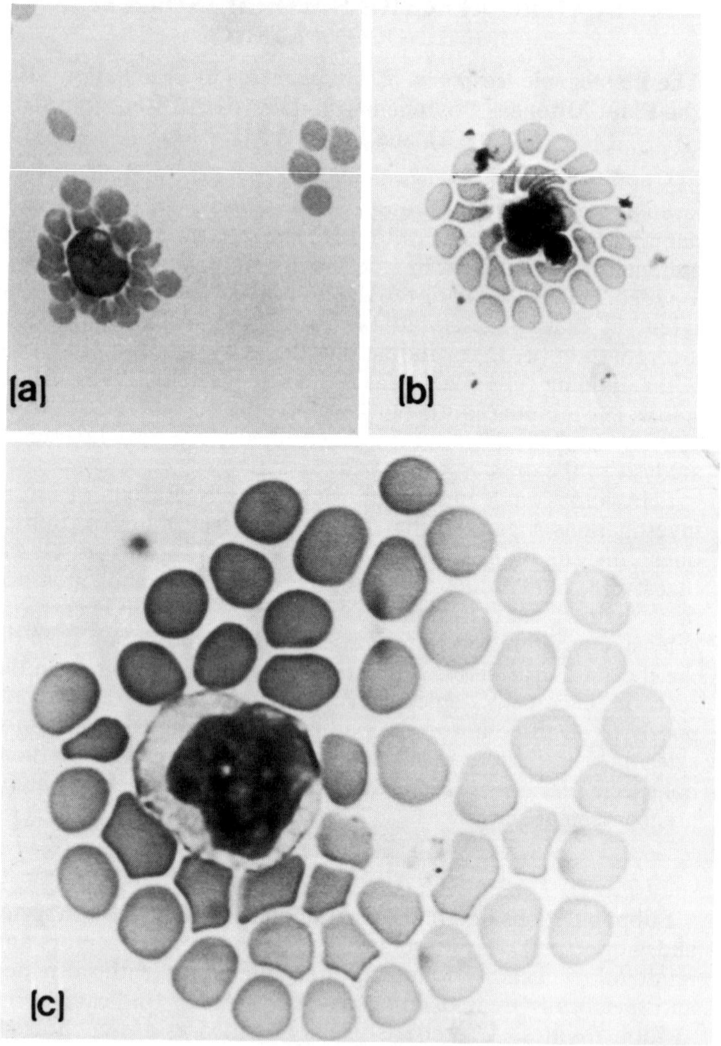

Figure 7.17 *Rosettes formed between sheep erythrocytes (E) and lymphocytes (T cells), referred to as E rosettes. (a) A single layer of indicator erythrocytes surrounding the T lymphocyte. (Original magnification ×400.) (b) A number of layers of indicator erythrocytes surrounding the T lymphocyte. (Original magnification ×400.) (c) Multiple layers of indicator erythrocytes surrounding the T lymphocyte. (Original magnification ×1,000.)*

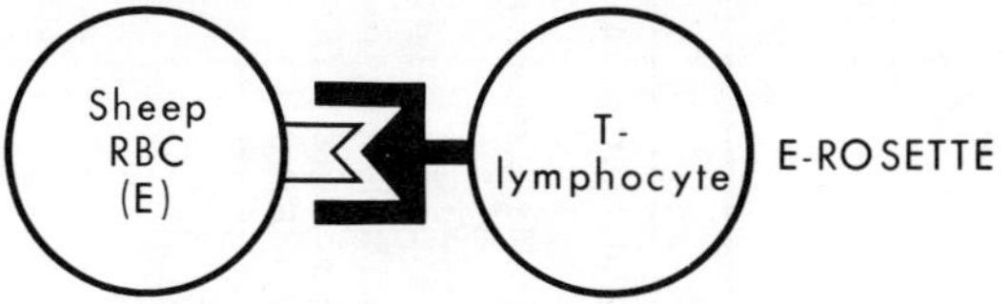

Figure 7.18 *A diagrammatic representation of the interaction of the T lymphocyte with sheep erythrocytes to form E rosettes.*

discontinuous density gradient. The nonrosetted cells remain at the interface, whereas the rosetted cells settle to the bottom of the tube as a pellet.

A rosette is formed as a result of the interaction between surface receptors on the mononuclear cells and specific surface configurations on the indicator erythrocytes. The three indicator cells conventionally used and the circulating cells which interact with the indicator cells are as follows:

1. E or sheep red blood cells (SRBC) form rosettes with lymphocytes which possess surface receptors for as yet unidentified configurations on the surface of the SRBC (Fig. 7.18, Table 7.3). The lymphocytes involved are thymus-derived or T cells as defined by their susceptibility to lysis in the presence of T cell-specific antiserum and complement and their absence from the circulation in individuals with thymic alymphoplasia.

2. EA or IgG antibody (A)-sensitized ox red blood cells (E) form rosettes with a population of mononuclear cells which have receptors for the Fc region of the IgG antibody molecule of the EA complex (Fig. 7.19). The mononuclear cells consist of monocytes and lymphocytes devoid of surface immunoglobulins and receptors for the SRBC. The lymphocytes are, therefore, neither B nor T cells which, by definition, possess surface membrane-bound immunoglobulins and receptors for SRBC, respectively. The EA-rosetting cells are referred to as "null" cells (Table 7.3).

3. EAC or IgM antibody (A)-sensitized ox red blood cell (E) to which is complexed the C′3 component of complement (C). Rosettes are formed with monocytes and lymphocytes which possess surface receptors for activated C′3 (Fig. 7.20). The majority of these lymphocytes bear surface immunoglobulins and are, therefore, considered to be B cells (Table 7.3).

The rosettes formed are referred to as E, EA, and EAC rosettes, and the mononuclear rosette-forming cells (RFC) are referred to as E, EA, and EAC rosette-forming cells or E-RFC, EA-RFC, and EAC-RFC. The presence of normal numbers of circulating E-RFC, EA-RFC, and EAC-RFC indicates a normal immuno-

Table 7.3
Classification of Lymphocytes on the Basis of Surface Membrane Receptors

T cell	B cell	Null cell
1. Possesses receptor for sheep RBC membrane antigen, facilitating rosette formation with sheep erythrocyte (E-rosette-forming cell or E-RFC)	1. Possesses surface immunoglobulins 2. Possesses receptor for C′3 component of complement facilitating rosette formation with erythrocyte (E)-antibody (A) (IgM)-complement (C) complex (EAC-RFC)	1. Does not possess detectable surface immunoglobulins 2. Does not possess detectable receptor for sheep RBC 3. Possesses receptor for Fc region of IgG antibody molecule, facilitating rosette formation with erythrocyte (E)-antibody (A) complex (EA-RFC)

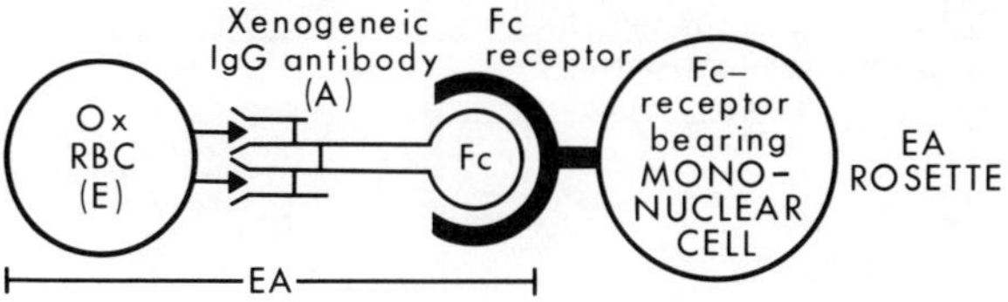

Figure 7.19 *A diagrammatic representation of the interaction of the Fc receptor-bearing mononuclear cell with the IgG antibody-sensitized erythrocyte (EA) to form EA rosettes.*

competent state. Conversely, a low number of these circulating cells, especially E-RFC and/or EAC-RFC, is indicative of a state of potential or actual cell-mediated or humoral immunoincompetence, respectively.

Important

1. It is important for the reader to realize that the receptors for Fc and C′3 are able to interact with the Fc region of the IgG antibody molecule and the C′3 component of the complement system, respectively, only after the antibody has reacted with the antigen and C′3 has reacted with the antigen-antibody complex. Obviously, lymphocytes could not normally circulate if they could interact with native circulating IgG molecules and noncomplexed C′3.

2. Only rosettes formed between lymphocytes and the indicator erythrocytes are usually considered in the evaluation of immunocompetence. However, the reader must be cautioned to the fact that cells other than lymphocytes possess surface receptors capable of interacting with the indicator erythrocytes to form rosettes. These cells include circulating monocytes, neutrophils, and eosinophils, as well as unexpected cells like the glomerular endothelial cells (Table 7.4).

Rosette formation with, or more precisely the adherence of the indicator red blood cells to, cells in a fixed tissue specimen can also be utilized in the determination of the relative numbers and location of T and B cells without disturbing the architecture of the tissue. Frozen sections are overlayed with the E and EAC indicator cells (to identify T and B cells, respectively) for 30 minutes at room temperature. The nonadherent indicator cells are then carefully washed off, leaving behind E and EAC adherent to the T and B cells.

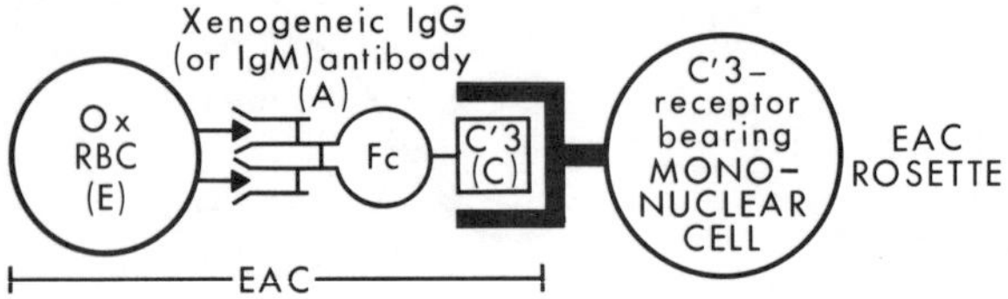

Figure 7.20 *A diagrammatic representation of the interaction of the C'3 receptor-bearing mononuclear cell with C'3 complexed to antibody-sensitized erythrocytes (EAC) to form EAC rosettes.*

The Mixed Leukocyte Culture Reaction (MLR)

Lymphocytes of one individual, when cultured with lymphocytes of an unrelated individual, respond with blastogenesis and mitosis to the alloantigens on the latter cells. These antigens are referred to as HLA (human leukocyte antigens) or transplantation antigens. The reaction takes place in culture over a period of 5 days. The responder cells which proliferate and divide in this reaction are primarily T cells, although a small proportion of the dividing cells may also be B cells recruited into a proliferative state by T cell-derived factors. The identity of the stimulator cells is less clear. Initially, the evidence pointed to the B cell as the stimulating cell; however, the results of recent investigations suggest that stimulation in the MLR may also be provided by the monocyte.

Responsiveness in the MLR is one of the criteria indicative of general T cell immunocompetence. The blastogenic response can be quantitated by the degree of incorporation of ^{3}H-thymidine into the DNA of the dividing cells. As for the mitogen-induced blastogenic reaction, the ^{3}H-thymidine is added to the cells 2 to 18 hours prior to the termination of culture. The extent of the blastogenic response is determined by the ratio of the counts per minute (cpm) in the culture of the cells of the two unrelated individuals divided by one-half of the sum of the cpm of the cultures of the cells cultured individually.

When the lymphoid cells of both individuals are co-cultured without any prior treatment, lymphoid cells of both parties proliferate in the MLR, and it is not possible to determine the extent of the response of each of the lymphoid cell populations (Fig. 7.21*a*). In practice, the cells of one of the individuals are inactivated by treatment with mitomycin-C prior to their co-culture with the cells of the second individual (Fig. 7.21*b*). Cells so treated are not killed, but they lose the ability to divide in culture. The untreated cells are, therefore, referred to as the

Table 7.4
Cells Possessing Surface Receptors

Cell	Receptor for		
	E	Fc	C′3
Lymphocyte	X	X	X
Monocyte		X	X
Neutrophil		X	X
Eosinophil		X	
Glomerular endothelial cell		X	
Postcapillary venule endothelial cell		X	

responder cells and the mitomycin-C-treated cells are referred to as the stimulator cells. The reaction is referred to as the one-way MLR reaction, and it was first introduced by Bach and Voynow in 1965. Thus, one can determine the blastogenic response of the cells of each of the cell donors toward each other.

The proliferative response of the circulating lymphocytes in the MLR, like the mitogen-induced proliferative response, requires the participation of monocytes. These cells can be supplied in either of the allogeneic cell suspensions, that is, the responder or stimulator cells. The monocytes do not in themselves respond, nor do they provide the stimulation for the proliferative response when they are syngeneic to the responder cells. They apparently function in an accessory or helper cell capacity to facilitate the blastogenic response by the T lymphocytes in the responder cell population.

The blastogenic response in the MLR reaction reflects the cell surface antigenic (HLA) dissimilarities between the cells of the two donors. This test is utilized in the Renal Transplantation Service along with other tests, i.e. the lymphocytotoxicity assay using commercially available antisera and complement, to establish or predict the immunologic reactivity of the cells of a potential renal allograft recipient toward the cells of a potential kidney donor. A marked blastogenic response by the cells of the potential recipient to the mitomycin-C-treated cells of the organ donor in the one-way MLR is indicative of certain rejection of a graft from this particular donor, should allografting be attempted.

Important

1. A blastogenic response in the one-way MLR should discourage consideration of a graft from the donor of the stimulator cells to the donor of the responder cells. However, the absence of

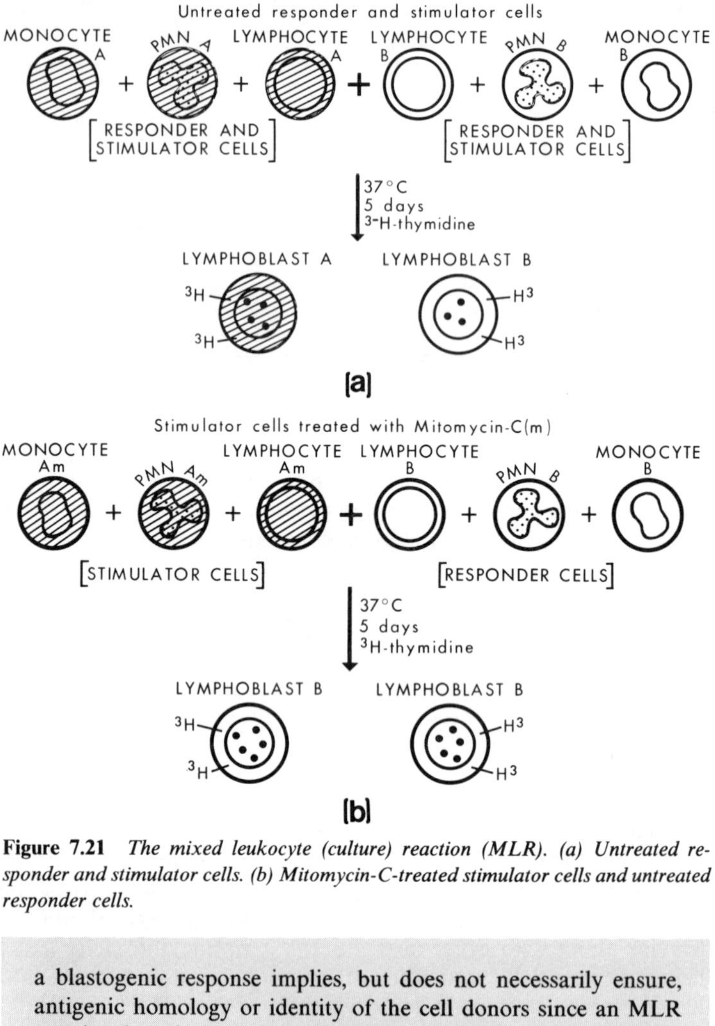

Figure 7.21 *The mixed leukocyte (culture) reaction (MLR). (a) Untreated responder and stimulator cells. (b) Mitomycin-C-treated stimulator cells and untreated responder cells.*

a blastogenic response implies, but does not necessarily ensure, antigenic homology or identity of the cell donors since an MLR reaction is only indicative of strong, not weak, antigenic differences. Thus, an allograft between two individuals even in the absence of a blastogenic response in the 5-day one-way MLR reaction may still result in chronic rejection of the allograft.

2. The monocytes are essential for the MLR reaction, although they do not proliferate in the reaction. Should both of the participating cell populations be deficient in monocytes, a poor or no MLR reaction will result, suggesting antigenic identity when this is not at all the case.

The Inhibition of Migration of Mononuclear Cells in Vitro

Lymphocytes of normal individuals stimulated to blastogenesis and mitosis by nonspecific mitogenic agents (phytohemagglutinin, pokeweed, concanavalin-A), and lymphocytes of individuals previously immunized to give a delayed hypersensitivity (cell-mediated immune) response incubated with the immunizing antigen, secrete a number of biologically active factors into their microenvironment which are collectively referred to as lymphokines (or products of lymphocyte activation). The **lymphokines** are designated on the basis of activity demonstrable under controlled in vitro conditions. In spite of the artificiality of the in vitro assay system, results of numerous in vivo and in vitro investigations strongly indicate an in vivo role for many, if not all, of the lymphokines.

Although in excess of 20 lymphokines have been identified in recent years, the conclusive existence of some still requires experimental verification. Artifacts must be ruled out. Furthermore, only a small number of lymphokines have been incorporated into procedures to assay the immunocompetent state. Only these will be referred to in this text, and they have been classified as follows:

1. Migration inhibition factor (MIF)
2. Macrophage chemotactic factor (MCF)
3. Mitogenic factor (MF)
4. Macrophage-activating factor (MAF)
5. Cytotoxic factor (CF)
6. Transfer factor (TF)
7. Osteoclast-stimulating factor (OSF)
8. Interferon

Only one of these factors, MIF, has been investigated to any significant extent in the assessment of the immunocompetent state. This factor is secreted by the sensitized lymphocytes following their interaction with the sensitizing antigen. MIF can be detected in vitro by its ability to inhibit the migration of mononuclear cells (macrophages, monocytes, and lymphocytes) from capillary tubes (Fig. 7.22).

Normally, the circulating mononuclear cells migrate out of the capillary tube in a concentric fashion to a distance of about 0.25 to 0.5 cm during overnight incubation at 37°C in 5% CO_2 in air. However, mononuclear cells of the sensitized or immunized individual will be inhibited from migrating out of the capillary tube if they are placed in medium containing the suspected antigen (Fig. 7.22). Furthermore, the supernatants of 24-hour cultures of sensitized cells and antigen are capable of inhibiting the migration of normal allogeneic mononuclear cells, thus dem-

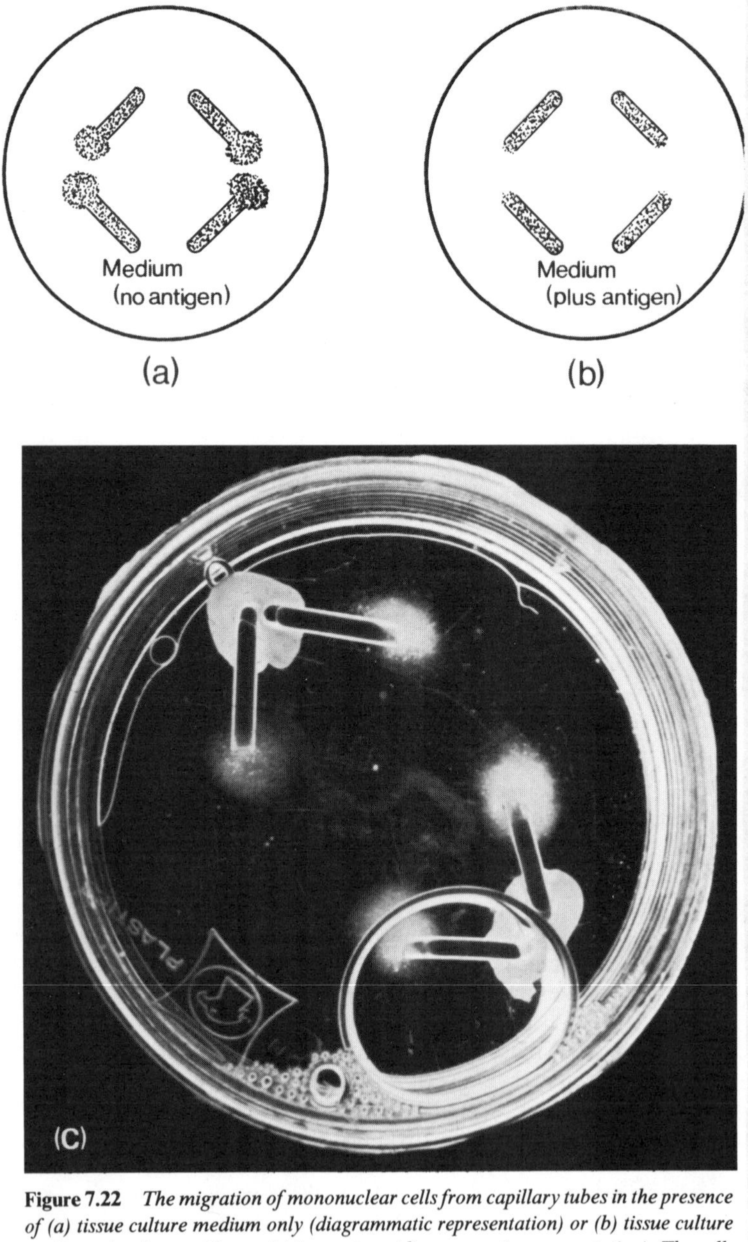

Figure 7.22 *The migration of mononuclear cells from capillary tubes in the presence of (a) tissue culture medium only (diagrammatic representation) or (b) tissue culture medium plus the specific sensitizing antigen (diagrammatic representation). The cells are inhibited from migrating in the presence of the antigen originally used to sensitize the donor of the cells. (c) Photograph of normal circulating human cells migrating out of capillary tubes (incubation time 20 hours).*

onstrating the soluble nature of this lymphokine and its secretion by the sensitized cells following interaction with the antigen.

Although it is not possible at this time to define precisely the pathology which would ensue in the absence of normal lymphokine synthesis and/or secretion, there does appear to be a relationship between a defect in the synthesis of these factors, especially MIF, and the appearance of certain forms of the immunodeficiency syndrome, such as chronic mucocutaneous candidiasis and chronic granulomatous disease (CGD).

The role which the lymphokines may play in the induction of the cell-mediated immune response is discussed in depth in Chapter 6.

Antibody-dependent Cellular Cytotoxicity (ADCC)

Mononuclear and polymorphonuclear cells capable of inducing lysis of randomly selected target cells in vitro continually circulate in the normal individual. One of these lytic reactions involves the cytolysis of target cells sensitized with IgG antibodies (allogeneic or xenogeneic) directed toward the target cells (Fig. 7.23). This reaction can be quantitated if the antibody-sensitized target cells are labeled with ^{51}Cr. Following lysis of the cells, the ^{51}Cr released into the supernatant fluid can be counted in a gamma counter. The result is usually expressed as the cytotoxic index, which is the ratio of the counts per minute in the culture of the target cells and effector cells divided by the counts per minute in the culture of the target cells alone.

The mononuclear cell which carries out the ADCC reaction, referred to as a killer or K cell, possesses a receptor for the Fc region of the IgG antibody molecule. This cell is referred to as the Fc receptor (Fc-R)-bearing cell. This does not mean that all Fc receptor-bearing cells are necessarily cytotoxic cells. Evidence

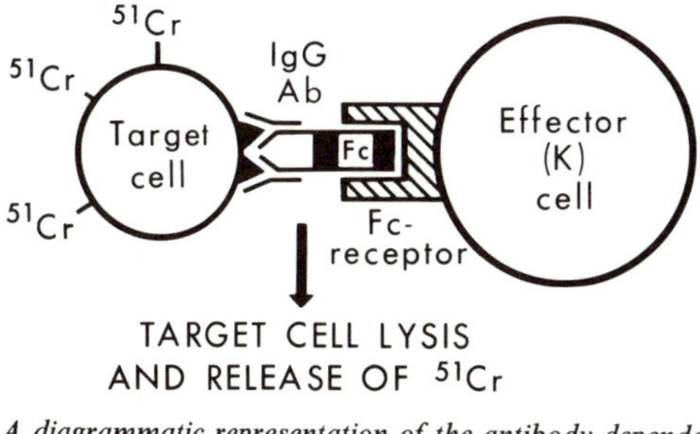

Figure 7.23 *A diagrammatic representation of the antibody-dependent cell-mediated cytotoxic (ADCC) reaction.*

has been presented demonstrating that only a small percentage of Fc-R-bearing cells are cytotoxic. Therefore, it is not enough to quantitate the number of Fc-R-bearing cells by the rosette assay (EA-RFC). It is essential to demonstrate whether these cells are also capable of mediating the ADCC cytotoxic reaction.

It is probable that the polymorphonuclear cells also mediate the ADCC reaction via their Fc receptors since they can only lyse antibody-sensitized, but not unsensitized, target cells. The ADCC activity would appear to be related to the presence of Fc receptors and indicates the existence of subpopulations of polymorphonuclear cells.

The Naturally Occurring (Antibody-independent) Cellular Cytotoxic Reaction (NOCC)

This reaction is mediated by circulating cells different from those which participate in the ADCC reaction. An important distinction between these two reactions is the state of the target cell. In contrast to the target cell in the ADCC reaction, the target cell here does not require adherent antibodies to impart to it the susceptibility to be lysed by the effector cells (Fig. 7.24). In fact, this cytotoxic reaction can be carried out in a serum-free or gamma globulin-free medium. In practice, however, the culture medium is supplemented with serum to facilitate optimal cytolysis and decrease spontaneous lysis of the target cells. The target cells used here can be any of a number of apparently unrelated cells, i.e. fetal cells, parenchymal lymphoid cells, malignant cell lines, chang cells, red blood cells, etc. Like the ADCC reaction, the NOCC reaction is carried out with ^{51}Cr-labeled target cells, and cytotoxicity is measured after a culture period of 24 hours.

The NOCC reaction described here is also referred to in the current literature as the spontaneous lymphocyte-mediated cytotoxic (SLMC) reaction and the natural killer (NK) reaction.

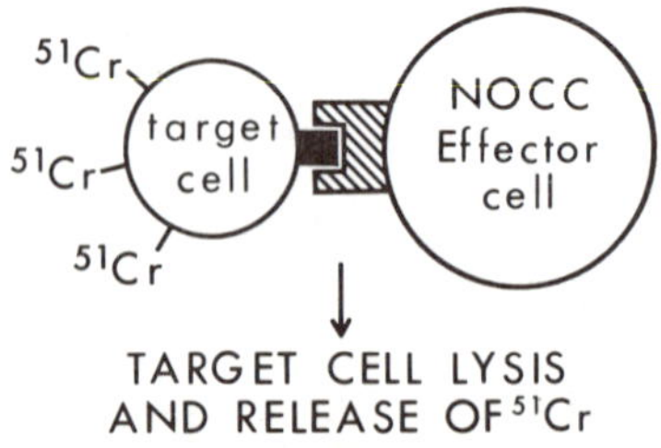

Figure 7.24 *A diagrammatic representation of the naturally occurring (antibody-independent) cell-mediated cytotoxic (NOCC) reaction.*

The term SLMC designates only naturally occurring cytotoxic lymphocytes. It was proposed on the assumption, since proven to be incorrect, that only normally circulating lymphocytes can mediate the antibody-independent cytolysis of selected target cells in vitro. In the broader perspective, however, the term SLMC is too restrictive to define the cytolysis of target cells by normally circulating cells since monocytes and neutrophils, as well as lymphocytes, are capable of lysing a variety of target cells in vitro independent of anti-target cell antibodies. Therefore, the term NOCC is proposed as a more appropriate term to define this cytotoxic reaction. The author further proposes that the term NK be reserved to designate the naturally occurring antibody-independent effector or cytotoxic cell, rather than the cytotoxic reaction per se. In this way, uniformity of the terms used to designate nonantigenically activated cytotoxic cells is preserved—the K cell for the cytotoxic cell in the ADCC cytotoxic reaction and the NK cell for the cytotoxic reaction in the NOCC cytotoxic reaction.

Important

In comparing and contrasting the properties of the ADCC and NOCC reactions, the following points should be stressed:

1. The target cell for the ADCC reaction must be intentionally coated with anti-target cell antibodies of the IgG class. These antibodies are not present in normal human serum but must be prepared by immunizing a rabbit or a goat. On the other hand, the target cell for the NOCC reaction can still function in that capacity in spite of all attempts to eliminate antibodies as participants in this reaction.

2. The effector cells in the ADCC reaction, often referred to as K cells, are morphologically heterogeneous, as activity has been attributed to lymphocytes, monocytes, neutrophils, and eosinophils. A common property of all these cells is the Fc receptor. Present evidence indicates that the nature of the target cell may play a role in determining the identity of the effector cell. This matter is far from resolved.

3. The effector cells in the NOCC reaction, referred to as NK cells, are also morphologically heterogeneous, their identity also appearing to depend on the nature of the target cell. Monocytes, lymphocytes, and neutrophils have variously been identified as the effector cells. The precise identity of the lymphocyte in terms of its surface receptors is also unresolved, as T cells and non-T cells bearing one or more of the primary receptors, as well as cells without any detectable receptors, have been implicated.

The Mitogen-induced Cellular Cytotoxic Reaction (MICC)

In this reaction, the target cell is lysed by circulating cells in the presence of the plant mitogen PHA, PWM, or Con-A (Fig. 7.25). The susceptibility of the target cell to lysis by the effector cell appears to be directly related to the capacity of both cells to interact with different sites on the mitogen molecule. This finding suggests that the effector cell interacts with the target cell via a receptor for the mitogen fixed to the target cell, but this has not yet been confirmed.

As in the case of the ADCC and NOCC reactions, the effector cells appear to be heterogeneous and include neutrophils, monocytes, and lymphocytes. The identity of the effector cell appears to be a function of the target cell selected for the assay.

This reaction is quantitated in the same way as is the ADCC reaction.

Important

The reader should be impressed with the fact that the MLR, ADCC, NOCC, and MICC reactions are all mediated by seemingly immunocompetent cells normally present in the circulation. It is important to stress that these effector cells have *not* been previously exposed to or sensitized with the target cells.

What is the relevance of these reactions in the assessment of immune responsiveness or immunocompetence? The ADCC reaction partially falls into the category of immunologically mediated reactions, as it can only be triggered following sensitization of the target cell by the antibody. The ADCC reaction may be considered as either a forerunner of the humoral immune response, as a protective reaction to pathogenic invasive agents in accordance with Darwinian evolutionary theory, or conversely as

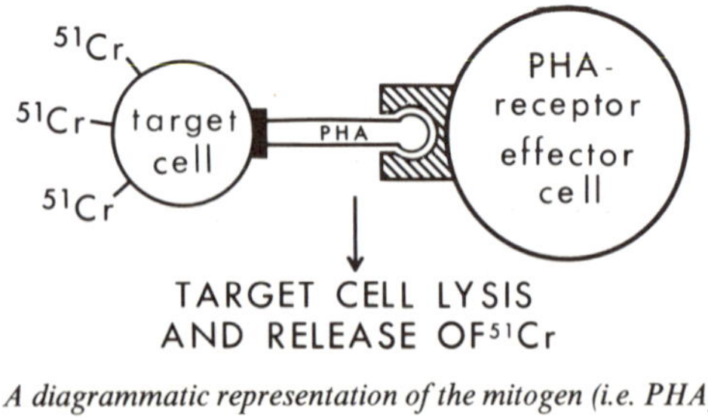

Figure 7.25 *A diagrammatic representation of the mitogen (i.e. PHA)-induced cell-mediated cytotoxic (MICC) reaction.*

an adaptation of humoral immunity in accordance with Lamarckian evolutionary theory.

In support of the Darwinian theory, investigations concerned with the phylogeny of the immune response have disclosed that antibodies of the IgG type appear to have evolved prior to the appearance of complement. Antibodies are capable of interacting with the invader but are incapable of lysing or killing it. However, the Fc receptor-bearing lymphocytes can carry out the lysis of the antibody-sensitized target cell. Once the complement system made its appearance, it probably displaced the Fc receptor-bearing cell as the major naturally occurring, nonimmunologically induced protagonist in antibody-mediated lysis. Complement and the IgG antibody molecules can gain access to compartments of the body which are inaccessible to the Fc receptor-bearing cells. This latter property would impart a greater survival value to antibodies and complement than to Fc receptor-bearing lymphocytes. Furthermore, the energy required for the synthesis of antibody molecules and the complement components is probably far less than that required for the synthesis of Fc receptor-bearing cells. Thus, the ADCC effector cell may represent a primitive improvisation by nature to serve as a stop gap, in an evolutionary sense, between the appearance of circulating antibodies and the later appearance of the complement system needed to facilitate lysis of antibody-sensitized target cells.

On the other hand, the ADCC effector cell may be considered to represent a more highly evolved immune system. In accordance with Lamarckian theory, nature has permitted the synthesis of some IgG antibody molecules which are not capable of fixing complement or do so to a limited extent. These are the IgG-2 and IgG-4 immunoglobulins. The Fc receptor-bearing cells may have been retained during the evolution of the humoral immune response in order to facilitate lysis of target cells sensitized with non-complement-fixing IgG antibodies. In the long run, evolution may dictate the cessation of synthesis of non-complement-fixing antibodies, which would then make the Fc receptor-bearing lymphocytes redundant in an immunologic sense. However, it may be that the non-complement-fixing antibodies have other roles to play which are not yet understood. For example, non-complement-fixing antibodies protect allografts from rejection by sensitized cells (enhancing antibodies). They may also protect autologous parenchymal cells from destruction by sensitized cells and thus prevent autoimmune disease.

It is instructive to note that the target cell need be sensitized with very few antibody molecules in order to be susceptible to lysis by Fc receptor-bearing lymphocytes. The number of antibody molecules required for ADCC-mediated lysis is 100 to 1,000 times less than is required for complement-mediated lysis. Thus, lysis by Fc receptor-bearing cells, or ADCC lysis, is very effective in the presence of a limited antibody response and could conceivably have great survival value in individuals in whom antibody synthesis takes place sluggishly or to a limited extent. Thus, the ADCC effector cell may provide an adequate defense toward pathogenic microorganisms in the event of a limited immune response, in which case antibodies, even if capable of fixing complement, would be synthesized in insufficient numbers to eliminate the invasive organisms by complement-dependent lysis. It may, therefore, be that nature, in its wisdom, has retained both of these antibody-dependent effector systems to ensure survival of the host in the event that one of these immune mechanisms may not function optimally.

The NOCC and MICC reactions are presently difficult to put into perspective as protective mechanisms insofar as current knowledge permits. Undoubtedly the reactions are detecting and identifying cells whose functions in vivo remain to be elucidated. Current speculation is that the NOCC effector cells provide the "immunologic surveillance" to tumorigenesis in view of their capacity to kill selected tumor cell lines in vitro, but this remains to be proven.

IN VIVO IMMUNE REACTIONS (SKIN REACTIONS)

There are three types of skin tests which are currently used in the differential diagnosis of immunologically mediated disease (Table 7.5). These are the immediate skin reaction, the delayed hypersensitivity skin reaction, and the Arthus reaction.

These reactions are discussed individually in detail in Chapter 14. However, it is appropriate to compare and contrast them at this point in order to appreciate the different properties which characterize each of these reactions in terms of the etiology, pathogenesis, reactants, and mediators involved.

Immediate Skin Reaction

The immediate skin reaction is pathognomonic for an IgE-mediated allergic state. In fact, as discussed in Chapter 14, 95% of clinically allergic individuals give an immediate skin reaction upon challenge epicutaneously (by scratch) or intradermally with the allergen. Conversely, less than 5% of normal individuals give an immediate reaction following challenge with the allergen. This may indicate a latent or subclinical allergic state and/or dermo-

Table 7.5
Characteristic Properties of the Different Skin Reactions Used in Diagnostic Immunology

Skin Reaction	Reactants		Pharmcologic Agents Involved	Temporal Aspects of the Reaction			Clinical Condition
	Extrinsic Factor	Intrinsic Factor		Time of First Appearance	Time of Maximum Reaction	Time of Resolution of Reaction	
				hr	*hr*	*hr*	
Immediate skin reaction	Allergen (innocuous nonreplicating, nonpathogenic, nontoxic), i.e. pollen, dust particles	Reagins or IgE antibodies	Histamine Serotonin	0.1	0.25	1–2	Allergy, especially respiratory (Type I)
Arthus reaction	Foreign serum Proteins (i.e. ATS)	Precipitating IgG antibodies	Activated complement components, enzymes	2–3	4–8	8–12	Immune complex disease (Type III)
Delayed hypersensitivity skin reaction	Fungi, most viruses, some bacteria (i.e. *M. tuberculosis*)	Sensiztized lymphocyte	Lymphokines	12–18	24–72	72–120	Cell-mediated immune reaction (Type IV)

graphism which can be ruled out by the simultaneous challenge with saline. The reaction which ensues is essentially identical to the triple response histamine-mediated reaction first described by Cannon. The reaction begins almost immediately with a sharply defined induration around the site of administration of the allergen accompanied by intense pruritis. Within minutes a wheal (a localized hive) will be formed centered about the point of application of the allergen (on the site of the original induration) consisting of a protein transudate low in gamma globulin. This raised lesion can be depressed by the application of finger pressure (pitting edema). The wheal is due to increased capillary permeability which permits the escape of fluid into the tissue spaces. As the wheal increases in size, it gradually becomes paler due to compression of the minute vessels. The wheal usually reaches its maximum height in about 5 to 15 minutes and may project 1 to 2 mm above the surface of the skin.

The wheal will generally be surrounded by a flare (or erythema or widespread flush) attributable to arteriolar dilatation. The flare actually precedes the wheal by up to several minutes. Unlike the wheal, the flare has an irregular shape corresponding to the distribution of the arterioles in the skin. The color is red, proving that rapid flow of blood is occurring.

The flare depends on an intact nerve supply to the skin and results from a local axon reflex. The wheal, composed of a transudate of protein-rich fluid, is attributed to the effects of histamine liberated as a result of the interaction between the mast cell-bound IgE antibodies and the allergen.

The reaction usually resolves by resorption of the fluid within 1 hour, leaving no sign of a reaction having taken place.

Delayed (Hypersensitivity) Skin Reaction

In contrast with the immediate skin reaction, this reaction does not even begin to make an appearance until 24 to 36 hours (the latent period) following challenge of the skin with the antigen (i.e. tuberculin). The reaction evolves very slowly, almost imperceptibly, over the next 24 to 36 hours. The hallmark is a firm, nonpitting, well-demarcated induration not accompanied by pruritis. In the normal course of events, the reaction will reach maximum intensity within 24 hours after its appearance and will subside over the next 24 to 48 hours. The induration is due to an exudate composed of fluid rich in gamma globulin and protein in general accompanied by a large number of variously shaped mononuclear cells. There is normally no residual tissue damage as a result of the reaction. Should the reaction be very intense, however, ulceration of the skin may occur due to thrombosis of the small vessels followed by ischemic necrosis. The result is fibrosis and scar formation.

This reaction is initiated by the interaction of the antigen with circulating sensitized mononuclear cells. The latter secrete a number of very potent pharmacologically active agents or mediators referred to collectively as lymphokines which are the responsible agents in the induction of this reaction (see Chapter 6).

Arthus Reaction

This reaction, named after Maurice Arthus who first described it in 1903, is relatively delayed in comparison with the immediate skin reaction, as it only becomes evident within 4 to 6 hours following challenge of the skin with the antigen. In contrast with the delayed skin reaction, it is initiated by the interaction of the antigen with circulating antibodies rather than with sensitized cells.

Due to the sluggish circulation in the small blood vessels, immune aggregates enlarge and eventually precipitate out and/or adhere to the vessel wall. Interaction of the immune aggregates with the complement system leads to the activation of anaphylatoxin and neutrophil chemotactic factor. The former causes the release of histamine from mast cells and the latter the accumulation of neutrophils which release potent blood-clotting agents and proteolytic enzymes. The result is an acute local inflammatory response, characterized by extensive nonpitting edema. The reaction reaches its climax within 6 to 12 hours following its initiation and gradually subsides without inflicting serious damage.

It must be stressed that, although the reaction is initiated as a result of the interaction between the soluble antigen and circulating antibodies, both complement and neutrophils must be present in normal concentrations in order for the reaction to take place. This reaction, like the immediate and delayed reactions, is a mediator-driven reaction. The mediators involved in the immediate reaction are histamine, serotonin, slow-reacting substance of anaphylaxis (SRS-A), bradykinin, and possibly acetylcholine. The mediators involved in the delayed reaction are lymphocyte-derived lymphokines. The mediators implicated in the Arthus reaction are complement-derived anaphylatoxin, neutrophil chemotactic factor, and proteolytic and blood-clotting factors released from the infiltrating neutrophils.

Schwartzman (or Sanarelli-Schwartzman) Reaction

The initial (or sensitizing) intradermal injection of a bacterial endotoxin (the lipopolysaccharide constituent(s) of gram-negative bacteria) results in a mild, localized, innocuous inflammation of short duration. In contrast, the second (or challenge) injection of the same or a different nonimmunogenic or antigenically non-cross-reactive endotoxin 24 to 48 hours later results in a rapidly evolving intense inflammatory reaction at the site of the initial administration of the endotoxin. Petechial hemorrhages becomes apparent within 1 hour which quickly merge into ecchymotic hemorrhages. The entire area takes on a purplish color (cyanosis) indicative of stasis, and this is followed by necrosis of the tissue, ulcer formation, and fibrosis. Histologic investigation reveals infiltration with polymorphs in various stages of degranulation and degradation, platelet thrombi, and necrosis of vessel walls. This reaction was described by Schwartzmann in 1928 and is referred to as the localized Schwartzman reaction.

It the animals are injected intravenously with the endotoxin on both occasions (sensitizing and challenge injections), many will succumb within a few hours of the challenge injection. The immediate cause of death will invariably be vascular collapse and shock. Postmortem examination will often reveal bilateral cortical necrosis of the kidneys and focal hemorrhagic necrotic lesions in the spleen and liver due to occlusion of the capillaries and sinusoids with fibrin and/or platelet-fibrin thrombi. This systemic reaction was first described by Sanarelli in 1924 working with the endotoxin of *Vibrio cholerae,* and it is referred to as the Sanarelli-Schwartzman reaction or the generalized Schwartzman reaction.

Neither the localized nor the generalized reaction is considered to be an immunologic reaction. Although many attempts have been made to demonstrate an immunologic etiology for this reaction, no evidence has been presented to support this view. The criteria which are universally accepted to define an immunologic reaction—(a) a latent period of sufficient duration to permit the formation of antibodies (minimum 3 to 5 days), (b) the detection of antibodies directed specifically to the sensitizing antigen, and (c) the necessary identity of both the sensitizing antigen and the challenge antigen—do not apply to this reaction. Nevertheless, the Schwartzman reaction is discussed here in order to underline the nonimmunologic nature of this reaction which is often incorrectly classified as an immunologically mediated reaction.

A number of acute, often life-threatening, conditions which appear unexpectedly and with sudden onset following extensive surgery, severe stress, hemorrhage, or difficult childbirth (often accompanied by gram-negative bacterial infection) present with a clinical picture similar to that observed in the Schwartzman reaction. These conditions are: (a) vascular collapse and shock concurrent with or following diagnosis of gram-negative septicemia; (b) the Waterhouse-Friderichsen syndrome or acute bilateral hemorrhagic necrosis of the adrenal glands; (c) bilateral cortical necrosis of the kidneys; (d) panhypopituitary syndrome (clinically referred to as Simmond's disease) as a consequence of ischemic or hemorrhagic necrosis of the anterior lobe of the pituitary gland (pathologically referred to as Sheehan's syndrome); (e) abruptio placentae; and (f) preeclampsia.

Sporadic reports or hemorrhagic necrosis of the ovaries, parathyroid and thyroid glands may also constitute instances of Schwartzman-like reactions in these endocrine glands.

Although these diverse clinical conditions would appear to be totally unrelated in terms of etiology and pathogenesis, a common feature is intravascular coagulation followed by necrosis of the tissue distal to the occluded vessel(s). In many instances, septicemia with gram-negative bacteria (i.e. *Neisseria meningitidis*, *Haemophilus influenzae*, *Salmonella typhi*, *Proteus vulgaris*, *Escherichia coli*, *V. cholerae*) can be documented. Disseminated intravascular coagulation (DIC), initiated by endotoxin, is a hallmark of the generalized Schwartzman reaction. The mechanism whereby endotoxins induce DIC is only slowly becoming understood. Endotoxin can interact with and activate C′3 via the alternate pathway of complement fixation. Endotoxin-C′3b complexes or possibly endotoxin-C′3b-conglutinin complexes may be bound to platelets via receptors for C′3b and Fc, respectively, resulting in platelet aggregation and lysis, especially along the intima of small blood vessels. Several highly potent pharmacologic agents released from these damaged platelets can accelerate endogenous thromboplastin formation, decrease coagulation time, and increase prothrombin consumption, all of which contribute to DIC. It is instructive to note that decomplementation of the experimental animal prior to the administration of the challenge dose of the endotoxin prevents the ensuing DIC and shock. The severity of the clinical state may reflect the sensitivity of the vasculature of the different potential target organs to the endotoxin.

Important

The differential diagnosis of shock should always include endotoxin-induced shock (Table 7.2). Anaphylatoxins, generated by the fixation of C′ via the alternate pathway by endotoxin, can directly induce liberation of histamine and serotonin from mast cells. It is essential to distinguish this form of shock from anaphylactic (allergic) shock mediated by histamine and serotonin liberated from mast cells and basophils following interaction of cell-bound IgE antibodies with the allergen (see Chapter 14).

Schick Test

This skin test is used to demonstrate the existence of circulating antibodies to diphtheria toxin. It was pioneered by Bela Schick more than 60 years ago and is still carried out in the differential diagnosis of immunodeficiency disease.

The basis of this test is that the intradermal injection of a small amount of diphtheria toxin is normally followed by a relatively innocuous inflammatory response within a few days which usually heals by resorption of the exudate. However, it may progress to a frank dermonecrotic reaction in some individuals. The reaction may be detected within 8 to 24 hours following the injection of the toxin, and it usually reaches maximum intensity within 3 to 6 days. This is referred to as a positive Schick test. The reaction is the result of a direct action of the toxin on the tissues. In the presence of circulating antibodies to diphtheria toxin, no skin reaction occurs due to the neutralization of the toxin by the antibodies. This is referred to as a negative Schick test.

Over the past 20 years, it has become increasingly recognized that an immediate (allergic) skin reaction, an Arthus reaction, and/or a delayed skin reaction, all immunologically mediated, may also occur at the site of injection of the diphtheria toxin. This is a result of often-repeated immunization with diphtheria toxoid as a prophylatic measure in North America and Europe. Although the immediate skin reaction occurs too early to be confused with the toxic reaction, the Arthus skin reaction may not reach its maximum intensity until 18 to 24 hours and, therefore, may be mistaken for an early positive Schick test. On the other hand, the delayed reaction may be truly delayed and may not attain maximum intensity until 3 to 4 days have elapsed from the time of challenge. It may be wrongly mistaken for the inflammatory reaction induced by the direct actions of the toxin.

To avoid an error in judgment, it is prudent to inject diphtheria toxoid into the contralateral arm as a control. Diphtheria toxoid cannot induce the toxin-related inflammatory reaction, but it can induce the immediate allergic wheal-and-flare reaction (in the presence of circulating specific IgE antibodies), the Arthus skin reaction (in the presence of circulating IgG antibodies), and/or a delayed skin reaction (in the presence of sensitized cells). The immediate reaction is early (minutes to 1 hour) and cannot be confused with the toxin-induced reaction. The absence of an Arthus or a delayed skin reaction in the control site removes any doubt as to the nature of the inflammatory reaction at the site of administration of the toxin. Furthermore, failure to detect circulating antibodies by the passive hemagglutination technique, using diphtheria toxoid-sensitized erythrocytes, effectively rules out the Arthus reaction as the etiologic mechanism for the inflammatory reaction.

With respect to the histopathology of the reaction, a positive reaction begins (at 8 to 24 hours) as a circumscribed area of redness (erythema) 1 to 3 cm in diameter. The redness may increase in intensity and reach its maximum by 3 to 6 days. There is no itching (pruritis) or marked swelling (edema), and the reaction gradually fades and disappears by 7 to 10 days. However, in more violent reactions, localized necrosis may occur with desquamation, slight ulceration, and healing by fibrosis and scar formation. Vesiculation may occur in very intense reactions. The reaction site may be marked by brownish pigmentation for weeks or months.

The usefulness of the Schick test is based on the fact that the intensity of the reaction is inversely related to the concentration of antitoxic antibodies in the blood. That is, it is marked in the absence of antibodies and minimal or absent in the presence of antibodies. This test may, therefore, be used where serologic techniques for determination of antibody titers to diphtheria toxin are not available. A negative Schick test (in an immunized individual) indicates the presence of at least 0.01 unit of antibodies per ml of serum—an amount sufficient to provide immunity to infection with *Corynebacterium diphtheriae.*

Dick Test

This skin test is used to determine the presence (or absence) of antibodies to the erythrogenic toxin of *Streptococcus pyogenes.* It is rarely used today in view of the fact that it only indicates whether a rash will accompany an infection with *S. pyogenes* (scarlet fever). It does not indicate the existence of protection or the degree of susceptibility to infection with the pathogenic strains of the streptococcal organisms (strep throat).

The intradermal injection of culture fluid containing the erythrogenic toxin is followed by an acute localized inflammatory reaction within 4 to 12 hours. The reaction attains maximum intensity by 18 to 24 hours and then gradually fades. A reaction is considered positive if the area of redness exceeds 1 cm in diameter.

Pseudoreactions, that is the immunologically mediated skin reactions which may occur following injection of the strep toxin (immediate Arthus and delayed skin reaction), are encountered very infrequently due to the fact that individuals are not intentionally immunized to streptococcus toxins as they are to diphtheria toxin. Therefore, the opportunity to develop an allergic (IgE) sensitivity, Arthus reactivity or sensitized cells is minimal.

CHAPTER 8

Suppressor Cells and Suppressor Antibodies

Alice to Humpty Dumpty: "If I say something, it means exactly what I wish it to mean, nothing more and nothing less."

Humpty Dumpty to Alice: "But Alice, how can the same words have so many different meanings at different times?"

—*Alice in Wonderland* by Lewis Carroll

The evidence that nature has assigned the role of modulating the immune response to suppressor cells and suppressor factors is overwhelming, but it is also overwhelmingly confusing. The confusion arises out of the failure of immunologists, up to the most recent times, to clearly and unequivocally (a) explain the inhibition of a specific immune response by nonspecific suppressor cells; (b) explain, in unambiguous terms, why the failure to demonstrate suppressor cells in in vitro assays is not accompanied by a panautoimmune syndrome in vivo; (c) demonstrate whether suppressor cells are homogeneous or heterogeneous; (d) demonstrate whether the suppressor cells which inhibit an antibody response are identical to those cells which suppress a cell-mediated immune response; and (e) demonstrate that the results obtained with the highly unphysiologic in vitro assays for suppressor cells can be extrapolated to the in vivo situation.

A large array of substances have been shown, over the past two decades, to be capable of inhibiting the immune response. These include plant extracts (such as phytohemagglutinin and concanavalin-A), mammalian cell extracts, hormones (both naturally occurring and synthetic analogues), antibiotics, other antigens (the inhibition of an immune response to a second antigen several days following the administration of the first antigen is referred to as antigen competition; the antigens do not necessarily have to be related nor can they be randomly selected, either; the interval of time which must elapse between their administration is crucial for the response to the second antigen to be abrogated), and a host of biologically derived and synthetic agents unrelated to each other which have been grouped under the umbrella term "immunosuppressive drugs." Only several of these immunosuppressive agents have been utilized in the human. They have been used in, and their activities documented in, the experimental animal, primarily the inbred mouse. Nevertheless, in spite of the controlled, highly unphysiologic and artificial conditions which have marked their utilization, their immunosuppressive activity is still controversial.

Two naturally occurring nontoxic agents which have been shown to exhibit immunosuppressive activity under esssentially physiologic conditions are antibodies and suppressor cells. The ensuing discussion will, therefore, be concerned with the immunosuppressive drugs, antibodies, and suppressor cells as potential and/or actual immunochemotherapeutic agents in humans.

IMMUNOSUPPRESSIVE DRUGS

The immunosuppressive drugs fall into a number of categories based on their composition, mode of action, toxicity, and source. They are described in detail in Chapter 16. Suffice it to say that the success attained with these drugs in the human, individually or in combination, is muted relative to the anticipated success at the time of their introduction and promotion as imunosuppressive agents. Azathioprine, thiouracil, actinomycin-D, cyclophosphamide, chlorambucil, antilymphocyte globulin (ALG), and the steroids are all toxic if used in quantities equivalent (mg per kg of body weight) to their effective doses in the experimental animal. Used in homeopathic doses, these agents are nontoxic but neither do they express immunosuppressive activity. Unfortunately, their immunosuppressive activity only increases at the expense of increased generalized toxicity. In the experimental animal, the pinnacle of immunosuppression with most of the drugs is attained at LD_{50} doses, a situation which cannot conceivably be tolerated in the human. For this and other reasons discussed at length in Chapter 16, the present coterie of "immunosuppressive drugs" will enjoy a very short life-span as chemotherapeutic agents.

ANTIBODIES

Antibodies have been shown to be capable of both enhancing and suppressing the immune response. This situation was clarified in the 1960s when it was observed that IgM antibodies stimulate or potentiate antibody formation but that IgG antibodies tend to limit, terminate, or suppress further synthesis of antibodies. It will be recalled (see Chapter 5) that the IgM antibodies are synthesized first in the primary immune response and the IgG antibodies are detected in the circulation only 1 to 3 days later. The IgM antibodies stimulate the synthesis of IgG antibodies, and the latter, as they increase in concentration, suppress the further synthesis of IgM antibodies. This feedback stimulation of antibody synthesis by IgM antibodies and feedback inhibition by IgG antibodies appeared to be the major physiologic control mechanism in the regulation of the humoral immune response until the discovery of suppressor cells. The latter appear to provide at least a second mechanism for the regulation of the antibody response and the primary mechanism for the regulation of the cell-mediated immune response.

Another mechanism whereby the humoral (antibody) immune system may inhibit antibody formation is via the synthesis of anti-idiotype (auto) antibodies. The reader will recall from the discussion on the structure of antibody molecules (Chapter 3) that the antigen-binding sites (at the amino terminal region of the Fab) on any two antibody molecules directed toward different non-cross-reacting antigens differ respect to composition (amino acid sequence) and/or spatial configuration. In other words, the antigen-binding sites on an IgG antibody molecule directed toward one antigen, i.e. diphtheria toxoid, must possess a unique composition and/or configuration different from the antigen-binding sites on an IgG antibody molecule directed toward a second non-cross-reacting antigen, i.e. pneumococcal polysaccharide. If this were not the case, then either antigen would be able to interact with both antibodies which clearly does not happen. Further evidence of the distinctness of the antigen bindings sites is provided by the fact that the antigen bindings sites on the human IgG antibody molecules express antigenic specificity following the injection of the IgG antibodies into the xenogeneic animal (i.e. rabbit) and this property is referred to as the idiotypic specificity (or idiotype) of the human IgG antibody molecule (see Chapter 3). It follows, therefore, that the number of idiotypes is approximately equal to the number of antigens (or more specifically antigenic determinants) to which the individual responds with antibody formation. Since the composition and/or configuration of any one idiotype is different from every other idiotype and many idiotypes are not synthesized and therefore will not appear in the circulation until many years after birth, it may logically be asked why the immune system does not recognize the idiotypes as foreign and synthesize antibodies to them.

In point of fact, it has been demonstrated in the experimental animal that antibodies can indeed be induced toward autologous antibody molecules and that the reactivity and specificity of these autoantibodies are directed toward the idiotype on the autologous antibody molecule. It has also been demonstrated that anti-idiotype antibodies suppress the in vivo and in vitro secondary response to the specific immunizing antigen and can facilitate the induction of a state of immunologic tolerance to the specific antigen. The ability of anti-idiotype antibodies to suppress antibody formation must surely be related to the fact that the anti-idiotype antibodies and the antigenic determinant sites on the antigen molecules compete for the same (antibody?) receptors on the antibody-forming cell; however, interaction of the cell with the anti-idiotype antibodies generates an inhibitory signal for antibody formation whereas the interaction of the cell with the antigen generates a stimulatory signal for antibody formation.

The synthesis of anti-idiotype antibodies prior to initial exposure to the immunizing antigen (by injecting purified allogeneic antibodies) would result in interaction of the anti-idiotype antibodies with the surface membrane antigen-specific receptors on the virgin immunocompetent antigen-recognizing cells (ARC) with respect to ARC-dependent antigens, and the precursor AFC cells with respect to the ARC (or T)-independent antigens, thus neutralizing them and preventing them from interacting with the antigen once it is administered. In the absence of a competent antigen recognition mechanism, no antibody synthesis can take place and a state of immunological tolerance will result (see Chapter 11).

In light of these results obtained in the experimental animal, it may not be inappropriate to predict that the normal individual, following an antibody immune response toward an exogenous bacterial antigen, synthesizes IgG antibodies directed toward the idiotype of the specifically-formed autologous anti-bacteria antibodies. The anti-idiotype antibodies would be in exceedingly low concentration and would therefore be very difficult to detect by current conventional assay systems. These anti-idiotype (auto) antibodies could function to bring about cessation of the immune response in the human in the manner described above for the experimental animal.

Whether the immunoinhibitory role of the IgG antibodies is strictly a reflection of the activity of the anti-idiotype antibodies, or whether there exist multiple mechanisms to account for the negative feedback regulatory function of the IgG antibody molecules, remain to be determined.

SUPPRESSOR CELLS

The term "suppressor cells" did not appear in the immunology literature until the late 1960s. The impact of the revelation of the existence of such cells was so immediate and intense that a new subdiscipline evolved concerned primarily with the identification and mechanism of action of suppressor cells in the immune response.

An important feature of the immune response in the experimental animal is a seemingly uncontrolled proliferation of lymphoid cells which generate numerous lymphoblasts, plasmablasts, and plasma cells. Obviously, if there were no brakes applied to this response, the ultimate result would be a malignant process the very first time the cells would be stimulated to carry out an immune response. Since the immune response as such would, therefore, have very little survival value, it obviously had to be modified through evolutionary processes to eliminate its life-threatening features before it could function as a defense mechanism. The suppressor cell (among other mechanisms which remain to be discovered) probably evolved to terminate the immunologically induced (or antigenically driven) proliferation of antibody-forming cells at a point beyond which further proliferation is unnecessary to provide the appropriate level of immunity.

If the reader considers the arguments presented above to be logical, if not necessarily totally valid, then the role of the suppressor cell may be seen in a different light—that is, a more general role in the reestablishment of homeostasis following the "pathologic" deviation from homeostasis incurred as a result of the induction of an antibody response or a cell-mediated response to an external stimulus encountered naturally, i.e. infection, or deliberately, i.e. immunization or allograft implantation.

Definition

A suppressor cell may be defined as a cell capable of aborting an otherwise anticipated immune response and of terminating an ongoing immune response. However, there are instances when inhibition or absence of an immune response may be wrongly attributed to the activity of suppressor cells. Specific immunosuppression must be distinguished from:

1. Those mechanisms which regulate **normal** physiologic functions required to maintain homeostasis
2. Failure of the immune response to occur due to factors other than suppressor cells, i.e. failure of helper cell function, in vivo lysis of helper cells by cytotoxic antibodies, or disturbance

in the microscopic architecture of lymphoid tissues concurrent with disease states

3. Failure of the immune response to occur due to disturbance of and distortion within the microscopic architecture of the lymphoid tissues as a consequence of the injection of a great excess (100 to 1,000 times the immunogenic dose) of a conventional antigen

4. Failure of the immune response to occur due to the induction of suppressor cell-independent immunologic tolerance.

The results of the vast majority of investigations carried out in humans clearly indicate that the suppressor (immunosuppressor or immunoinhibitory) cells are T cells, distinct from the other immunocompetent, immunoresponsive T and non-T cells involved in inducing, mediating, augmenting, and sustaining the immune response. The nonsuppressor T cells are highly heterogeneous functionally (see Chapters 5, 6, and 9) and may be classified as follows: (a) **helper cells** in the humoral immune response; (b) **helper cells** in the cell-mediated immune response; (c) **sensitized cells** in the cell-mediated immune response; (d) **effector cells** in the cell-mediated immune response; (e) **memory cells** in the cell-mediated immune response; (f) **cytotoxic cells** in the cell-mediated immune response; and (g) **responder cells** in the cell-mediated immune response.

Until the mid-1970s, it was assumed that the suppressor cells constitute a homogeneous family of cells and that the same cells act to suppress the humoral and the cell-mediated immune responses (Fig. 8.1). It was not clear whether the target cells for

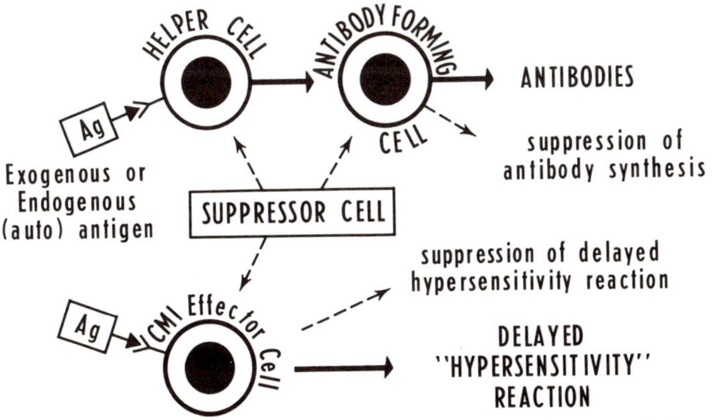

Figure 8.1 *The suppressor cell and the mechanism of its action in the regulation of humoral and cell-mediated immune responses.*

the suppressor cells in the humoral immune response were the helper cells, the antibody-forming cells, or both.

However, on the basis of experiences with the immunocompetent T cells, which were also considered at one time to be homogeneous and later demonstrated to be highly heterogeneous and to constitute myriads of different cell types, it could have been safely predicted that the suppressor T cell population is also highly heterogeneous. Such is, in fact, the case. Suppressor cells only appear to be homogeneous by light microscopy, as they all present morphologically as small, mature lymphocytes. However, they are highly heterogeneous in terms of function. Within the past few years it has been shown that there exist suppressor cells which are specific for the humoral (or antibody) immune response and other suppressor cells specific for the cell-mediated immune response. Furthermore, the suppressor cells for each immune response (although it has been definitely demonstrated only for the humoral immune response thus far) may be categorized as antigen-specific and non-antigen-specific (Table 8.1). The majority of investigations have consistently implicated only T lymphocytes, specifically T_G lymphocytes, as suppressor cells. Nevertheless, results of a not insignificant number of investigations have presented evidence which implicates the monocytes as suppressor cells as well. The monocytes are, therefore, included in Table 8.1. An in-depth discussion as to the identity of the suppressor T cells in terms of their surface membrane receptors is presented in Chapter 9.

Table 8.1
Classification of Circulating Suppressor Cells

I. Humoral (Antibody) Immune Response
   A. Perenially circulating suppressor cells
      1. Non-antigen-specific T lymphocytes
         a. Do not require additional signal(s) to be activated
         b. Require additional signal(s) to be activated
      2. Non-antigen-specific monocytes
   B. Transiently circulating suppressor cells
      1. Antigen-specific T lymphocytes
      2. Antigen-specific monocytes
II. Cell-mediated Immune Response
      1. Antigen-specific T cells
      2. Non-antigen-specific T cells?
      3. Monocytes?

Important

1. The distinction between T_G suppressor cells and monocyte suppressor cells may prove to be more academic than real in view of the evidence supporting an ontogenic relationship between these cells. The T_G cells stain for nonspecific esterase, a characteristic considered to be specific for monocytes, and they possess surface membrane configurations or structures which induce antibodies in the xenogeneic animal which cross-react with monocytes but not other classes of T cells. It may, therefore, be speculated that the T_G lymphocytes are the progeny of the same stem cells which generate the monocytes or that the T_G lymphocytes are transformed monocytes of a particular class (see Chapter 9).

2. Although monocytes (or circulating phagocytic cells) have been shown by numerous investigators to have suppressor cell activity, it is necessary to recognize that the suppressor nature of these phagocytic cells may be more apparent than real. It has been shown that immune responses in vitro are highly susceptible to inhibition by excessive numbers of normal phagocytic cells. The mechanism of this type of immune suppression is not understood. It is, therefore, necessary to distinguish between true (antigen-specific) suppressor cell activity and the apparent immunoinhibitory activity of excessive numbers of normal phagocytic cells. The latter may be confused with specific immunosuppression by the uncritical or unwary investigator.

Suppressor Cells and the Humoral (Antibody) Immune Response

How might the suppressor cells act to bring about cessation of an already ongoing immune response? Let us initially confine ourselves to the primary antibody immune response. An understanding of the mechanism which regulates specific antibody synthesis may be facilitated by an understanding of the mechanism which maintains a homeostatic balance with respect to the circulating concentration of nonantibody gamma globulins. For many years, it was assumed that a mechanism must exist in vivo to maintain the gamma globulins at an almost constant concentration throughout the adult life-span (approximately ages 15 to 65). Only after Rittenberg, in the 1940s, administered isotopically labeled gamma globulin into the isologous animal and demonstrated that gamma globulin has a finite half-life in vivo was it appreciated that the circulating concentration of gamma globulin represents the balance between gamma globulin synthesis (anabolism) and gamma globulin degradation (catabolism). It was suggested, during the 1940s to the 1960s, that the synthesis and secretion of gamma globulin are governed by the concentration of gamma globulin in the circulation. The mechanism for the regulation of gamma globulin synthesis was considered to be a feedback or servomechanism. As the concentration of these proteins decreases in the circulation, the cells are signaled to synthesize and secrete gamma globulin; whereas, when the concentration of gamma globulin increases beyond the established norm for the individual, the cells cease to synthesize and secrete these proteins.

However, this theory failed to provide an explanation for the induction and cessation of synthesis of specific antibodies or for the marked elevation in nonantibody gamma globulins which accompanies specific antibody synthesis. In the late 1940s, Bjorneboe and Kabat demonstrated, in the experimental animal, that the sharp increase in the concentration of gamma globulin in the circulation following antigen stimulation cannot be accounted for by the concentration of specific antibodies. By far the major portion of the excess gamma globulins synthesized consisted of nonantibody molecules. The mechanism for maintaining a constant concentration of gamma globulins in the circulation eluded investigators until the concept of suppressor cells emerged in the late 1960s and was immediately accepted, as there was a void to be filled. It was demonstrated that cells normally exist in the circulation capable of regulating the synthesis and secretion, and, therefore, the circulating concentration, of the normal gamma globulins. Investigations by Moretta initiated in the mid-1970s demonstrated the existence of two types of T cells in the circulation—T_G and T_M cells. T_G cells possess receptors for the Fc of the IgG molecule, and T_M cells possess receptors for the Fc of the IgM molecule. Although neither T_G nor T_M cells are capable of antibody or immunoglobulin synthesis, a property characteristic of the B cells, T_G cells are capable of inhibiting immunoglobulin synthesis by the normal B lymphocytes, whereas T_M cells are capable of stimulating excessive immunoglobulin synthesis by the otherwise normal circulating B lymphocytes. In other words, when normal B cells are provided with the appropriate signals to initiate immunoglobulin synthesis, the synthesis is regulated by the interacting T cells and is a result of the relative proportion and functional states of the T_G and T_M cells.

In the conventional in vitro assay routinely used to demonstrate the immunoglobulin synthetic capacity of B cells and the suppression/helper activity of T cells, immunoglobulin synthesis does not take place unless a second signal in addition to that from the T_M cell is provided to the B cell. This second signal is provided in vitro by pokeweed mitogen. Thus, B cells incubated with T_M cells and pokeweed synthesize immunoglobulins, but B cells by themselves, or in the presence of only pokeweed mitogen or T_M cells, do not synthesize immunoglobulins. Furthermore, the addition of T_G cells to B cell-T_M cell-pokeweed mitogen cultures inhibits immunoglobulin synthesis. The T_M cells are, therefore, referred to as the helper cells since they furnish one of the signals to the B cells, and the T_G cells are referred to as the suppressor cells since they transmit a negative (or feedback inhibition) signal (Fig. 8.2). The evidence to date strongly indicates that the T_G cell exerts suppressor activity by inhibiting the helper cell from transmitting its positive signal to the B cell; the T_G cell does not act on the B cell proper.

Important

1. It is essential for the reader to realize that the terms helper and suppressor T cells, which define subclasses of circulating cells in the normal individual, refer to cells which function to maintain homeostasis, and in that context they should be referred to simply as regulator cells. It is one thing to define cells which inhibit specific antibody synthesis as suppressor cells; it is highly questionable whether this same term should be utilized to refer to a normal cell which under normal conditions functions to maintain homeostasis. It is necessary to differentiate between physiologic regulating mechanisms and newly induced or newly activated cells by antigens which function to limit the immune response. The latter presents as a pathologic change from the morphologic point of view.

2. The assumption is made that the functions of the T and B cells and their proportion in the circulation mirror their interrelationship within the lymphoid tissues. However, it should be stressed that immunoglobulins and specific antibodies are normally synthesized by the B cells in the spleen and lymph nodes and not by the B cells in the circulation. The circulating B cells may represent immature or spent immunoglobulin-synthesizing cells. It is probably for this reason that the circulating B cells must be stimulated with two signals—one provided by pokeweed mitogen, which probably mimicks one of the in vivo signals, and the second given by the T_M cells—to synthesize immunoglobulins.

Suppressor cells are generally detected by their ability to inhibit the mitogen (phytohemagglutinin or concanavalin-A)-induced blastogenic response or mitogen (pokeweed)-driven immunoglob-

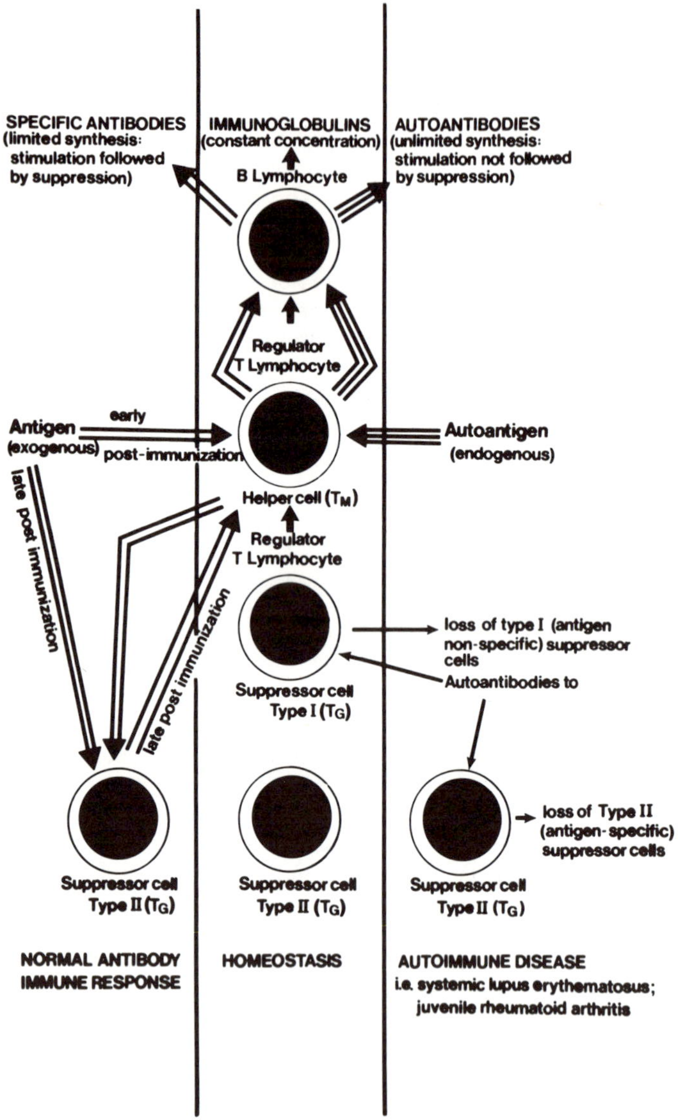

Figure 8.2 *Suppressor cells and their regulatory roles in the induction of (antigen) nonspecific immunoglobulins, antigen-specific antibodies, and autoantibodies.*

Table 8.2
Assays to Detect Suppressor Cells

A. Nonspecific assays
   1. Inhibition of the T cell blastogenic response to mitogen (PHA or Con-A) stimulation in vitro
   2. Inhibition of immunoglobulin synthesis by B cells stimulated with pokeweed in vitro

B. Specific assays
   1. Inhibition of the blastogenic response upon stimulation with specific antigens in vitro
   2. Inhibition of synthesis of specific antibodies in vitro
   3. Inhibition of the induction of plaque-forming cells to specific antigens in vitro
   4. Capacity to prevent, following transfer to a syngeneic host, the otherwise normal immune response in vivo

ulin synthesis by normal circulating B cells in vitro (Table 8.2). The suppressor cells which inhibit or markedly reduce the antigen- or mitogen-induced blastogenic response must first be activated by prior incubation with the antigen or mitogen (usually concanavalin-A) for 24 to 48 hours, respectively. Inhibition of this blastogenic response to antigen or mitogen stimulation in vitro is indicative of suppressor cells capable of inhibiting the cell-mediated immune response (the T cell blastogenic response is considered to be indicative of the capacity to mount a cell-mediated immune response). In constrast, the suppressor cells which inhibit or significantly diminish immunoglobulin synthesis by normal B cells do not require prior activation; they demonstrate suppressor activity immediately following their isolation. The inhibition of immunoglobulin (or antibody) synthesis is indicative of suppressor cells capable of inhibiting the humoral (antibody) immune response. Immunoglobulin synthesis can be detected in two ways—intracytoplasmic immunoglobulins by immunofluorescence and immunoglobulins secreted into the medium by radioimmunoassay. It is essential that the reader realize that, in fact, no correlation exists beween the percentage of the cells which stain for intracytoplasmic immunoglobulins and the amount of immunoglobulins secreted by these cells into the medium. In other words, a suspension of B cells may secrete copious amounts of immunoglobulins but stain very faintly and only in small numbers for immunoglobulins, whereas another suspension of B cells may secrete very little immunoglobulin but stain in large numbers for intracytoplasmic immunoglobulins. Usually, it is the quantity of immunoglobulins secreted into the medium which is clinically relevant and not the presence or absence of intracytoplasmic immunoglobulins. The entire assay system is highly unphysiologic, as it is artificially and empirically contrived. That is not to say that suppressor cells which regulate immunoglobulin synthesis do not exist. Suppressor cells undoubtedly exist, but their detection and assessment in this assay system are fortuitous.

Types I and II Suppressor Cells

If the T cell which normally appears to function in a regulatory capacity with respect to immunoglobulin synthesis in vivo and which inhibits immunoglobulin synthesis in the assay system in vitro is defined as a suppressor cell, then there exist two distinct classes of suppressor cells—non-antigen-specific and antigen-specific suppressor cells. The suppressor cells which inhibit total immunoglobulin synthesis by B cells represent polyclonally active non-antigen-specific T suppressor cells, whereas the suppressor cells activated by the specific antigen represent the monoclonally active antigen-specific suppressor cells which act very specifically to inhibit the synthesis of antibody molecules with a particular antigenic specificity. The nonspecific suppressor cells are referred to as Type I T suppressor cells, and the antigen-specific suppressor cells are referred to as Type II T suppressor cells in Figure 8.2. The Type II T suppressor cells have recently been shown to possess surface receptors for histamine (Table 8.3).

The Type I suppressor cells appear to be functionally heterogeneous (Table 8.3) in that there are two distinct types of suppressor cells in this category. One of these suppressor cells, referred to as a Type Ia suppressor cell, is capable of inhibiting immunoglobulin synthesis by B cells without requiring prior stimulation. In other words, it is already "turned on" in vivo. The other suppressor cell is referred to as a Type Ib suppressor cell. It can inhibit immunoglobulin synthesis by B cells only if it is first incubated with the mitogen concanavalin-A, which provides the signal for the conversion of the innocent bystander T cell to a functional suppressor cell (Table 8.3). These cells may be the precursors of the Type Ia suppressor cells.

The Type II suppressor cells are normally absent from the circulation of the normal unimmunized individual. They can be detected for only a short time at a particular period following immunization, usually after the peak of antibody synthesis has been attained. Investigations in the experimental animal have disclosed the appearance of cells in the spleen and lymph nodes

Table 8.3
Properties of Circulating Suppressor Cells Which Regulate the Humoral (Antibody) Immune Response

A. Perennial lymphoid suppressor cells (non-antigen-specific) (Type Ia)
  1. Constantly circulate
  2. Do not require stimulation to be activated
  3. Can inhibit total synthesis of immunoglobulins in pokeweed-stimulated B cells (assay requires 6 to 7 days of culture)
  4. Appear to act nonspecifically
  5. Possess cell surface receptors for Fc(IgG)
  6. Possess surface membrane receptors characteristic of T cells

B. Perennial lymphoid pro-suppressor cells (non-antigen-specific) (Type Ib)
  1. Constantly circulate
  2. Can only function as suppressor cells following preculture for 24 to 48 hours with a particular stimulating agent, i.e. concanavalin-A
  3. Appear to act nonspecifically
  4. Possess cell surface receptors for Fc(IgG)
  5. Possess surface membrane receptors characteristic of T cells

C. Transient lymphoid suppressor cells (antigen-specific) (Type II)
  1. Detected only following antigenic stimulation
  2. Stimulated or activated by specific antigens
  3. Can suppress immune response to a specific antigen only
  4. Appear to act specifically
  5. Possess cell surface receptors for Fc(IgG) and histamine
  6. Possess surface membrane receptors characteristic of T cells

D. Monocyte suppressor cells
  Properties are too vague and ill-defined to permit their listing at this time.

within several weeks following maximum antibody synthesis which, following their transfer into syngeneic normal recipients, are capable of suppressing an antibody response to the antigen used to immunize the donor of these cells. Thus they are true antigen-specific suppressor cells. These cells appear to inhabit the spleen and lymph nodes only transiently after antibody synthesis has reached its peak, following which they can no longer be detected.

It has been known for many years that a secondary or anamnestic immune response in animals and in humans cannot be successfully induced until a finite time has elapsed following the primary immune response (1 to 2 months). Presumably, the inability to mount a secondary immune response immediately following a primary immune response may be attributed to antigen-induced Type II suppressor T cells activated during the latter (postantibody) phase of the primary response. These suppressor cells would, therefore, appear to have a functional life-span not in excess of 1 to 2 months. Furthermore, their antigenic specificity can be easily demonstrated by the fact that only the secondary response to the original immunizing antigen is affected by these cells, not the response to any other non-cross-reacting antigen.

We can now return to the discussion of the manner whereby the suppressor cells inhibit the antibody immune response. A proposed mechanism, presented diagrammatically in Figure 8.2, takes into account current findings with respect to both general immunoglobulin and specific antibody synthesis. The scheme attempts to present a unified mechanism to account for the maintenance of homeostasis, the induction and cessation of antibody synthesis, and the induction and progression of autoimmune diseases. In the unimmunized normal individual, immunoglobulin synthesis by B cells is regulated by a signal which emanates from the "nonspecific" T_M helper cells. This T_M helper cell is held in check by the "nonspecific" T_G regulatory Type I suppressor cell. Thus, when the T_G Type I suppressor cell is activated following synthesis of excessive numbers of "nonspecific" immunoglobulins, it inhibits the transmission of a positive signal from the "nonspecific" T_M helper cell to the immunoglobulin-synthesizing B lymphocyte. This inhibitory signal from the T_G Type I suppressor cells appears to result from activation of these cells by aggregates of immunoglobulins. Aggregated as well as nonaggregated nonantibody immunoglobulins circulate in the normal individual, and the aggregated immunoglobulins may play a regulatory role to dampen synthesis of immunoglobulin molecules by activating the "nonspecific" T_G Type I suppressor cells. The synthesis of immunoglobulins in the normal unimmunized individual appears, therefore, not to be regulated by positive and negative signals transmitted alternately or sequentially by the T_M and T_G cells, respectively, as was originally perceived, but by a positive signal and the absence of a positive signal coming from the "nonspecific" T_M helper cell. The Type II suppressor cell probably exists in an inactive or dormant state in the normal unimmunized individual.

Following immunization with an exogenous antigen, "antigen-specific" T_M helper cells are immediately stimulated and they facilitate synthesis of specific antibodies by the appropriate B lymphoid cells. The T_G Type II suppressor cells are normally activated later in the immune response by circulating antibody-antigen complexes, and these T_G suppressor cells act on the "antigen-specific" T_M helper cells in such a manner as to shut off the positive signals to the B cells, resulting in cessation of cellular proliferation and antibody synthesis. Furthermore, these "antigen-specific" T_M helper cells, when induced in excessive numbers as a result of hyperimmunization, can directly activate the Type II suppressor cells, completing a feedback loop which imposes negative feedback regulatory functions to the T_M helper cells and the T_G Type II suppressor cells. Thus, there exist two mechanisms for the activation of the Type II suppressor cells in the immunized individual—activation by antigen and activation by "antigen-specific" T_M helper cells.

Recent findings suggest, however, that the mechanism of suppressor cell activation and function, with respect to both polyclonally-stimulated immunoglobulin synthesis and antigen-induced specific antibody formation, is more complex than is alluded to above. It would appear that both T cell-T cell interaction and secreted soluble factors are involved.

Functionally-active T suppressor cells are generated from inactive precursor pre-suppressor T cells as a result of transformation and/or proliferation. The pre-suppressor cells are stimulated subsequent to their interaction with a soluble suppressor cell activating factor(s) (mediator? hormone?) secreted by pro-suppressor (or suppressor cell activating) T cells following their interaction with the suppressor-inducing stimulant (antigen in the case of the specific immune response and probably some form of aggregated immunoglobulin in the case of "non-specific" immunoglobulin synthesis). Both the pro-suppressor and pre-suppresor T cells can be distinguished from the helper T cells since the former are relatively radiosensitive in vitro while the helper cells are radioresistant. The suppressor cell activating factor secreted by the stimulated pro-suppressor cells exhibits genetic restriction as it can only induce the generation of suppressor cells from pre-suppressor T cells syngeneic to the pro-suppressor cells.

The overtly active or effector suppressor cells secrete a soluble suppressor factor (antigen-specific in the case of an immune response) which, as a consequence of its interaction with the (antigen-specific) helper T cells, is capable of suppressing immunoglobulin and/or antibody synthesis by the B cells. This suppressor factor(s) appears to be different from the suppressor cell activating factor in that it does not exhibit any obvious genetic restriction as it can induce suppression of B cells allogeneic to the suppressor T cells which synthesized the suppressor factor.

The reader will undoubtedly conclude, after reading the foregoing discussion, that the regulatory mechanism for antibody and immunoglobulin synthesis is very complex and ill-understood, involving a number of T cell subsets and several distinct soluble factors. Whether the predominant role in the induction of immunosuppression should be attributed to strictly cell-cell interaction or to soluble suppressor factors, or to both, remains to be determined. The precise composition of the soluble factors, and the mechanism of action of these suppressor factors and the suppressor cells, must be precisely defined before attempts at eliminating, inhibiting or enhancing these immunosuppressive agents can be rationally contemplated in order to re-establish the normal immunocompetent state.

Suppressor Cells and Immunodeficiency and Autoimmune Diseases

Suppressor cells are intimately involved in the etiology and pathogenesis of immunodeficiency and autoimmune disease. Should there be a deficiency of the "nonspecific" polyclonal T_M helper cells in the normal unimmunized individual, or should these cells be rather sluggish in attaining a responsive state, then the Type I suppressor cell activity will be dominant. The result is hypo- or agammaglobulinemia (panaimmunoglobulinemia) (Table 8.4). Should "antigen-specific" T_M helper cells be deficient or defective, the patient will present clinically with an immunodeficiency disease, either generalized to include all antigens (due to the absence of all clones of "antigen-specific" helper cells) or specific to a single antigen (due to the absence of a single clone of "antigen-specific" helper cells or clonal deletion). On the other hand, the immunodeficiency disease may be attributed to hyperresponsive T_G Type II suppressor cells in spite of normal numbers of "antigen-specific" T_M helper cells (Table 8.4). In these circumstances, the patient will present clinically with immunodeficiency disease in spite of essentially normal levels of "nonspecific" immunoglobulins.

It is also proposed that the antibody-mediated autoimmune diseases result as a consequence of deficiencies of or defects in both the Type I suppressor cells which inhibit the synthesis of "normal" immunoglobulins and the Type II suppressor cells which inhibit the synthesis of antibody immunoglobulins, in this case autoantibodies to autoantigens (Table 8.4). Under these circumstances, not only can autoantibodies by synthesized, but their synthesis will not be inhibited or shut off, allowing the autoimmune disease to progress in the absence of feedback-inhibition.

The scheme presented in Figure 8.2 and Table 8.4 is supported by clinical findings in patients afflicted with immunodeficiency and autoimmune diseases. As is discussed in Chapter 10, at least some forms of immunodeficiency diseases appear to be characterized by the presence of excessive numbers of suppressor cells capable of inhibiting antibody and immunoglobulin synthesis by otherwise normal B cells. On the other hand, there appears to be a deficiency of suppressor cells in patients with autoimmune diseases, a situation which permits an immune response by the host toward (selective?) autoantigens (see Chapter 12). For example, it has recently been demonstrated that patients with active systemic lupus erythematosus (SLE) possess very few or no circulating suppressor T cells, thus permitting their B cells to synthesize autoantibodies continuously. This is the result of lysis of T suppressor cells by antibodies present in the sera of these individuals. A similar situation has been found to exist in patients afflicted with rheumatoid arthritis. The immunologic defect in these patients is restricted to the suppressor T cell compartment since circulating T cells of normal individuals, but not T cells of patients with SLE or rheumatoid arthritis, are able to suppress autoantibody synthesis by B cells of these patients. Furthermore, the T cells of patients with SLE or rheumatoid arthritis are unable to limit immunoglobulin synthesis by normal allogeneic B cells.

Obviously, a delicate balance must be achieved and maintained in the normal individual between the different immunocompetent and immunosuppressor T cell populations to ensure that the immune response to the stimulus will be of benefit to the host.

Suppressor Cells and the Cell-mediated Immune Response

Although there is no question but that antigen-specific suppression of the cell-mediated response can be induced, the mechanism whereby this state is achieved is not well understood. Chase and Sulzberger, in the late 1940s, demonstrated in the guinea pig that ingestion of the sensitizing antigen could successfully prevent any subsequent induction of a cell-mediated immune response to this antigen by conventional means. However, the mechanism whereby the immune response is suppressed by ingested antigen is still not understood. It is possible that suppressor cells are activated by this unusual exposure to the antigen, but this has not yet been proven. Certainly, suppressor cells can be detected in animals sensitized with contactants such as oxazolone, trinitrophenyl (TNP), and dinitrochlorobenzene (DNCB). Results of recent investigations have shed some light on the mechanism of suppression of a cell-mediated immune response by suppressor cells. As was discussed in Chapter 6,

Table 8.4
Helper and Suppressor Cells in the Induction of Immunodeficiency and Autoimmune Disease*

Absence of or Defect in				Increase in Number or Hyperactivity in				
Ag-specific T_H	Non-Ag-specific T_H	Ag-specific T_S (Type II T_S)	Non-Ag-specific T_S (Type I T_S)	Ag-specific T_H	Non-Ag-specific T_H	Ag-specific T_S (Type II T_S)	Non-Ag-specific T_S (Type I T_S)	Clinical Syndrome
No	No	No	No	No	No	No	No	Homeostasis (no disease state)
No	Yes	No	No	No	No	No	No	Hypo- or agammaglobulinemia
No	No	No	No	No	No	No	Yes	Hypo- or agammaglobulinemia
								Postsurgery or postinjury immunodeficiency
No	No	No	No	No	Yes	No	No	"Essential" hypergammaglobulinemia
No	No	No	Yes	No	No	No	No	"Essential" hypergammaglobulinemia
								Panautoimmune disease
Yes	No	No	No	No	No	No	No	Ag-specific immunodeficiency
								Normal gamma globulins
No	No	No	No	Yes	No	No	No	Ag (or organ)-specific autoimmune disease

No	No	Yes	No	No	No	No	No	Ag (or organ)-specific autoimmune disease
No	No	No	No	No	No	Yes	No	Ag-specific immunodeficiency Normal gamma globulins
No	No	No	No	Yes	No	No	Yes	Hypo- or agammaglobulinemia and Ag-specific autoimmune disease

* Ag = Antigen
T_H = helper T cell (T_M)
T_S = suppressor T cell (T_G)

sensitized cells, following interaction with the sensitizing antigen, secrete a large number of mediators referred to collectively as lymphokines. It is generally accepted that the lymphokines function to attract, trap, and prevent the emigration of cells from the challenge site, thus initiating the sequence of events which culminates in a reaction which exhibits the morphologic features characteristic of the delayed skin reaction.

One of the lymphokines is mononuclear cell migration inhibitory factor (MIF). This lymphokine supposedly initiates the train of events which leads to the characteristic mononuclear cell infiltrate following intradermal challenge with the antigen by preventing emigration of mononuclear cells, especially monocytes, which accidentally or by chemotaxis infiltrate the challenge site "just to have a look at what is going on." However, these cells are impeded from departing the challenge site by the MIF secreted by the few sensitized cells, and these cells become active participants in the production of the cell-mediated delayed skin reaction. Recent investigations have disclosed that a factor which acts antagonistically to MIF is secreted by suppressor cells and their precursors. This factor is termed migration stimulation factor (MSF). Thus, if suppressor cells are activated either before or concurrent with sensitized cells, the MSF which they release upon exposure to and interaction with the antigen will interfere or totally negate the effects of MIF liberated from the sensitized cells. Thus, the infiltration of mononuclear cells into the challenge skin site would not take place, and the pathologic lesion characteristic of the delayed skin reaction would not be evident.

It is unlikely that MSF provides the basis for our total understanding of the mechanism of suppressor cell inhibition of the cell-mediated immune reaction. However, it provides a beacon for continued active investigations which will undoubtedly result in the demonstration of more mediators released from suppressor cells capable of abrogating the cell-mediated immune response.

Suppressor Cells and the Anergic State following Trauma, Severe Burns, and/or Surgery

Suppressor cells are also emerging as an important factor in the consideration of the mechanism of the anergic state which characterizes patients following trauma, severe burns, and surgery. This general anergic state is blamed for the life-threatening episodes of sepsis which occur and recur in such patients during the initial period of recovery and convalescence. In fact, septicemia is the major cause of morbidity and death following severe thermal injury. Such affected individuals have been shown to possess hyperactive and/or excessive numbers of suppressor cells in the circulation. The suppressor cells are of the Type I variety in that they do not require prior stimulation to inhibit total immunoglobulin synthesis by normal B cells in vitro. They also have the ability to inhibit the normal T cell blastogenic response. Thus, polyclonally active suppressor cells for both the humoral and cell-mediated immune responses characterize these patients. Although it is neither feasible nor appropriate to screen all trauma, burn, and surgical patients for excessive circulating suppressor cell activity, those patients who have infectious complications and are unable to contain their infections should be investigated for excessive generalized suppressor cell activity. These patients will often give a history of a generally decreased resistance to infections. They should be treated very aggressively with antibiotic chemotherapy and the appropriate fluids.

The identity of the suppressor cells in these patients has not been unequivocally established. Evidence has been presented favoring both T_G cells and monocytes as the suppressor cells. As discussed previously, the distinction between the T_G suppressor cells and monocyte suppressor cells may be illusory in view of their probable ontogenic relationship.

Can an explanation be offered to account for the presence of activated Type I T_G suppressor cells in the circulation of patients following extensive trauma, severe burns, or surgery? As was discussed previously, Type I suppressor cells require interaction with immune complexes or gamma globulin aggregates to become activated. It is possible that there is excessive aggregation of immunoglobulins following a traumatic accident, burns, or surgery, with the result that Type I suppressor cells are inappropriately activated. It is possible that this response by the host has a protective function. Undoubtedly, the generalized inflammatory response which is triggered by a traumatic or burn injury is accompanied by the liberation of organ-specific and non-organ-specific autoantigens into the circulation. The presence of autoantigens in the circulation coupled with the inflammatory response is considered to be conducive for the induction of autoantibodies and autoimmune disease (see Chapter 12). Thus, it may be speculated that the activation of Type I T_G suppressor cells in these patients at the time of the injury inhibits any autoimmune response which would otherwise take place to the long-term detriment of the host. The transient phase of relative immunodeficiency may, therefore, have long-term benefit for the host and have great survival value. Nevertheless, since the primary concern of the physician is usually focused on management of the patient during the crisis period, the state of apparent immunodeficiency which often presents in the patient is considered a liability, highly detrimental to the patient's welfare. Therefore, it is not surprising that numerous attempts are being made to prevent the generation of suppressor cells following surgery and, failing that, to correct the imbalance among the T cells and to neutralize or disarm the spontaneously generated suppressor cells.

Vitamin A administered in large doses preoperatively and postoperatively is capable of preventing activation of suppressor cells and of maintaining the circulating immunocompetent cells in a normal state of activity. The mechanism of action of vitamin A in this situation is not known; it may inhibit nonspecific aggregation of the circulating immunoglobulins, thereby preventing activation of the Type I T_G suppressor cells. Immunodeficiency under other circumstances can apparently be corrected and immunocompetence reestablished following administration of naturally occurring nutrients such as the trace metals (i.e. zinc) and essential fatty acids which may be deficient in these patients (see Chapter 13). It may, therefore, be anticipated that systematic investigations involving the administration of vitamins, fatty acids, and/or trace metals pre- and postoperatively and as soon as possible following trauma or extensive burns will establish their efficacy in the maintenance of the immunologic status quo which characterizes the normal state.

Suppressor Cells and Malignant Disease

If the immune system plays a role in the control, eradication, or suppression of malignant disease, it is necessary to postulate that a humoral and/or cell-mediated immune response is initiated in response to specific antigens characteristic of the cancer cell (see Chapter 16). Suppressor cells would be activated only later, thus allowing sufficient time for the immune system to eliminate the malignant (or mutant or potentially neoplastic) cells. The failure of the immune system to eliminate or control a malignant growth may be a reflection of (a) rapidly activated suppressor cells, (b) the emergence of inappropriately large numbers of suppressor cells, or (c) a sluggish or delayed immune response to the cancer-specific antigens, possibly attributable to their poor antigenicity, which is prematurely terminated by activated suppressor cells.

For whatever reason that suppressor cells are activated to the detriment of the host, present investigations suggest that it may be possible to preferentially eliminate suppressor cells without affecting the immunocompetent cells, thus permitting the latter to exercise their role in the eradication of the malignancy. It has been shown that suppressor cells can be preferentially eliminated by exposure of the host to low doses of irradiation and/or cyclophosphamide. These initial findings will surely encourage large-scale investigation and application of these findings to the benefit of the patient.

It is necessary, however, to sound a cautious note in the haste to attribute to suppressor cells all regulatory (or negative feedback) functions insofar as the spontaneous emergence of autoimmune disease or malignant disease is concerned. In attributing etiologic and pathogenetic roles in the induction of specific diseases to suppressor cells, a fundamental and implicit assumption is that these cells are clonally selected, or generalized disease would be the rule. In other words, only those suppressor cells directed toward designated organ-specific antigens should be affected. The imbalance between these specific suppressor cells and the normal immunocompetent B or T cells which they regulate, due to either the absence of or a defect in the function of the suppressor cells, results in the "spontaneous" emergence of a specific autoimmune disease. The presence of excessive numbers of suppressor cells may inhibit the immune response to newly emerging mutant cells, resulting in the development of overt malignant disease. These suppressor cells or their immediate precursors must be monoclonally selected or unipotent and not polyclonally selected or pluripotent, otherwise it would be very difficult to entertain the emergence of a specific autoimmune disease due to the immune response to a single organ-specific antigen (i.e. thyroglobulin or intrinsic factor) in the absence of generalized autoimmune disease, or a specific malignant disease. It has so far not been demonstrated whether suppressor cells detected in patients with autoimmune and malignant diseases are pluripotent or unipotent. This fundamental issue must be resolved, one way or the other, before suppressor cells can be taken seriously as participants in the induction of disease.

CHAPTER 9

The Classification and Immunologic Functions of the Circulating Lymphocytes, Monocytes, and Neutrophils

THE HETEROGENEITY OF LYMPHOCYTES, MONOCYTES, AND NEUTROPHILS

Until the 1960s, the circulating leukocytes were classified primarily on the basis of morphologic characteristics following staining and examination by light microscopy, and secondarily on the basis of the ability of the cells to phagocytose iron or carbon particles. Thus, the leukocytes were classified by morphologic criteria as mononuclear and polymorphonuclear cells. The former include lymphocytes (small, medium, and large) and monocytes, and the latter include the neutrophils, eosinophils, and basophils. The primary phagocytic cells are the monocytes and the neurtrophils.

By the mid-1960s, a third criterion, that of specific cell surface structures which are antigenic in the xenogeneic animal (and are incorrectly referred to as cell surface antigens since they are not antigenic in the human), was applied in the further characterization of the circulating lymphocytes. It was demonstrated that a relatively large percentage of the circulating lymphocytes (55 ± 10%) possess surface structures characteristic of thymus (T) cells, and a lesser percentage (15 ± 5%) exhibit surface structures and surface membrane immunoglobulins (SmIg) characteristic of bone marrow (B) lymphoid cells. These circulating lymphocytes are, therefore, not inappropriately referred to as T and B cells. The circulating lymphocytes which are neither T nor B cells are referred to as null cells. The T and B cells were shown to possess distinct roles in the immune response (see Chapters 5, 6 and 10). Conventional wisdom dictated the acceptance of functionally distinct circulating lymphocytes and, therefore, the heterogeneous nature of these cells. Nevertheless, even as recently as the late 1960s, the circulating monocytes and neutrophils were still considered to be essentially homogeneous populations of cells.

By the early 1970s, a fourth criterion was utilyzed to categorize the leukocytes. Normal circulating cells were shown to be able to lyse target cells in the (a) antibody-dependent cell-mediated cytotoxic (or ADCC) reaction; the effector cell is referred to as the killer (or K) cell; (b) the antibody-independent cell-mediated cytotoxic (or AICC) reaction or the naturally occurring cell-mediated cytotoxic (or NOCC) reaction; the effector cell is referred to as the natural killer (or NK) cell; and (c) the mitogen-induced cell-mediated cytotoxic (or MICC) reaction. Depending on the target cells selected in the different assays, normal lymphocytes and/or monocytes and/or neutrophils can be shown to possess cytotoxic activity. However, these assays do not distinguish between cells within each class of leukocytes.

The demonstration of specific receptors on the surface membranes of the freshly isolated circulating lymphocytes in the early 1970s finally laid to rest the battered but still adhered to concept of lymphocyte, monocyte, and neutrophil homogeneity. The circulating lymphocytes can be characterized and fractionated on the basis of surface receptors for (a) a structure on the sheep erythrocyte (SRBC), (b) the Fc of the IgG molecule [Fc(IgG) or FcG], and (c) the C′3 component of complement (Fig. 9.1, Table 9.1). Cells with each of these receptors can be separated from each other on the basis of their ability to form rosettes with SRBC (or E), IgG antibody-sensitized ox erythrocytes (or EA), and C′3-IgM antibody-sensitized ox erythrocytes (or EAC) (please review discussion of rosette-forming cells, Chapter 7). Only the T lymphocytes form rosettes with E (E rosettes). The B lymphocytes form the majority of rosettes with EAC (EAC rosettes), and the null lymphocytes (the non-T, non-B cells) form the majority of the rosettes with EA (EA rosettes) (Fig. 9.1). It was originally postulated that a cell could possess only one of these unique markers. Although initial evidence favored this assumption, it has more recently been recognized that some lymphocytes may carry two or even all three of these receptors. It is, therefore, possible to distinguish about 10 distinct lymphoid cell populations on the basis of surface membrane receptors (Fig. 9.1).

Whether the multireceptor-bearing cells are the precursors for the single receptor-bearing cells or whether they constitute the progeny of the single-receptor bearing cells is not known at the present time. It is of more than academic or philosophic importance to determine whether a lymphocyte with receptors for both

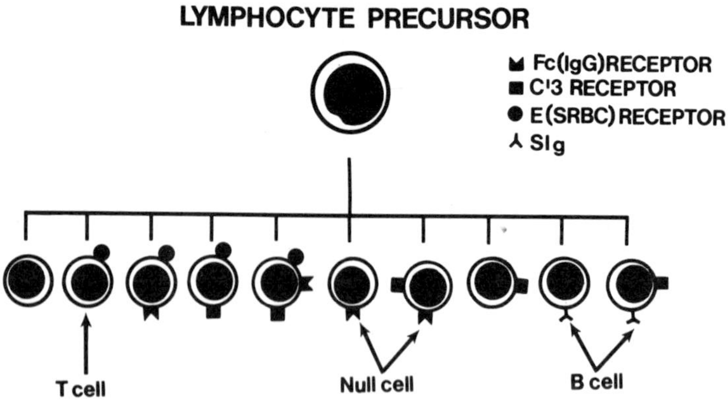

Figure 9.1 *The different classes of freshly isolated human circulating lymphocytes as defined on the basis of cell surface receptors for SRBC or E, Fc(IgG) or EA(G), and C'3 or EAC.*

the SRBC and the Fc of IgG is a T cell which incidentally also possesses a receptor for the Fc of IgG or whether it is an FcG receptor-bearing null cell which incidentally also happens to possess a receptor for the SRBC. In the final analysis, the classification of these cells as T or null cells is a reflection of the prejudice or inclination of the investigator since existing evidence precludes an objective assessment. If the investigator is primarily interested in the isolation and characterization of different T cell populations, then he/she will consider all cells which possess receptors for the SRBC to be T cells and those cells which also carry receptors for FcG and C'3 to be subclasses of T cells. On the other hand, if the investigator is primarily interested in demonstrating the heterogeneity of FcG receptor-bearing null lymphocytes, then he/she will consider all cells with receptors for the FcG to be null cells and those cells which also carry receptors for SRBC and C'3 to constitute subclasses of null cells. Until precise functional criteria can be applied along with receptors toward the identification of lymphoid cell populations, this area of the field will remain poorly defined.

Monocytes have also been shown to be heterogeneous on the basis of cell surface receptors. Four subclasses of monocytes can be isolated on the basis of surface membrane receptors for FcG and C'3 (Fig. 9.2).

Table 9.1
Percentages of the Freshly Isolated Normal Circulating Lymphocytes Exhibiting Surface Membrane Receptors

Cells with Receptors for	Pseudonym for Receptor	Pseudonym for Cells	Percentage of Circulating Lymphocytes
SRBC or E	E receptor	T cells	50–70
Antibody (IgG)-sensitized erythrocytes or EA	Fc (IgG) receptor	Null cells	10–25
Complement-antibody (IgM)-sensitized erythrocytes or EAC	C′3 receptor	B cells	10–30

Equally surprising is the demonstration that neutrophils are also heterogeneous, with the cells possessing either no receptors or receptors for FcG and/or C′3 (Fig. 9.3).

One may, therefore, conclude that the normal circulating lymphocytes, monocytes, and neutrophils are highly heterogeneous classes of cells on the basis of surface membrane receptors, antigens, and immunoglobulins.

As stated previously, the circulating B lymphocytes are defined by convention as cells with surface membrane immunoglobulins (SmIg), primarily IgM, IgD, and IgG. It is considered coincidental that these cells also possess the receptor for C′3 which allows them to rosette with the EAC indicator cells. However, the reader is cautioned that the reverse is not true. Although the majority of the EAC rosetting cells are B cells, a not insignificant proportion of the EAC rosetting cells is composed of T cells and null cells which also bear the receptor for C′3. T cells also display certain surface configurations in addition to the characteristic receptor for SRBC. Thus "activated" T cells, i.e. cytotoxic T cells generated in the MLR and T cells which undergo blastogenesis in response to specific antigen stimulation, bear the Ia antigen on the surface. The Ia antigen(s) is antigenic only in the xenogeneic animal, not in the isologous or syngeneic host and, therefore, should be referred to as a surface configuration or structure and not an antigen. The Ia antigens are the protein expressions of the immune response or Ir genes which appear to be part of the major histocompatibility complex (MHC) which codes for transplantation antigens (the HLA antigens) as well as for the fundamental capacity to respond to particular exogenous antigens. Ia

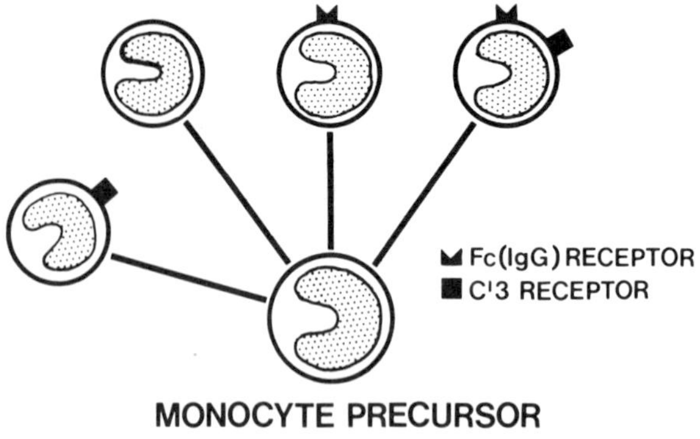

Figure 9.2 *The different classes of freshly isolated human circulating monocytes as defined on the basis of cell surface receptors for Fc(IgG) or EA (G), and C′3 or EAC.*

antigens were originally considered to be restricted to cells which participate directly in the humoral immune response, i.e. B cells and macrophages. However, they have now been demonstrated as well on activated T cells which participate in the humoral and cell-mediated immune responses but not on immunologically unresponsive T cells nor on the circulating T cells in the normal unimmunized individual. Although it has been suggested that one function for the Ia antigen(s) is to facilitate cell-cell interaction and cooperation in the immune response, definitive evidence in support of such a role is still being awaited. It has, however, been demonstrated in animals that T cell activation in vitro, i.e. blastogenesis in response to antigen stimulation, can only occur in the presence of histocompatible Ia antigen-bearing macrophages. Presumably, the Ia antigen on the macrophage facilitates the macrophage-T cell interaction in the T cell blastogenic response to antigen stimulation.

Do the receptors impart a functional role to the cells? The FcG and C′3 receptors certainly appear to do so. The FcG receptor-bearing lymphocytes, monocytes, and neutrophils are capable of mediating cytolysis of target cells sensitized with even modest numbers of specific IgG antibody molecules in the ADCC reaction (see Chapter 7). This is a specific cytolytic reaction, as the target cells are not affected if they are passively coated with normal nonimmune IgG immunoglobulins. It is now accepted that the ADCC reaction constitutes the basis for the opsonization reaction (or the antibody-enhanced phagocytic reaction), as originally described by Sir Almroth Wright in 1904 (see Chapter 2).

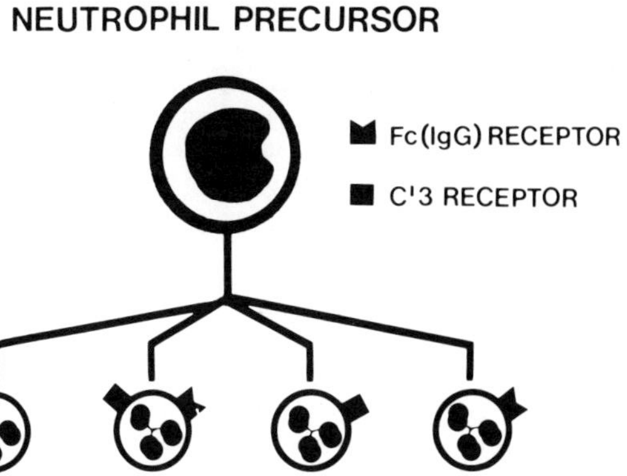

Figure 9.3 *The different classes of freshly isolated human circulating neutrophils as defined on the basis of cell surface receptors for Fc(IgG) or EA(G),* and *C′3 or EAC.*

If the antibody-sensitized target is a bacterium or a virus particle, it will be more quickly eliminated by the ADCC mechanism then via the "normal" nonimmune phagocytic route. The receptors for C′3 on monocytes and neutrophils also unquestionably enhance the phagocytic activity of these cells. Thus, immune complexes which are capable of fixing complement will be phagocytosed by the C′3 and FcG receptor-bearing lymphocytes, monocytes, and neutrophils. Therefore, the receptors for FcG and C′3 impart survival value to the species, and they should be considered to be the result of evolutionary development and not a haphazard occurrence.

Important

Up to the present time, only the FcG receptor-bearing circulating null lymphocytes, and not the SRBC receptor-bearing T lymphocytes and C′3 receptor-bearing B lymphocytes, have been shown to be capable of lysing the appropriate indicator erythrocytes. Thus, the freshly isolated null cells can lyse the EA indicator cells, but the freshly isolated T and B cells cannot lyse the SRBC and EAC indicator cells. From a phylogenetic point of view, it may be that the receptor-bearing lymphocytes have not evolved or been selected by evolution to be naturally cytotoxic. The FcG receptor-bearing lymphocytes may be the evolutionary progeny of a subclass of lymphocytes which are capable of lysing suitably sensitized targets. Thus, in addition to antibody formation and cell-mediated immunity as specific protective mechanisms to invasive pathogens, nature also provides a subclass of lymphocytes

Table 9.2
Immunologic Functions of T Cells

1. **Helper cells** in the humoral immune response
2. **Helper cells** in the cell-mediated immune response
3. **Responder cells** in the cell-mediated immune response
   a. Cells which respond with blastogenesis and mitosis in the MLR reaction in vitro
   b. Cells which respond with blastogenesis and mitosis in the presence of the specific immunizing antigen in vitro
4. **Cytotoxic cells** in the cell-mediated immune response
   a. Specific cytotoxic cells induced in the MLR reaction in vitro
   b. Nonspecific cytotoxic cells generated within cultured T cells (24 hours at 37°C) (ADCC, NOCC, and MICC cytotoxic cells)
5. **Memory cells** in the cell-mediated immune response
6. **Sensitized cells** in the cell-mediated immune response
   a. Specific sensitized cells which characterize the delayed (hypersensitivity) skin reaction
   b. Specific sensitized cells which characterize the infiltrating cells in a rejected allograft
7. **Effector cells** in the cell-mediated immune response
   These are the cells to which is attributed the capacity to reject the allograft.
8. **Suppressor cells** in the humoral immune response
9. **Suppressor cells** in the cell-mediated immune response

capable of lysing antibody-sensitized targets should the antibodies themselves be insufficient to eliminate the offensive target (pathogen) (see Chapter 7).

THE HETEROGENEOUS NATURE OF THE T LYMPHOCYTES

By the mid-1970s, it had been amply verified that the SRBC receptor-bearing T cells actively initiate and participate in the different forms of cell-mediated immunity, provide helper cells for the humoral immune response, and provide suppressor cells with respect to both the humoral and cell-mediated immune responses (Table 9.2). It is evident from Table 9.2 that T cell participation in the antibody response appears to involve a singular form of activity, that of the antigen-specific ARC helper cell, whereas a large number of different types of activities characterize T cell participation in the cell-mediated immune response. Thus, with respect to the cell-mediated immune response, T cells provide:

1. The antigen-specific helper cells in the induction of the cell-mediated immune responses
2. The cells which undergo blastogenesis and mitosis and the

cells which are transformed to cytotoxic cells in the mixed leukocyte reaction (MLR)

3. The cells which undergo blastogenesis and mitosis upon exposure to the specific sensitizing antigen in vitro

4. The sensitized cells which characterize the mononuclear cell infiltrate in the delayed (hypersensitivity) skin reaction and in the various organs with ongoing cell-mediated immune reactions (i.e. the lungs in tuberculosis)

5. The effector cells which interact with and kill allogeneic cells in an allograft implant

6. The memory cells which permit for a rapid anamnestic response following a second exposure to the antigen

It may be that the helper cells are identical to the cells which undergo blastogenesis in response to stimulation with allogeneic cells in the MLR or soluble antigens in vitro. It is also possible, if not probable, that the cytotoxic cells induced in the MLR reaction in vitro are the identical counterparts of the effector cells assigned the role of killing the allografted cells in a transplanted tissue or organ. It is not known whether the memory cells are the progeny or transformed products of the cells which participate in this immune response or whether they constitute a new series of cells. It is unlikely that the induction, maintenance, cessation, and reinitiation of the cell-mediated immune response can be the functions of a single subclass of T cells; rather, different subclasses of T cells express the different roles in the cell-mediated immune response.

The investigations initiated by Moretta and his associates in 1975 and extended by Richter in 1980 utilizing specific surface membrane receptors as cell markers provided evidence for the heterogeneity of the normal circulating T lymphocytes. Freshly isolated T cells were shown to consist of cells with receptors for FcG (T_G cells) and C′3 (T_C cells). Incubated (24 hours) T cells exhibit, additionally, large numbers of T cells with receptors for the Fc of IgM or FcM (T_M cells) and increased numbers of cells with receptors for C′3 (T_C cells) (Table 9.3). In addition to the T cells bearing single receptors for FcG, FcM, or C′3 (the T_G, T_M, and T_C cells, respectively), a significant proportion of the incubated T cells are multireceptor cells which bear surface membrane receptors for FcM and C′3 (T_{M+C} cells). A small percentage of the T cells bear receptors for both FcG and C’3 (T_{G+C} cells). The remaining T cells do not bear detectable surface receptors for FcG, FcM, and C′3 and are designated as T null cells or T_N.

As discussed previously, the capacity to facilitate and suppress the humoral and cell-mediated immune responses is a property

Table 9.3
Classification of the Normally Circulating T Cells

Cells*	Percentage of Circulating T Cells	Function
T_G cells (= T_H cells?)	5–15	ADCC cytotoxic cells† MICC cytotoxic cells† NOCC cytotoxic cells† Suppressor cells
T_M cells	10–20	Helper cells
T_C cells	10–20	?
T_{M+C} cells	15–25	?
T_{G+C} cells	Very few	?
T_N cells	40–50	?

* T_G cells are cells with receptors for Fc(IgG). T_H cells are cells with receptors for histamine. T_M cells are cells with receptors for Fc(IgM). T_C cells are cells with receptors for C′3. T_{M+C} cells are cells with receptors for both Fc(IgM) and C′3. T_{G+C} cells are cells with receptors for both Fc(IgG) and C′3. T_N cells are cells with no detectable receptors.
† These activities of the T_G cells are markedly enhanced after the cells are incubated at 37°C for 24 hours.

of the T cells. The facilitating or helper cells were shown by Moretta to possess receptors for FcM, and they constitute a subclass of the T_M cells. The suppressor cells (see Chapter 8) were shown by Moretta to possess receptors for FcG, and they constitute a subclass of the T_G cells. More recently, suppressor T cells have also been shown to possess receptors for histamine, and these cells have been designated as T_H cells. The T_G cells may, therefore, be considered to embrace suppressor and nonsuppressor populations of T cells, with a proportion or all of the suppressor T cells bearing receptors for histamine. Thus, the circulating T cells consist of at least seven distinct populations of cells (Fig. 9.4).

Do the cells of one subclass of T cells constitute the precursors of the cells of another subclass of T cells? It is tempting to speculate that the T_N cells constitute the precursors for the cells in all the other subclasses of T cells, but there is no evidence in favor of this assumption. Furthermore, it must be borne in mind that the classification of T cells described above is based upon analyses of T cells under essentially static in vitro conditions. In point of fact, cells of one subclass of T cells do transform into cells of another subclass of T cells in tissue culture, or they at least synthesize and/or express receptors characteristic of cells of

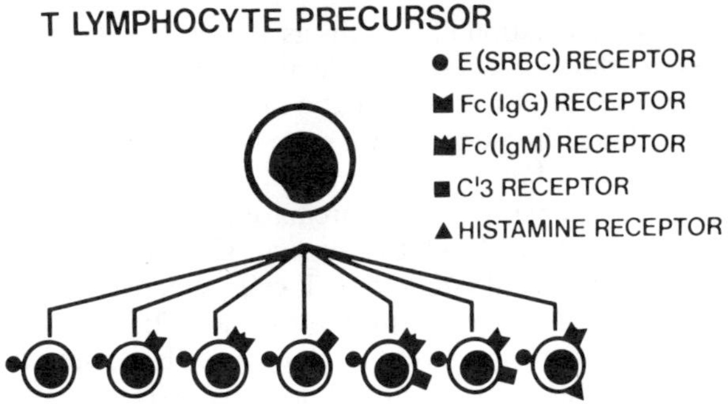

Figure 9.4 *The different populations of human circulating T lymphocytes as defined on the basis of cell surface receptors detected on the freshly isolated, 24-hour-incubated T cells.*

another subclass of T cells. Thus, T_G cells synthesize or express receptors for FcM and C′3, T_M cells synthesize or express receptors for FcG and C′3, and T_C cells synthesize or express receptors for FcG and FcM. The freshly isolated circulating T cells display minimal ADCC, NK, and MICC cytotoxic activity; however, the cytotoxic activity increases markedly following overnight incubation at 37°C (Table 9.3), and it appears to be primarily the property of the relatively few T_G cells, and to a lesser extent of the T_{G+C} cells, in the circulation. The T_M and T_{M+C} cells do not exhibit significant cytotoxic activity. These activities of the incubated T cells were first reported by Richter in 1981. Of course, one can always criticize findings obtained under the highly unphysiologic conditions which pertain in tissue culture in vitro and consider that they may be totally artifactual. Nevertheless, results obtained in tissue culture strongly suggest that the circulating single receptor-bearing noncytotoxic T cells (the T_G, T_M, and T_C cells) represent T cells in transition and that these monoreceptor T cells emigrate from the circulation as they generate additional receptors and attain cytotoxic activity. One may, therefore, speculate that the infiltrating T cells (the thymus-derived cells in the peripheral lymphoid organs) constitute the in vivo counterparts of the in vitro incubated T cells.

It is interesting to note that many of the T_G cells isolated by rosetting with EA(G) stain for nonspecific esterase, a property considered to be characteristic for monocytes, suggesting that the T_G cells have evolved from monocytes and that these cells should be classified as monocytoid T lymphocytes. However, evidence has been presented recently which places serious doubt on the validity of the designation of T_G cells as T cells. Reinherz and his colleagues in 1980 succeeded in producing monoclonal antibodies toward a number of distinct T cell and monocyte surface constituents using cloned immune mouse spleen—mouse myeloma hybridoma cells. Antibodies were pro[illegible] toward three unique cell surface components on the circulating T cells which were designated as the T_3, T_4, and T_5 antigens. The T_3 antigen can be detected on virtually all circulating T cells, whereas the T_4 and T_5 antigens can be detected on 60 to 65% and 25 to 35% of the circulating T cells, respectively. Helper T cells possess the T_4 antigen, and the suppressor (and cytotoxic) T cells possess the T_5 antigen. However, this classification by Reinherz of T cells into T_4 helper and T_5 suppressor cells does not correlate with the Moretta classification of the T cells into T_M helper and T_G suppressor cells based on cell surface receptors for FcM and FcG, respectively. Although both isolation techniques yield two populations of functionally identical helper and suppressor cells, the identities of the cells are different depending upon the criteria (cell surface antigens or receptors) utilized for their isolation. The T cells designated T_M helper cells by Moretta on the basis of surface membrane receptors for FcM cannot be distinguished from the unfractionated T cells by Reinherz on the basis of their interaction with the anti-T_3, anti-T_4, and anti-T_5 monoclonal antibodies. Furthermore, the T null cells (the T cells depleted of T_G and T_M cells by rosette formation) cannot be distinguished from the unfractionated T cells either on the basis of cell surface T_4 and T_5 antigens. Reinherz has also demonstrated that only a small minority of the cells designated T_G suppressor cells by Moretta on the basis of surface membrane receptors for FcG react with any of the T cell-specific monoclonal antibodies, whereas a majority of the T_G cells react with the monocyte-specific monoclonal antibodies. It would, therefore, appear from the results of Reinherz that the majority of the T_G cells are either unconventional FcG receptor-bearing T cells with monocyte markers or transformed monocytes. However, it is not surprising that a high proportion of the T_G cells isolated by the technique described by Moretta stain as monocytes because monocytes are, in fact, carried down nonspecifically with the T_G-EA(G) rosettes during the isolation of the T_G cells. If the monocytes are eliminated from the mononuclear cells prior to the isolation of the T_G cells by rosetting with EA(G), then a much smaller number of T_G cells are recovered as compared to the isolation procedure of Moretta, and the majority of these cells would presumably be T_G cells. To further complicate matters, it has not yet been demon-

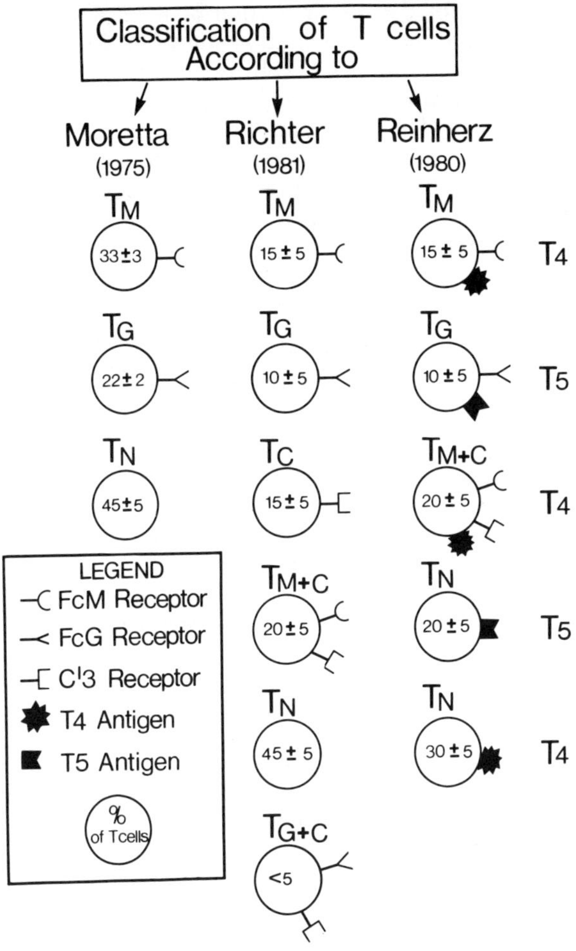

Figure 9.5 *Classification of the circulating T cells on the basis of receptors (Moretta, Richter) and surface membrane antigens (Reinherz).*

strated (at the time of submission of this chapter to the publishers) whether the T_5 cells isolated from T_G-depleted T cells and the T_4 cells isolated from T_G- and T_M-depleted T (null) cells display suppressor and helper activity, respectively, in any of the conventional assays, as has been intimated and implied but not proven by Reinherz. If the classification of T cells using monoclonal antibodies to T cells is to attain credibility and be accepted as the method of choice for the discrimination between and the demonstration and isolation of helper and suppressor T cells, it must be resolved whether or not the T_5 cells isolated from T_G-depleted T cells display suppressor cell activity and whether the T_4 cells isolated from T_M-depleted T cells exhibit helper cell activity.

It should be obvious from the foregoing discussion that this area of the discipline is rather muddled at the present time, and the findings are conflicting, controversial, and seemingly irreconcilable. It would seem prudent to await resolution of the various issues which have been addressed above and foolhardy to predict which of the classifications of T cells will survive the test of time. Nevertheless, the author considers it appropriate to present the various classifications of the T cells as they appear in mid-1981 (Fig. 9.5) in view of the universal interest in T cell typing procedures and the clinical relevance of T cells in health and disease. On the basis of existing data, the author considers that (a) the T_4 cells isolated from unfractionated normal mononuclear cells consist of helper (T_M) and nonhelper (T_N) cells, (b) the T_5 cells isolated from unfractionated normal mononuclear cells include suppressor (T_G) and nonsuppressor (T_N) cells, and (c) the T_N cells which carry the T_4 and T_5 antigenic markers constitute the precursors of the helper and suppressor cells, respectively (Fig. 9.5).

The concept of the homogeneity of the circulating lymphocytes, which appeared sancrosanct up to the 1960s, has been totally rejected and disbanded as a result of the demonstration of (a) functionally distinct T and B lymphocytes in the mid-1960s, (b) different lymphocytes bearing receptors for Fc(G), Fc(M), C′, and sheep erythrocytes in the early 1970s, and (c) unique surface antigens on different T lymphocytes utilizing monoclonal antibodies in the early 1980s. We can most assuredly anticipate the discovery of new receptors, antigenic cell surface configurations, and functions in the 1980s which will result in the demonstration of even greater diversity among these lymphoid cell populations.

CHAPTER 10

Immunodeficiency Diseases

The history of immunodeficiency disease dates back to the classical immunologic investigations of Waksman and Good in the United States, Taylor in England, and Miller and Nossal in Australia during the period of 1960 to 1970. Their investigations were concerned with unraveling the role of the then lightly regarded thymus in the immune response. Their findings attained unanticipated prominence in the light of the finding of Claman, Chaperon, and Triplett in 1966 of a synergism or cooperation required of a T cell and a B cell to effect an antibody response. This finding was momentous, as it constituted the very first proof for the requirement and active participation of at least two functionally distinct lymphoid cells in the immune response (see Chapter 5).

Another major finding which set the stage for the discovery of immunodeficiency disease was the demonstration by Glick of an immunologic role for the bursa of Fabricius in the bird. As discussed at length in Chapter 5, the findings can be summarized as follows:

1. Extirpation of the thymus in the neonatal mouse, rat, or rabbit leads to a moderate to marked impairment of the capacity to mount a cell-mediated immune response and a definite disturbance in the antibody synthetic mechanism.

2. Extirpation of the bursa of Fabricius in the neonatal chicken results in a marked impairment of the antibody response without a concomitant deleterious effect on the cell-mediated immune response. Although mammals do not possess a distinct organ like the bursa of Fabricius, it has been suggested that the gut-associated lymphoid tissues, especially the appendix and/or Peyer's patches, constitute the mammalian equivalent of the avian bursa and that they provide the precursors of the B cells which eventually inhabit the bone marrow.

Within several years following the experimental work on the thymus and bursa of Fabricius, it became apparent to a number of immunologically oriented physicians that clinical states similar to the immunodeficient state induced in the thymectomized chicken, rat, or rabbit and the bursectomized chicken occur spontaneously in humans.

Immunodeficiency disease must be contrasted with the laboratory-defined immunodeficiency state diagnosed on the basis of in vitro criteria. A diagnosis of immunodeficiency may be indicated on the basis of results of a number of immunologic tests which define the immune state. Thus, the absence of a mitogen or MLR-induced blastogenic response, the absence of normal levels of rosette-forming cells, and the failure to give ADCC and NOCC reactions all indicate a potential or actual immunodeficiency state. The failure to detect immunoglobulins in general and/or specific antibodies in the circulation points to a humoral immunodeficiency syndrome. The presence of low levels of circulating lymphocytes, the absence of a thymic shadow in an anteroposterior film or tomogram, the absence of lymphoid tissues in Waldeyer's ring (tonsils, adenoids), and the failure to give a delayed hypersensitivity skin reaction following appropriate sensitization all point to a defect in cellular immunity. However, it should be stressed that the major criterion defining immunodeficiency disease is the clinical condition of the patient—if he/she is consistently well, then he/she does not suffer from immunodeficiency disease even if the laboratory data indicate a most definitive diagnosis of immunodeficiency.

It is important to stress that an individual with a condition diagnosed as immunodeficiency disease is one who lacks the capacity to respond with an immune response and/or one in whom the beneficial manifestations of the immune reaction cannot be properly expressed or are ineffective. The reader should recall that antibodies by themselves are not cytotoxic but require the assistance of complement. Sensitized cells may be incapable of synthesizing one or more of the lymphokines. Furthermore, certain microorganisms are eliminated primarily via their phagocytosis by macrophages. The following defects in one or more of the cellular and humoral components of the immune system will be reflected as immunodeficiency diseases in the patients so affected:

1. Diminished or absent neutrophil and monocyte or macrophage phagocytic and/or chemotactic activity
2. Diminished or absent complement (C′1 to C′9) hemolytic activity
3. Failure of precursors of immunocompetent B cells to generate committed unipotent antibody-forming cells (humoral immunity)
4. Failure of precursors of immunocompetent T cells to generate sensitized cells with the capacity to synthesize the necessary

lymphokines (cell-mediated immunity)

5. The absence or sharply diminished concentration of certain intracellular enzymes, such as adenosine deaminase (humoral and cell-mediated immunity)

6. An imbalance of suppressor and immunoresponsive (and/or potentiating and/or enhancing and/or augmenting) cells in favor of suppressor cells

7. The absence of certain clones of cells programmed to interact with a particular antigen or set of antigens via surface receptors; such a situation will be revealed by the inability of the individual so affected to respond to a particular pathogen while his resistance to other pathogenic microorganisms remains essentially intact (clonal deletion).

Numerous new syndromes have been described and proposed in rapid succession over the past 10 years, but the hoped-for orderly advancement of knowledge in this field has not taken place. Instead, we have been witness to an explosion in the number of syndromes with the majority bearing the names of the investigators credited with their description. Investigators have in general succumbed to the temptation to designate syndromes as distinct entities in spite of the fact that the different syndromes are distinguished on the basis of only subtle, often ill-understood differences in the presenting symptomatology and even less well-defined defects in the immune system. This situation is aggravated by the absence of appropriate methods for the detection and evaluation of these defects. The situation today regarding the classification of the different immunodeficiency diseases can at best be charitably described as confusing and at worst as chaotic.

Since the field is still evolving and distinctions between the more recently classified syndromes are becoming blurred, the following discussion will deal only with those syndromes which are well-defined and have withstood the test of time.

The normal ontogenic development of the immune system and the major defects which may arise and present as immunodeficiency diseases are presented in Figure 10.1 and described in Table 10.1.

CLASSIFICATION OF IMMUNODEFICIENCY DISEASES

Primary

1. Congenital
   A. Bruton syndrome or sex-linked hypogammaglobulinemia
   B. Di George syndrome or thymic hypoplasia

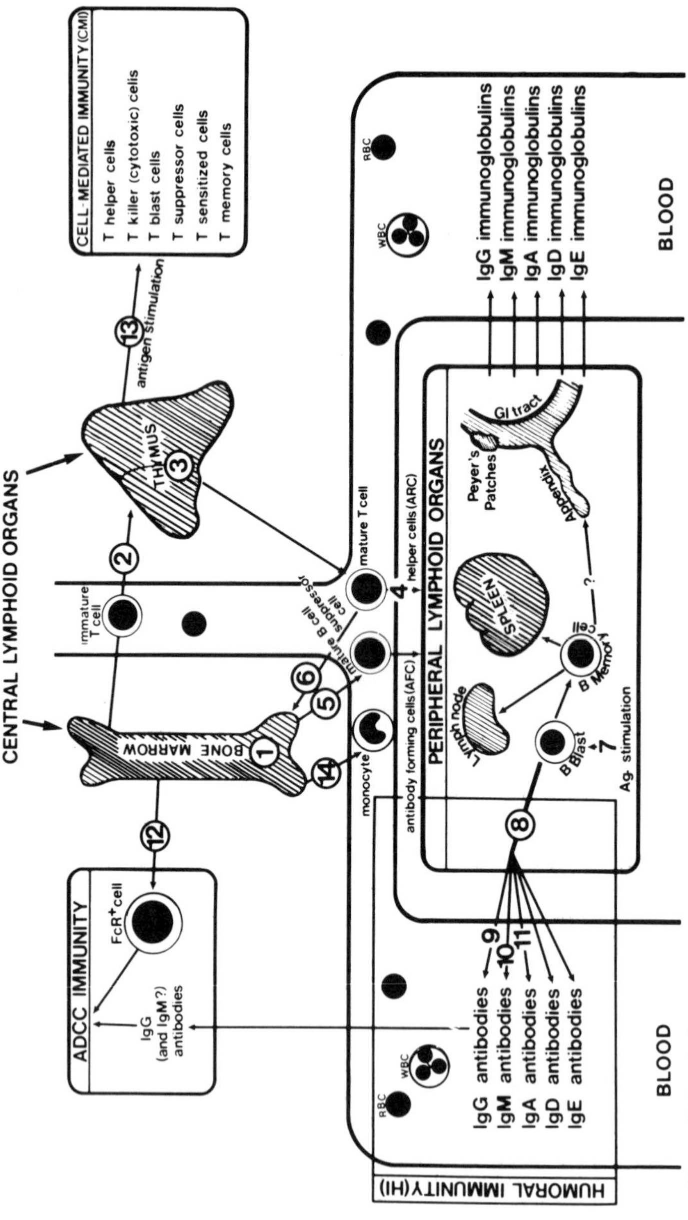

Figure 10.1 *Defects which may arise during the ontogeny of the immune system (congenital defects) or later in life (acquired defects) which present as immunodeficiency diseases.*

Table 10.1
Sites of Pathologic Lesions or Maturation Arrest (Already Defined or Not Yet Defined) in the Pathogenesis of Immunodeficiency Diseases

1. Reticular dysgenesis
   a. Aplastic anemia
   b. Pancytopenia
   c. Primarily neutropenia or thrombocytopenia
2. Thymic alymphoplasia (Nezelof syndrome)
3. Thymic aplasia (Di George syndrome)
4. Selective defect in antibody synthesis to T- or ARC-dependent antigens only (NYD)
5. Panaimmunoglobulinemia (absolute agammaglobulinemia) (also Bruton sex-linked agammaglobulinemia)

2 + 5. Lymphopenic agammaglobulinemia (Swiss-type agammaglobulinemia)

6. a. Nezelof syndrome
   b. Recurrent transient neutropenia
7. Clonal deletion—failure to respond with antibody formation to a specific antigen(s). Immune response to other antigens is intact.
8. Agammaglobulinemia with normal numbers of B cells. Specific B cell defect, possible maturation block, at the preimmunocompetent stage level.
9. Specific IgG hypoimmunoglobulinemia
10. Specific IgM hypoimmunoglobulinemia (Wiskott-Aldrich syndrome)
11. Specific IgA hypoimmunoglobulinemia
12. Failure to detect ADCC cytotoxic cells (NYD)
13. Defective cell-mediated immunity
    a. May be generalized in spite of normal numbers of circulating T cells and relatively normal thymus architecture
    b. May be specific with respect to a particular antigen (NYD)
14. Defect in monocyte function—chemotaxis and phagocytosis.
    a. Chronic granulomatous disease (CGD)
    b. Chédiak-Higashi syndrome

C. Nezelof syndrome
D. Severe combined immunodeficiency (Swiss type)
E. Wiskott-Aldrich syndrome
F. Chronic granulomatous disease
G. Chronic mucocutaneous candidiasis
H. Hypocomplementemic syndrome
I. Chédiak-Higashi disease

2. Acquired
   A. Acquired variable hypogammaglobulinemia

Secondary

1. Immunodeficiency diseases secondary to viral infections
2. Immunodeficiency diseases secondary to malignant disease,

especially of the lymphoid system, attributable to:
(a). Displacement and replacement of immunocompetent cells by malignant cells
(b). Inhibition of immunocompetent cells by immunosuppressive factors secreted by the malignant cells
3. Immunodeficiency diseases induced as a consequence of the treatment of malignant disease, autoimmune disease, and allograft rejection. The therapy used in each of these situations (irradiation and/or cytotoxic drugs and/or steroids) is immunosuppressive and often lympholytic. These are, therefore, iatrogenically induced immunodeficiency diseases.

TRANSIENT PHYSIOLOGIC HYPOGAMMAGLOBULINEMIA

Before embarking on a discussion of immunodeficiency diseases, it is necessary to caution the reader to the fact that a condition may evolve in the infant which could very easily be confused with the Bruton hypogammaglobulinemia syndrome. This condition is referred to as **transient physiologic hypogammaglobulinemia** and will usually be detected by 3 to 4 months of age. It occurs with an equal frequency in both male and female infants (compared with the Bruton syndrome which affects male infants only).

The newborn is normally immunlogically immature at birth; the peripheral lymphoid tissue is relatively aplastic with respect to lymphocytes, lymphoid follicles are very infrequently observed, and the synthesis of IgG immunoglobulins is almost nonexistent. The IgG immunoglobulins in the neonate circulation are totally maternal in origin, and they provide passive immunity to the infant. It should be noted that the failure of the immune system to function at this time is coupled with the immaturity of the gastrointestinal tract with respect to its absorptive properties. It has been observed, in a number of animal species, that a variety of protein molecules can be absorbed whole through the gut in the neonate (Fig. 10.2). Although this capability diminishes very rapidly with each passing day and ceases to exist by 7 to 10 days of life, it nevertheless provides the infant with an energy-saving mechanism to maintain and augment his serum IgG level by straight absorption of maternal IgG present in mother's milk (hence the benefits of breastfeeding). Nature, therefore, provides a mechanism allowing for the conservation of energy in the newborn, energy which would otherwise have to be diverted to degrade the proteins in the gut taken in as food into their constituent amino acids, transport them through the gut epithelium, and reutilize them in protein synthesis.

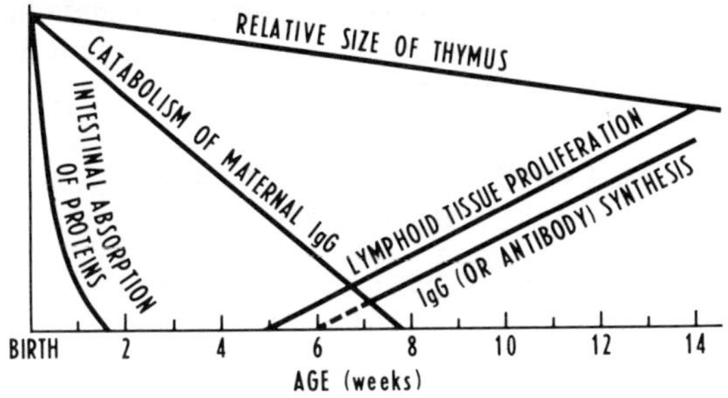

Figure 10.2 *The interrelationship between the development of the immune system, lymphoid cell proliferation, and maternal immunoglobulin catabolism in the early postnatal period.*

Under normal circumstances, maternal IgG is no longer absorbed undegraded by the 2nd week of life and begins to decrease in concentration due to its catabolism by the host. It reaches very low levels by 8 to 12 weeks of life (Fig. 10.2). At this point, the host's own lymphoid tissues begin to attain a mature status, and immunoglobulin (and antibody) synthesis is initiated. Usually the transition from the stage of passively mediated immunity to that of actively instituted immunity progresses smoothly and is undetected. However, there are occasions when the newborn immune system is rather sluggish to mature and does not respond quickly to the signal produced by the low level of circulating maternal immunoglobulins, with the result that a rather lengthy period of hypoimmunoglobulinemia may ensue. During this period the infant will be markedly susceptible to infections, especially gram-positive organisms, and will present with a short history of recurrent infections involving the respiratory tract, pharynx, and middle ear. Laboratory investigation at this time will reveal an abnormally low concentration of circulating IgG and IgM immunoglobulins. If the infant is a male and if the family history is difficult to assess or is noncontributory, then the condition could easily be mistaken for that of a congenital sex-linked hypogammaglobulinemia syndrome. Administration of gamma globulin is contraindicated at this point, as it will only exacerbate the condition by further delaying synthesis of autologous IgG and IgM immunoglobulins. In fact, one could conceivably induce a long-term agammaglobulinemia by the continuous administration of exogenous gamma globulin at this stage. The child should be treated symptomatically and the immunoglobulin level should be checked every 2 to 3 weeks. Should the infant fail to synthesize immunoglobulins over a further extended period of time (i.e. 3 to 4 months), then a diagnosis of congenital hypo- or agammaglobulinemia should be considered.

PRIMARY CONGENITAL IMMUNODEFICIENCY DISEASES

Bruton Hypogammaglobulinemia (X-linked Hypo- or Agammaglobulinemia)

This is a congenital condition, affecting only male children, the symptoms of which are not apparent until about 6 to 10 months of age. The history is one of recurrent respiratory infections responsive to antibiotic therapy but increasing in severity. The infectious organisms are usually pyogenic and include *Haemophilus influenzae, Pseudomonas aeruginosa,* streptococci, and staphylococci. Resistance to viruses and mycotic agents is not obviously impaired, and patients make a normal recovery from measles, mumps, and varicella. Smallpox vaccination is followed by a typical primary take.

Physical Examination. Essentially noncontributory. Lymph nodes are palpable.

Radiologic Examination. Thymus shadow is normal. Lateral x-rays of nasopharynx may reveal absence of tonsils and adenoid tissues.

Immunologic Investigations.

1. Immunoglobulins—Low serum IgG, IgM, and IgA. IgG usually less than 100 mg%.

2. Antibodies—Isohemagglutinins are low or absent. No or very poor antibody response to immunization with typhoid, influenza, polio, diphtheria toxoid, tetanus toxoid.

3. Skin tests for delayed hypersensitivity are normal. Schick test is positive (the reader is reminded that this skin reaction will be positive if there exist insufficient antibodies to neutralize the diphtheria toxin).

4. Complement hemolytic activity is normal.

5. Circulating white blood cells—(a) The white blood cell count and differential are usually normal, and the lymphocyte count in absolute numbers is normal. This is not surprising in view of the fact that about 70% of the circulating lymphocytes are normally T cells and this condition is a B cell dysfunction. (b) The phagocytic, chemotactic, and bactericidal activities of the circulating monocytes and neutrophils are normal. (c) The blastogenic response of the circulating lymphocytes to stimulation

with phytohemagglutinin, pokeweed, and concanavalin-A is normal.

6. Biopsy examination—(a) Examination of a lymph node biopsy will reveal absence of plasma cells, lymphoid follicles, and germinal centers in the B cell-dependent areas. (b) Examination of a bone marrow biopsy will reveal a deficiency of plasma cells. (c) Examination of a rectoanal (suction) biopsy will reveal a deficiency of plasma cells in the lamina propria.

Treatment. Treatment consists of aggressive antimicrobial chemotherapy and replacement therapy with human immune gamma globulin. Gamma globulin is administered in 5-cc volumes, intramuscularly in the thigh or deltoid region. Allow 18 to 24 hours for intravascular-extravascular equilibration, and check for levels of IgG, IgM, and IgA. Gamma globulin should be injected at 2-day intervals until the level of IgG is 300 to 400 mg%. Immunoglobulin levels should be checked at 2-week intervals at first, than at monthly intervals.

Important

1. Immunoglobulin catabolism is markedly increased at time of severe infection or stress. Therefore, it may be necessary to administer more gamma globulin more frequently.

2. Bacterial infections must be treated promptly and with high doses of antibiotics. Patients who have developed bronchiectasis may require continuous prophylaxis with tetracycline or penicillin. These patients are especially susceptible to infection with pyogenic microorganisms. On first suspicion of it, treat aggressively or patient will die with overwhelming infection (bacteremia followed rapidly by septicemia and abscess formation in any or all organs).

Differential Diagnosis.

1. Infantile x-linked agammaglobulinemia or hypogammaglobulinemia
2. Intestinal lymphangiectasis
3. Protein-losing gastroenteropathy
4. Cystic fibrosis
5. Physiologic hypogammaglobulinemia

A number of common clinical findings may be present, to varying degrees, in all of the conditions listed above and are, therefore, not specific for the Bruton syndrome. These are: recurrent respiratory infections; severe bacterial infections, i.e. pneumonia; recurrent diarrhea; failure to thrive; and paucity of lymph nodes, tonsils, and adenoid tissue.

Di George Syndrome (Congenital Thymic Hypoplasia or Congenital Pharyngeal Pouch Syndrome)

Infants with this condition tend to present with bouts of hypocalcemic tetanic seizures beginning within hours after birth or not for several days and with cardiac failure due to often inoperable congenital heart disease. If the latter condition does not result in death of the infant within the first 2 to 3 weeks after birth, the infant will probably survive, providing the hypothyroid and hypo- or euthymus conditions are treated. This somewhat confusing clinical picture is attributed to the fact that the thymus and the parathyroid glands develop from the 3rd and 4th pharyngeal pouches, as do other structures such as the aortic arch, ear, and facial structures. Failure of these pharyngeal pouches to develop normally will invariably result in abnormalities in the development of, or absence of, the structures or organs derived from these pouches, especially certain cardiovascular structures, the thymus, and the parathyroid glands. Abnormal embryogenesis of the thymus gland can result in complete or partial lack of the thymus or abnormal (ectopic) location of the thymus accompanied by failure of normal cell migration and maturation.

Physical Examination. Patients present with one or more of the following features to lesser or greater degrees—hypertelorism, shortened philtrum of the lip, micrognathia, low-set notched ear pinnae, aortic arch abnormalities (i.e. right-sided aortic arch), and tetralogy of Fallot. The patients are weak, fail to thrive, and are susceptible to sudden death. Should they survive infancy, they will present with a history of recurrent severe viral infections.

Other less frequent features include hypothyroidism, esophageal atresia, urinary tract infection and bifid uvula.

Radiologic Examination. Thymic shadow may or may not be detected. Ectopic thymus is difficult to identify.

Immunologic Investigation. (a) Normal levels of antibodies and immunoglobulins; (b) normal or low-normal levels of lymphocytes (lymphopenia is uncommon); although a common feature is a marked reduction in the number of circulating T cells, the total lymphocyte count will tend to be in the normal range due to a compensatory increase in the number of immunoglobulin-bearing B cells; (c) negative delayed hypersensitivity skin tests; (d) low serum calcium (5 to 7 mg%) and high level of phosphorous; (e) normal level of complement activity; (f) normal or slightly diminished response of the circulating white blood cells to in vitro stimulation with plant mitogens and allogeneic cells (MLR).

Treatment.

1. Control hypoparathyroidism. Administer calcium gluconate intravenously immediately to stop and prevent hypocalcemic seizures. The diet should be supplemented with vitamin D and calcium daily to maintain a normal circulating concentration of calcium.
2. Perform fetal (10- to 14-week-old) thymus transplant, which supplies the T cells deficient in the patient.
3. Treat infections aggressively.
4. Administer immune gamma globulin, if indicated (especially as prophylaxis for viral infections).

Nezelof Syndrome

This syndrome may be considered to be either a more severe variant of the Di George syndrome or a less severe variant of the severe combined immunodeficiency (SCID) syndrome. Lymphopenia is the most characteristic finding, accompanied by below normal immunoglobulin levels. In mild cases, the immunoglobulin level may be near normal, suggesting the Di George syndrome; in severe cases, the immunoglobulins may be absent, suggesting the SCID syndrome. There is absence of cell-mediated immunity with greater than normal susceptibility to gram-negative sepsis and Candida infections of the mouth, gastrointestinal tract, esophagus, and perianal region. Virus infections may be unduly severe and include adenovirus, varicella, measles, and progressive vaccinia.

The patient with Nezelof syndrome may experience severe recurrent episodes of the disease which may occur unpredictably in an almost cyclical fashion in the absence of any recognized predisposing or precipitating factors. These severe episodes are characterized by pancytopenia and are accompanied by severe infections. Abdou has demonstrated the existence of T suppressor cells in the bone marrow during these crises capable of inhibiting granulocytopoiesis. These T suppressor cells are transiently detected only during the periods of severe infections when the patient presents with pancytopenia. These activated T suppressor cells in the bone marrow may be responsible for the leukopenia and the ensuing severe infections which are experienced by patients with the Nezelof syndrome.

Physical Examination. The child will tend to be irritable, underweight, and poorly nourished (due to malabsorption syndrome). Thrush may be present.

Radiologic Examination. Absence of thymic shadow.

Immunologic Investigation. (a) Profound lymphopenia usually accompanied by normal immunoglobulin levels. (b) Disturbance of lymphoid architecture, especially depletion of the thymic-dependent area. (c) Markedly depressed response of the circulating lymphocytes to in vitro challenge with phytohemagglutinin, allogeneic cells (MLR), and other antigens.

Treatment. Treatment consists mainly of aggressive antimicrobial chemotherapy as the infections arise. A thymic graft (10- to 14-week-old fetus) may be attempted.

Severe Combined Immunodeficiency (Lymphopenic Agammaglobulinemia)

This is a congenital, inherited immunodeficiency disease affecting both the humoral and cellular immune systems. It is characterized by the early onset of severe infections and a rapidly progressive course with early demise. It is accompanied by lymphoid and plasma cell aplasia and thymic aplasia or dysplasia. The symptoms appear in the immediate postnatal period. Infections with respect to all pathogens and especially microorganisms with normally low pathogenicity, i.e. *Pneumocystis carinii,* become more devastating, protracted, and refractory to antimicrobial therapy. The child usually dies within a few months of birth.

Evidence presented over the past 5 years strongly suggests that the etiology and pathogenesis of at least one form of this disease may be attributed to a defect in intracellular purine metabolism. The cells of a number of patients appear to be deficient in the enzyme adenosine deaminase, thus permitting the accumulation of purine metabolites such as deoxyadenosine, adenosine, and deoxyadenosine triphosphate. These metabolites are released into the circulation and are cytotoxic to lymphocytes and inhibit the maturation of immunocompetent cells.

Physical Examination. The child may appear to be emaciated and underdeveloped and will cry continually. It will not gain weight and may suffer from recurrent bouts of diarrhea. Respiratory infection will be a constant feature. Lymph nodes are not palpable.

Radiologic Examination. (a) No thymus shadow; (b) no tissue in Waldeyer's ring.

Immunologic Investigation. (a) The most dramatic finding is an absolute or near absolute lymphopenia. (b) The concentration of immunoglobulins will be very low, or immunoglobulins may be undetectable by conventional assay procedures. (c) Examination of spleen and lymph node biopsies reveal a lack of cells in both the thymic-dependent and bursal-dependent areas. (d) No isoagglutinins are detected in the circulation. (e) The humoral immune response is poor or absent. (f) Schick test is positive (no circulating antidiphtheria toxin antibodies). (g) Delayed skin reactivity is absent. (h) The blastogenic responses of the circulating lymphocytes to the plant mitogens phytohemagglutinin and concanavalin-A, and to allogeneic cells in the MLR, are very low or absent. (i) Adenosine deaminase concentration in the circulating cells may be below normal or absent.

Treatment. Infections must be treated vigorously without delay. Hyperimmune gamma globulin should be administered at properly spaced intervals in order to maintain a concentration of 300 to 400 mg%. Specific antisera should also be administered as required. Transfer factor may be administered. The most appropriate but still experimental treatment is a fetal bone marrow allograft which provides the precursors of the immunocompetent B and T cells.

As discussed above, recent investigations suggest that at least one type of combined immunodeficiency may be the result of a diminished concentration or absence of intracellular adenosine deaminase. The immune reactivity of the circulating lymphocytes of some patients with this disease, as determined by in vitro tests, can be reconstituted by the addition of adenosine deaminase. The immune competence of the cells of other patients with this defect can be restored by the addition of adenosine deaminase and thymosin. Adenosine deaminase has been infused into patients with immunodeficiency disease associated with a deficiency in adenosine deaminase with very promising results.

Important

Patients with congenital immunodeficiency disease frequently require whole blood transfusions. Great care must be taken that no viable allogeneic lymphocytes are transfused into these patients because a graft versus host reaction may ensue. Blood earmarked for a patient with immunodeficiency disease, especially that affecting the cellular immune system, must be irradiated prior to its administration.

Wiskott-Aldrich Syndrome

This is a sex-linked recessive disease characterized by thrombocytopenia, eczema, and abnormally high susceptibility to many infections. The natural history of this disease is one of repeated infections with low-grade pathogenic, nonpyogenic microorganisms, the latter often characterized by normally highly antigenic carbohydrate antigens. There is a marked defect in cell-mediated immunity which leads to recurrent viral infections. Severe episodes of thrombocytopenia recur with increasing frequency during childhood and eventually present as a permanent thrombocytopenia. Eczema, the third of the triad of symptoms, also appears early in life and remains a constant feature.

Patients have a much higher than normal (100 times) predisposition to develop lymphoreticular malignancies, which often metastasize to the central nervous system.

Many of these affected individuals succumb during childhood from infections as a consequence of the immunologic deficiency, hemorrhage secondary to thrombocytopenia, or malignant tumors.

Physical Examination. Noncontributory.

Radiologic Examination. Thymus shadow normally present. Tonsils and adenoid tissues normally seen in x-ray of nasopharynx.

Immunologic Investigations.

1. Immunoglobulins—Low or absent IgM, often accompanied by low or absent IgA. IgG level is normal.

2. Antibodies—Isohemagglutinins are low or absent. Antibodies to polysaccharide antigens are absent. Antibody levels to a variety of protein antigens are either reduced or normal.

3. Skin reactions—Skin tests for delayed hypersensitivity are poor or absent. The Schick test is negative, denoting the presence of toxin-neutralizing antibodies in the circulation.

4. Complement hemolytic activity is normal.

5. Circulating white blood cells—(a) Moderate to severe lymphopenia. (b) The blastogenic response to stimulation with phytohemagglutinin, pokeweed, and concanavalin-A is depressed. (c) There appears to be a defect in monocyte-mediated antibody-dependent cytotoxicity, although the number of monocytes is normal.

6. Biopsy examination—The thymus is normal in size and architecture. There is a loss of lymphocytes in the T cell-dependent areas in the lymph nodes.

Treatment.

1. Transfuse platelets as required.
2. Administer gamma globulin high in IgM, if available, to maintain an IgM level of 50 to 100 mg%.
3. Treat infections vigorously.
4. Administer transfer factor, if available.
5. Investigate for malignancies frequently.

Chronic Granulomatous Disease (CGD)

This disease is due to an inherited defect of leukocyte bactericidal function characterized by widespread granulomatous lesions of the skin, lungs, and lymph nodes. Hypergammaglobulinemia is not uncommon. The disease makes its appearance in the first few months of life. Initial lesions are typically eczematoid reactions of the skin around the nose and ears which progress to prevalent skin lesions accompanied by enlarged, inflammed local lymph nodes. The skin lesions will frequently recur, producing tissue necrosis, granuloma formation, and suppurative adenopathy. Hepatosplenomegaly is a constant feature. Abscesses of the liver, spleen, lungs, and bones are frequent and severe.

Pulmonary involvement is almost a constant feature, with hilar enlargement, bronchopneumonia, and empyema. Lung abscesses may be present.

An indication of the pathogenesis of this disease is the failure to observe rapid clearing of symptoms and dissolution of lesions following intensive appropriate antimicrobial treatment. Lung infiltrates tend to persist for weeks.

Radiologic Examination. Reticulonodular densities in the lung fields will be seen which represent granulomas. In some patients, areas of bronchopneumonia resolve into discrete areas of consolidation referred to as "encapsulating pneumonia," diagnostic of CGD.

Hematologic Investigation. (a) Leukocytosis (compensatory), affecting both granulocytes and mononuclear cells; (b) elevated sedimentation rate; (c) anemia.

Immunologic Investigation. (a) Normal immunoglobulin levels or compensatory hyperimmunoglobulinemia; (b) skin tests for delayed hypersensitivity are normal; (c) phagocytosis by phagocytic cells is low or absent; (d) complement hemolytic titer is normal.

Bacteria normally killed by phagocytic cells survive intracellularly and eventually kill the cell, partly due to failure of the cell to synthesize H_2O_2 required for the intracellular bactericidal activity. The patient is, therefore, very susceptible to infections with organisms of low virulence and pathogenicity which do not themselves produce H_2O_2 intracellularly, such as *Staphylococcus aureus, Staphylococcus epidermidis, Serratia marcescens, Escherichia coli, Pseudomonas aeruginosa, Proteus vulgaris, Aerobacter aerogenes, Candida albicans,* and *Aspergillus fumigatus.*

On the other hand, infections with highly pathogenic organisms like *Streptococcus pyogenes* or *Diplococcus pneumoniae* are not encountered, as these organisms secrete H_2O_2 and, therefore, the bactericidal system in the phagocytic cells functions normally.

There may be a defect in the chemotactic activity of the phagocytic cells as well.

Treatment. No specific treatment exists at the present time.

Chronic Mucocutaneous Candidiasis

This condition presents as a persistent infection of the skin and mucous membranes by *Candida albicans.* The condition is often accompanied by severe endocrinologic disturbances, such as hypothyroidism, parathyroid deficiency, diabetes, and Addison's disease. Suffice it to say that the basic underlying cause of this distressing disease is not known, as the lymphocyte count is normal, immunoglobulin and antibody levels are normal, complement activity is normal, and thymic and lymph node architecture is normal. There is some evidence of a defect in the monocyte-macrophage system in terms of diminished phagocytic activity and/or response to products of stimulated lymphocytes (lymphokines). The cell-mediated immune response, in general, is depressed. The immunologic defect, if it exists, is often specific or selective for Candida and may constitute an example of clonal deletion.

Physical Examination. Essentially noncontributory. No inappropriate findings on physical examination.

Immunologic Investigation.

1. Immunoglobulins—Normal levels of IgG, IgM, and IgA.
2. Antibodies—Normal levels of isohemagglutinins and normal levels of antibodies following immunization.
3. Skin tests for delayed hypersensitivity are diminished or absent.
4. Complement hemolytic activity is normal.
5. Circulating white blood cells—(a) White blood cell count and differential are usually normal, and lymphocyte count in absolute number is normal. (b) The phagocytic and/or chemotactic activities of the circulating monocytes may be markedly diminished. (c) The blastogenic response of the circulating lymphocytes to stimulation with phytohemagglutinin, pokeweed, and concanavalin-A may be normal or reduced.
6. Assay for lymphokines—MIF and/or macrophage chemotactic factor may not be secreted by patients' lymphocytes following incubation with Candida antigen(s).
7. Biopsy examination—Thymus, spleen, and lymph node architecture is usually normal. However, a depletion of cells in the T-dependent areas of the lymph nodes and spleen will not infrequently be observed.

Treatment. The best treatment to date is vigorous administration of antifungal agents, both local and systemic. Transfer factor has been tried with enthusiastic endorsement and great publicity but with very limited clinical success. There is no specific cure for this disease at the present time.

Hypocomplementemia Syndrome

Some individuals are congenitally deficient in one or more of the constituents of the complement (C′) system. Under these circumstances, there is failure to lyse invading organisms even if antibodies are formed and phagocytosis is normal. It will be recalled that the interaction of bacteria with antibodies does not result in death of the organisms, but it is the subsequent interaction with the intact C′ system which produces lysis of the invader.

The patient may present with symptoms identical to those of a patient with primary x-linked agammaglobulinemia. A feature will be recurring infections with pyogenic organisms in spite of normal antibody and cell-mediated immune responses. Cell-mediated immunity is not affected by a defect in the complement system, as complement is not required for the cell-mediated immune reaction.

Radiologic Examination. Noncontributory.

Hematologic Investigation. Normal white blood cell differential and absolute lymphocyte count.

Immunologic Investigation. (a) Normal levels of immunoglobulins and isohemagglutinins; (b) normal antibody response; (c) normal cell-mediated immune response (delayed hypersensitivity skin reaction); (d) a loss of hemolytic complement activity. This is a consistent finding attributed to the congenital absence of one or more of the complement constituents.

Treatment.

1. Infections must be treated vigorously with antibiotics.
2. Transfusion with normal human serum with high hemolytic complement titer should be considered at the height of the infection.

Chédiak-Higashi Syndrome

The Chédiak-Higashi syndrome (CHS) is very infrequently encountered but must be considered in the differential diagnosis of immunodeficiency disease. This disease is similar to chronic granulomatous disease (CGD) discussed above in that it, too, is characterized by an increased susceptibility to bacterial infection attributed to defects in neutrophil migratory and bactericidal activities. The concentration of immunoglobulins in the circulation, the synthesis of antibodies to conventional antigens, the cell-mediated immune response, and the C′ hemolytic titer are all within the normal range. A major distinction between CGD and CHS is that there is a marked susceptibility to infection with minimally virulent bacteria in CGD, whereas there is an increased susceptibility to gram-positive pyogenic bacteria in CHS. Thus a characteristic feature of CHS is repeated febrile episodes due to staphylococcal infection of the skin, lungs, bronchi, middle ear, and upper respiratory tract. The disease may be localized, although multisystem involvement is the general rule. The patient may, therefore, present with lymphadenopathy, hepatosplenomegaly, peripheral neuropathy, neutropenia, and thrombocytopenia.

When neutrophils of patients with CHS are incubated with known numbers of common pathogenic bacterial, phagocytosis of the microorganisms appears to be normal but the ingested bacteria survive intracellularly for a prolonged period of time relative to their survival time following phagocytosis by normal neutrophils.

Characteristic findings in smears of these CHS neutrophils are large granular peroxidase-positive inclusions. Hydrogen peroxide formation is normal. It appears that microtubule function is abnormal, resulting in the defective release of lysosomal enzymes into the phagocytic vacuoles.

The poor migratory response to chemotactic stimuli by the CHS neutrophils (their movement appears more random than directionally oriented even when subjected to very effective conventional chemotactic stimuli) appears to be due, at least in some instances, to the presence in the circulation of IgG immunoglobulins (autoantibody?) which can attach to the neutrophils and specifically and irreversibly inhibit their locomotion. The possible autoimmune nature of this syndrome is suggested by the finding of massive infiltration of the bone marrow by lymphocytes capable of synthesizing autoantibodies to the neutrophils and megakaryocytes. Some of these lymphocytes may be suppressor cells capable of preventing the generation of granulocytes and thrombocytes.

CHS is, therefore, a syndrome characterized by defective neutrophils, the defects in which may be due to different etiologic mechanisms. These may vary from extracellular factors such as autoantibodies directed specifically to neutrophils and platelets and intracellular defects due to abnormal microtubular function, abnormal synthesis of intracellular proteolytic enzymes, etc.

Treatment. There is no specific treatment for the CHS syndrome. Aggressive antibiotic therapy is the rule when required. The hemorrhagic tendencies due to the thrombocytopenia usually respond to multiple blood or platelet transfusions. At times of crisis, prednisone administration is appropriate. Death usually results from infection unresponsive to antibiotic therapy or uncontrolled hemorrhage. Patients with less severe forms of the disease may survive well into the fifth and sixth decades.

ACQUIRED VARIABLE HYPOGAMMAGLOBULINEMIA

This immunodeficiency syndrome resembles x-linked Bruton hypogammaglobulinemia only in the sense that the most notable feature of both of these conditions is the low concentration of circulating gamma globulin. In contrast to the Bruton x-linked hypogammaglobulinemia syndrome, which invariably presents during the first year of life, the acquired variable hypogammaglobulinemia (or AVH) syndrome surfaces in the third or fourth decade of life and it occurs as frequently in males as in females. The AVH syndrome evolves very insidiously; the patient may exhibit signs and symptoms of autoimmune disease, malabsorption syndrome accompanied by a protein-losing enteropathy, and/or recurrent sinopulmonary infections with pyogenic microorganisms for several years before a diagnosis of AVH is made based on a laboratory finding of a low concentration of circulating gamma globulins, especially the IgG immunoglobulins.

A picture of frank or severe immunodeficiency rarely develops in AVH to the degree that it presents in the childhood Bruton hypogammaglobulinemia. The concentration of the immunoglobulins may be significantly below normal, but not exaggeratedly so. In fact, the concentration of total immunoglobulins may be only slightly below normal. However, determination of the concentration of the individual immunoglobulins generally reveals a low concentration for the IgG immunoglobulins, with somewhat depressed concentrations for the IgA and IgM immunoglobulins.

The symptom which most frequently presents initially consists of recurrent sinopulmonary infection with pyogenic bacteria such as *Diplococcus pneumoniae* and *Haemophilus influenzae*. Succeeding episodes of infection tend to be more severe, require more aggressive antimicrobial chemotherapy, and result in longer lasting, seemingly intractable sequelae. Chronic bronchiectasis may develop, as may chronic conjunctivitis, otitis media, and sinusitis. The malabsorption syndrome, which may be mistaken for sprue and thus wrongly diagnosed, may be severe and unresponsive to conventional therapy. It may be severe enough to present as a protein-losing enteropathy with its consequent dependent edema. However, examination of an intestinal biopsy would rule out a primary malabsorption syndrome such as sprue because the characteristic flattening of the villi seen in sprue is absent and the biopsy specimen appears to be essentially normal. This syndrome may be secondary to a low concentration of secretory IgA, although this has so far not been proven. In some instances, the generalized edema may be the primary presenting feature and may wrongly suggest cardiovascular disease, especially cardiac failure or valvular insufficiency. Some patients may present initially with splenomegaly or hepatosplenomegaly and/or lymphadenopathy. A lymph node biopsy may reveal a confused picture of lymphoid hyperplasia. However, closer examination will reveal excessive, almost compensatory, proliferation of cells in the T-dependent areas with either small but normal appearing follicles or a total absence of cells in the B cell (follicle) compartment.

Patients may also present with symptoms of autoimmune disease, which occurs with an unexpectedly high frequency in this syndrome. The most frequently presenting autoimmune diseases are hemolytic anemia, thrombocytopenia, pernicious anemia, rheumatoid arthritis-like syndromes, systemic lupus erythematosus, and dermatomyositis. The combination of a low concentration of IgG and autoimmune disease may appear to be an incompatible or contradictory picture, but it may occur and may be predicted on the basis of distinct defects within the different helper and suppressor T cell populations in the individual (see Chapter 8, suppressor cells).

As the AVH syndrome progresses, defects in the cell-mediated immune system surface as well, and a diagnosis of acquired variable hypogammaglobulinemia becomes evident.

The etiology and pathogenesis of this disease can be (apparently) directly attributed to an alteration in the ratio of the T_G suppressor cells to the T_M helper cells in the circulation and their states of immunologic activity. It has been repeatedly demonstrated that the circulating B cells of patients with the AVH syndrome behave normally in vitro when separated from the isologous T cells, and they can be induced to synthesize immunoglobulins in the presence of normal T cells. On the other hand, T cells of patients with the AVH syndrome can suppress immunoglobulin synthesis by normal B cells in vitro. These results strongly suggest that suppressor cells play a major role in the evolution of at least this type of immunodeficiency disease.

Physical Examination. Usually noncontributory during quiescent periods. Hepatosplenomegaly and/or lymphadenopathy may be apparent.

Radiologic Examination. Thymus shadow is normally present. Tonsils and adenoid tissues (unless previously excised) are normally seen in x-ray of nasopharynx.

Hematologic Investigation. Usually noncontributory. However, patients presenting with purpura and complaints of fatigue and weakness may present with thrombocytopenia and normocytic normochromic anemia, respectively. As the disease progresses, the absolute number of T cells in the circulation diminishes.

Immunologic Investigation.

1. Immunoglobulins—Low IgG (often less than 300 mg%). IgM and especially IgA may be very low as well or be present in below normal concentration. Whether the concentration of secretory IgA is abnormal is not known at the present time.
2. Antibodies—Isohemagglutinins are low in concentration or absent. Antibody levels to a variety of protein and bacterial antigens are reduced or absent.
3. Skin reactions—(a) The Schick test is usually positive, demonstrating a lack of antibodies to diphtheria toxin. This test is relevant only if it is carried out after deliberate immunization with diphteria toxoid has been attempted. (b) Reduced or absent delayed skin reactions.
4. Complement hemolytic titer is normal.
5. Circulating white blood cells—(a) Monocytes and neutrophils display normal phagocytic and chemotactic activity. (b) The blastogenic response of the lymphocytes to stimulation with the mitogens phytohemagglutinin, pokeweed, and concanavalin-A may be significantly reduced or absent. (c) The blastogenic response of the lymphocytes to stimulation with allogeneic cells in the MLR may be significantly reduced or absent.

Differential Diagnosis. Acquired variable hypogammaglobulinemia must be distinguished from (a) primary malabsorption syndrome; (b) autoimmune disease; (c) generally low-grade immunity; a slow responder to antigenic stimulation; and (d) chronic lung disease which may or may not be accompanied by such predisposing factors as perennial respiratory allergy or alpha-1 antitrypsin deficiency.

Treatment.

1. Aggressive antimicrobial (antibiotic) chemotherapy when necessary.
2. Pulmonary physical therapy when warranted.
3. Dietary restrictions to control the malabsorption problems.
4. Corticosteroids and immunosuppressive agents to control the autoimmune disease, should it reach crisis proportions.
5. Infusion of hyperimmune gamma globulin at defined intervals of time and in sufficient quantities to maintain a circulating IgG concentration above 300 mg%.
6. Oral administration of zinc sulphate. Recent investigations have disclosed that patients with this form of immunodeficiency

have low levels of zinc in the circulation. The ingestion of zinc sulphate, which is easily absorbed through the gut, may totally ameliorate the symptoms. The beneficial effects of zinc may be attributed to its requirement in the in vivo synthesis of prostaglandins which are capable of restoring the balance of the T_G and T_M cells in these patients and restoring normal immunologic functions to these cells (see Chapter 13, Nutrition and Immunity).

Important

The immunodeficiency diseases described above constitute the most clearly defined and understood of the many diseases classified in numerous books and current review articles as immunodeficiency diseases. As discussed above, the classification of immunodeficiency diseases has been witness to an uncontrolled proliferation of "titled" syndromes. The effect is to intimidate the reader, to persuade him that the increasing number of syndromes is a reflection of new knowledge. With a few exceptions, nothing could be further from the truth. Before accepting that a newly described syndrome is indeed a new form of an immunodeficiency disease, the reader would do well to compare its characteristics with those of the established syndromes described in this text.

CHAPTER 11

Immunologic Tolerance

MECHANISMS OF TOLERANCE

Immunologic tolerance is an induced state characterized by the failure of the host to synthesize antibodies or generate sensitized cells to a specific antigen while the response to all other antigens is intact and normally expressed. The terms **immunologic paralysis** and **immunologic unresponsiveness** are synonymous with **immunologic tolerance** and were coined by different investigators who were concerned with defining what appeared to be distinct phenomena. Immunologic tolerance dates back to the immediate post-World War II period when Felton, at the National Institutes of Health in Bethesda, Md., reported that mice injected with a suprathreshold dose of a Pneumococcus polysaccharide antigen failed to respond with antibody formation, even if they were subsequently reinjected with normal immunogenic doses of the antigen. Although immunologic tolerance was first described in mice, it can be induced as well in guinea pigs and rabbits with protein antigens. Tolerance can be induced with respect to both humoral and cell-mediated immunity. Immunologic tolerance should not be confused with the term **immunologic suppression**, which is used to designate a state of generalized (nonspecific) inhibition of immune responsiveness resulting from the administration of potent chemotherapeutic drugs. The latter are often immunosuppressive and highly toxic chemical agents, i.e. azathioprine (Imuran), cyclophosphamide, and chlorambucil. Irradiation will also bring about a state of generalized immune suppression or incompetence, as will the injection of nitrogen mustard or its analogues, folic acid antagonists, amino acid analogues, etc.

Important

The major properties which distinguish immunologic tolerance from immunologic suppression are:

1. There is no significant effect on the numbers and function of the circulating lymphocytes following the induction of a state

of immunologic tolerance. On the other hand, lymphopenia is characteristic of a state of immunologic suppression.

2. Immunologic tolerance is characterized by the absence of disturbance or alteration in the gross architecture or microscopic organization of the lymphoid tissues; on the other hand, immunologic suppression is characterized by marked disruption of lymphoid tissue architecture often accompanied by lymphocyte depletion.

3. Immunologic tolerance is specifically induced to a particular antigen. The immunologic response to other antigens is unaffected. In immune suppression, the immune response to all antigens is depressed or totally inhibited.

It is much easier to induce tolerance in a neonatal animal than in an adult animal. Furthermore, the more antigen that is administered, the more obvious and longer lasting will be the induced state of immunologic tolerance. The induction of a state of immunologic tolerance was, therefore, considered to be conditional upon the administration of a supraimmunogenic dose of the antigen, a dose equivalent to more than 100 times the normal immunogenic dose. Immunologic tolerance induced in this manner is referred to as **high dose** (or **high zone**) **tolerance**. Since the neonatal animal is very susceptible to the induction of tolerance, it was originally conjectured that potentially immunocompetent neonatal clonally selected cells, not yet having matured to immunocompetent status, are somehow more easily "turned off" by the antigen so as to be unable to respond with antibody formation to this antigen at a future date. Another theory was that these cells are somehow irreversibly damaged by the high dose of antigen. It was also observed that the number of phagocytic cells is low in the immediate postnatal period. It was, therefore, assumed that the absence of functional macrophages in the first few days of life enhances the susceptibility of the animal toward the induction of tolerance. Immunologic tolerance can be prevented in the neonatal mouse if it is given macrophages from adult syngeneic animals along with the antigen in even a tolerogenic dose.

How are immunocompetent cells so adversely affected by an antigen so as to be inhibited, rather than stimulated, in the synthesis of antibodies? Are the immunocompetent cells, in fact, functioning normally and is the reason we detect no antibodies due to their being "mopped up" by circulating antigen as rapidly as they can be secreted into the circulation by the antibody-forming cells? In point of fact, most investigators have concluded that antibody synthesis does not occur during the induction of the tolerant state. No antibody-forming cells can be detected by the immunofluorescence assay. However, there have been reports of specific antibodies in low concentration in the circulation during the induction of the tolerant state.

Any theory proposed to define the mechanism of immunologic tolerance must take into account the fact that the state of tolerance does not appear to last for the lifetime of the animal and is not transmitted to the offspring. It is a temporary state of specific nonreactivity which can be overcome or reversed by the host at a later date.

It is currently believed that the tolerant state is the result of activation of suppressor cells (T lymphocytes) which exert a specific inhibitory effect on otherwise competent antibody-forming cells. The injection of an immunogenic dose of the antigen tends to stimulate antibody-forming cells and does not appear to activate suppressor cells. However, suppressor cells are probably activated but much more slowly than are the antibody-forming cells, so that they are not functionally active until several weeks following the induction of antibody synthesis. These suppressor cells probably function by exerting a negative feedback on the immune response at a time when it would no longer be necessary anyhow. As the dose of antigen is increased, more suppressor cells become activated sooner. A very large supraimmunogenic dose of the antigen will, therefore, tend to activate the suppressor cells as rapidly as, or more rapidly than, the antibody-forming cells, resulting in a state of tolerance or absence of antibody synthesis (Fig. 11.1).

The suppressor cell theory, however attractive, does not explain how the state of immunologic tolerance is maintained when suppressor cells can no longer be detected, nor does it explain the mechanism of induction of immunologic tolerance following the administration of the antigen in a very small (subimmunogenic) amount. This state of tolerance is referred to as **low dose** (or **low zone) tolerance**.

One explanation for **low dose tolerance** is that the antigen, administered in a very low dose, interacts with the normally present precommitted ARC cells, initiating proliferation of these cells and their release of receptors or antigen-receptor complexes. Having carried out their function, the ARC cells disappear. However, the concentration of antigen-receptor complexes is too low to initiate antibody synthesis, and the result is failure of activation of the AFC cells. A later injection of the same antigen,

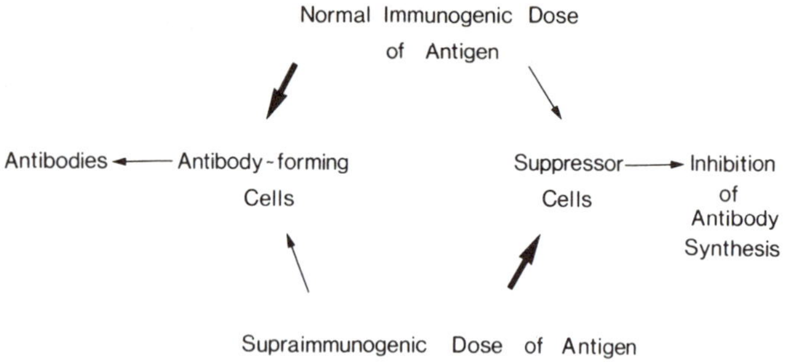

Figure 11.1 *The induction and inhibition (tolerance?) of the immune response as a function of the dose of antigen administered.*

in an immunogenic dose, will fail to stimulate antibody synthesis due to the absence of specifically precommitted ARC cells. For antibody synthesis to occur, a sufficient period of time must elapse between the induction of the state of low dose tolerance and the later administration of the antigen in an immunogenic dose in order to allow for the regeneration of the specific ARC cells from precursor stem cells. Thus, the duration of low dose tolerance may be short-lived or long-lived, or it may last for the lifetime of the host, depending upon the capacity of the host to regenerate ARC cells from precursor stem cells.

It appears, therefore, that two different mechanisms exist to facilitate the establishment of the immunologically tolerant state. One mechanism is activated when a large dose of the antigen is administered, and the other mechanism appears to operate when a very small amount of the antigen is administered.

As stated above, immunologic tolerance may exist in the apparent absence of suppressor cells. It is, therefore, necessary to theorize the existence of tolerant cells in addition to suppressor cells. What is the identity of the cells which are tolerized in the tolerant host? Since the immune responses to both T cell-dependent and T cell-independent antigens are inhibited in the tolerant host, one could logically conclude that either B cells alone or both T cells and B cells are induced to a state of active tolerance in the tolerized host. With respect to T-dependent antigens, it has been demonstrated that both B and T cells are induced into active tolerant states. With respect to T-independent antigens, the B cells are converted to actively tolerant cells following injection of the antigen in the tolerance-inducing dose. The T cells appear to be more susceptible to the induction of tolerance than are the B cells because tolerant T cells can be detected within 24 hours following antigen administration whereas tolerant B cells are not detected until several days to a week following antigen administration. Furthermore, T cell tolerance lasts longer than B cell tolerance.

A note of caution must, however, be sounded. All of the above evidence in favor of tolerant T and B cells emanates from experiments in the inbred mouse. Tolerant T and B cells are demonstrated by their ability (or lack of) to transfer immune responsiveness to a designated antigen in a syngeneic immunoincompetent host mouse. This type of tolerance is referred to as **infectious tolerance** because it can be transferred with cells from a tolerant animal to a nontolerant recipient animal. With respect to T-dependent antigens in the mouse, it has been shown that either the bone marrow (B) cells or the thymus (T) cells, but not both, need come from the tolerant mouse in order to suppress antibody formation in the immunoincompetent recipient. With respect to T-independent antigens, the bone marrow (B) cells must come from the tolerant donor. However, it has not been unequivocally demonstrated that the tolerant bone marrow (B) cell is not, in fact, an infiltrating suppressor T cell. Furthermore, it must also be firmly established that the transferred tolerant cells are not in fact mixtures of tolerant and immunocompetent cells, with the tolerant (suppressor?) cell activity predominating over and suppressing the immune responsiveness of the immunocompetent cells.

Although these experiments have facilitated an understanding of the mechanism of induction of immunologic tolerance in the inbred mouse, it does not necessarily follow that tolerance in other animal species, especially the human, is similarly effected. Nevertheless, the results from the mouse experiments provide food for thought for those investigators primarily concerned with the immune response in humans and its inhibition intentionally as a result of the induction of a state of immunologic tolerance.

Important

The reader should be aware that the term immunologic tolerance takes on a totally different meaning when used to define the acceptance of an allograft (a tissue or organ from a genetically nonidentical or unrelated individual). As will be discussed in Chapter 16, an allograft is normally rejected within 7 to 12 days following its implantation into the host in the absence of intervention with immunosuppressive drugs. However, it has been reported by numerous investigators that antibodies to the allograft induced in the host protect the allograft from rejection by the cell-mediated immune system. This protection afforded the allograft by antibodies is referred to as allograft tolerance or enhancement. Used in this context, tolerance denotes the formation of "protective" antibodies directed toward the specific transplantation antigens, whereas, when used to define the induced absence of an immune response with respect to a specific exogenous or autoantigen, tolerance implies the absence of antibody synthesis.

CLINICAL RELEVANCE AND APPLICATION OF IMMUNOLOGIC TOLERANCE

Immunization Procedures

In the immediate postnatal period, the infant is essentially immunologically immature and generally immunoincompetent. The circulating immunoglobulins are maternally derived (IgG traverses the placental barrier; the other immunoglobulins do not). The infant does not possess mature peripheral lymphoid tissues (spleen, lymph nodes), nor does it synthesize its own IgG antibodies. This state is usually referred to as **immunologic immaturity**. Within 12 weeks the peripheral lymphoid tissues enlarge and there is proliferation of lymphoid cells and synthesis of IgG. The infant is now immunologically mature. At times, there may be a lag in the maturation of the peripheral lymphoid tissues with a resultant delay in the capacity to synthesize antibodies. Under these conditions, the transition from a dependence on maternally acquired antibodies to a dependence on autologous antibodies is not as smooth as it should be, and the infant may go through a phase referred to as **transient physiologic hypogammaglobulinemia** (see Chapter 10). The immunoglobulin concentration may remain very low for several weeks to several months, and the infant will, of course, be highly susceptible to infectious agents. At this stage, the condition could be easily misdiagnosed as a congenital agammaglobulinemia. During this phase of its life the infant is also much more susceptible to the induction of immunologic tolerance, if immunization is attempted.

It is, therefore, not advisable to immunize infants prior to 2 to 3 months of age, as a state of tolerance to the antigen could conceivably be induced if the infant is still in the state of immunologic immaturity. The antigens commonly administered at this age are diphtheria toxoid (D), tetanus toxoid (T), and *Bordetella pertussis* (P). These three antigens are given simultaneously as DPT vaccine. It is indeed fortuitous, and a reflection of our luck rather than intelligence or knowledge, that we can inject DPT even in the early postnatal period and successfully immunize to these antigens. The reason why tolerance is not produced to any of the components of DPT when all three are given together is that the pertussis constituent of the DPT vaccine is an endotoxin and adjuvant. The latter actually suppresses the induction of a state of immunologic tolerance even if it could occur with respect to the D and/or T components of the DPT vaccine. How the adjuvant inhibits the induction of tolerance is not understood, but it is a reproducible finding. Therefore, it is safe to immunize a neonate within the first 3 months of age providing an adjuvant is administered along with the antigens. Pure protein antigens should not be administered prior to 3 months of age.

Transplantation

Current techniques aimed at forced acceptance of vascularized allografts by the host (i.e. kidney, skin, heart) are primitive, and their application usually results in illness in the host and generalized immunosuppression. Treatment includes irradiation and/or the administration of alkylating agents (i.e. nitrogen mustard) and/or chemical "immunosuppressive" drugs—actinomycin-D, Imuran, and steroids and/or antilymphocyte globulin. Not only does this treatment often result in a generalized state of immune suppression, but it also increases the incidence of malignancies.

Many attempts are being made to induce a state of immunologic tolerance of a long-term nature toward the transplantation antigens. This would ensure survival of the graft with none of the deleterious and life-threatening consequences of nonspecific therapy. Once a state of tolerance is induced to the transplantation antigens of the allograft, the individual should accept the graft without requiring chemotherapy, and acceptance of the graft should be permanent.

The Prevention of Erythroblastosis Fetalis or Hemolytic Disease of the Newborn

Erythroblastosis fetalis results from the synthesis of anti-Rh antibodies by the Rh-negative mother toward Rh antigens present on the fetal cells. This immune response does not affect the first Rh-positive pregnancy because the fetal-maternal placental barrier is not normally breached to a significant degree until expulsion of the infant during the act of parturition. At this time, concurrent with the trauma of placental separation, there is some spilling of fetal Rh-positive erythrocytes into the maternal circulation, with subsequent formation of anti-Rh antibodies of the IgG immunoglobulin class. In point of fact, some fetal erythrocytes do invade the maternal circulation as early as the second trimester of pregnancy but in insufficient numbers to trigger off an immune response. The IgG anti-Rh antibodies can circulate for long periods of time (up to several years), and their synthesis can be stimulated by the few erythrocytes (review the characteristic properties of the primary and secondary response, Chapter 5) which penetrate the maternal circulation during the first and second trimesters of a second pregnancy. These antibodies will invade the fetal circulation, react with the fetal erythrocytes, lyse them in the presence of complement, and contribute toward their phagocytosis and intracellular lysis by macrophages.

In the early 1960s, it became apparent that IgG and IgM antibodies function in the regulation of antibody synthesis, with IgM antibodies stimulating IgG antibody production and IgG antibodies suppressing further IgM antibody synthesis. Thus, IgG antibodies may be considered as specific immunosuppressive agents with respect to a particular antigen. Freda in New York seized upon this observation and was the first to apply it in a clinical setting. Freda and his associates injected allogeneic anti-Rh antiserum into Rh-negative women immediately following the birth of the first Rh-positive infant (gravida 1, para 1) and observed that these passively transferred antibodies were able to suppress the synthesis of anti-Rh antibodies by the mother. Anti-Rh antiserum is now commercially available under the name **Rhogam** and, when administered at the appropriate time, is effective in inhibiting active synthesis of anti-Rh antibodies.

CHAPTER 12

Autoimmunity and Autoimmune Diseases

The term **autoimmunity** implies the induction of an immune response, humoral or cellular, to autologous or self antigens. Until the early 1950s it was very unwise to suggest that such a thing as an autoimmune response could occur. In fact, when Ehrlich in 1898 predicted with amazing accuracy (that is, his predictions conform with our present concepts) the mechanism of antigen triggering of antibody synthesis and secretion, he considered it blasphemous to suggest that an immune response could be triggered by anything but an exogenous agent. Ehrlich coined the term "horror autoxicosis," which implies the inability of the body to respond to an autoantigen, in 1903 and it was accepted by the world as dogma, although attempts were made to discredit it from time to time. One must be reminded that Donath and Landsteiner reported the existence of autoantibodies (to red blood cells) as long ago as 1904. Dameshek and Schwartz reported the existence of autoantibodies in patients with hemolytic anemia in 1938. However, it was not until Witebsky demonstrated, in a series of investigations carried out between 1937 and 1957, the experimental induction of autoantibodies and autoimmune disease in the guinea pig following the administration of extracts prepared from autologous (or homologous) organs, such as thyroid, that the dogma of horror autoxicosis was laid to rest. By the middle 1950s, autoimmune responses had been successfully induced in mice, rats, guinea pigs, hamsters, and rabbits to a large number of autoantigens, both organ (parenchymal) and nonorgan (connective tissue) specific. Furthermore, autoantibodies and sensitized cells were detected with increasing frequency in patients suspected of being afflicted with autoimmune diseases. By the late 1950s, autoimmunity became an accepted discipline in the field of clinical immunology.

THEORIES OF THE MECHANISM OF AUTOIMMUNITY

In his proposed mechanism of immunologic tolerance, Burnet postulated that cells exist in the embryo capable of responding immunologically to all antigens at a future, postnatal date and that these cells are clonally selected. He speculated that the clones of cells programmed to interact postnatally with autoantigens are somehow destroyed upon contact with autoantigens in utero (clonal suicide) and no longer exist following birth. Since exogenous (i.e. bacterial, viral) antigens would normally not penetrate the fetal circulation, the clones of cells programmed to interact with these antigens postnatally would be unaffected in utero and would, therefore, be present in the immunologically mature animal. This theory, propounded and elaborated upon in the early 1960s, had a plausible ring to it and appeared to provide a satisfactory answer to a very compelling question, which is why only the clones of immunocompetent cells directed toward autoantigens appear to be eliminated at birth whereas the clones of cells precommitted to interact with exogenous antigens survive and provide us with the mechanism to eliminate pathogenic invasive agents.

Burnet considered that autoimmunity could only occur postnatally following the generation and proliferation of "forbidden clones" of lymphoid cells with specificity directed toward specific autoantigens. However, Burnet's clonal selection theory for antibody formation, and clonal deletion theory for the lack of autoantibody formation in the normal individual, ignored the experiments initially begun by Witebsky in the 1930s and continued by Rose, Weigle, and many other investigators who demonstrated the unequivocal induction of experimental autoimmune disease in the young and adult animal. These results in the experimental animal would appear to invalidate Burnet's hypothesis of clonal suicide in utero, since the clones of immunocompetent cells directed toward autoantigens are obviously not obliterated in utero and can be stimulated in the postnatal state. There is today no doubt that the capacity to respond to autoantigens is always present but lies dormant in normal animals and humans. One may, therefore, ask why autoimmunity does not occur more frequently than it does in the immunologically mature individual. The first and, therefore, classic explanation is that the autoantigens are normally sequestered within anatomically distinct, encapsulated organs. Thus, thyroid-specific antigens, for example, do not normally circulate to the spleen and/or lymph nodes where they could stimulate the specific immunoresponsive cells.

Has this explanation withstood the test of time? One would have to say no. Circulating cells and serum proteins are not sequestered; yet autoimmune diseases appear to evolve spontaneously toward circulating white blood cells, erythrocytes, platelets, and gamma globulin. Furthermore, irradiation, trauma, or surgery causes the release of organ-specific, potentially autoantigenic, proteins into the circulation (i.e. irradiation of the neck causes damage to thyroid follicles and release of thyroglobulin into the circulation); yet autoimmunity does not result under these circumstances.

A second explanation propounded recently is that suppressor cells exist normally in vivo and that their function is to inhibit the synthesis of autoantibodies or the induction of sensitized cells directed toward autoantigens. The suppressor cell theory dictates that suppressor cells, like antigen-reactive cells, are clonally precommitted and are capable of selectively inhibiting the immune response to specific antigens. Since the immune response to exogenous antigens is not exaggerated in the patient with autoimmune disease, it would appear that only those suppressor cells directed toward the specific autoantigens are absent or are defective in the patient with autoimmune disease. Systemic lupus erythematosus (SLE), a collagen disease, is characterized by the presence of circulating antibodies to autologous erythrocytes, leukocytes, not infrequently platelets, and DNA. The renal complications in SLE stem from the deposition of immune complexes (antibody-DNA complexes) along the glomerular basement membrane. It has been shown by a number of investigators that there is a deficiency of circulating suppressor cells capable of inhibiting the synthesis of these autoantibodies in patients with SLE.

A condition similar to SLE occurs spontaneously in the NZB/NZW mouse. This mouse appears to be normal in the immediate postnatal period. However, as it matures (4 to 6 months), it develops any of a number of autoimmune diseases, such as autoimmune hemolytic anaemia. It also displays renal symptoms characteristic of SLE and possesses circulating anti-DNA antibodies. The animal dies with a lymphoma or monoclonal macroglobulinemia syndrome or renal failure. The disease process can be halted or prevented by the administration of syngeneic young thymus cells which presumably contain the normal complement of suppressor cells or their immediate precursors.

It has also been reported that a disease similar to autoimmune thyroiditis occurs spontaneously in chickens of the obese strain. Neonatal thymectomy results in an earlier onset and increased severity of the thyroiditis, suggesting that these neonatally thymectomized chickens are deprived of thymus-derived suppressor cells which would ordinarily delay the onset of the disease.

However, as discussed in Chapter 8, one would anticipate that the neonatal extirpation of the thymus (in the obese chicken) or the premature involution of the thymus (in the NZB mouse) would deprive the animal not only of suppressor cells which would normally inhibit the synthesis of anti-DNA antibodies (NZB mice) and antithyroglobulin antibodies (obese chickens), but also of suppressor cells directed to all other autoantigens (whether the suppressor cells are clonally selected or not is irrelevant since the source of all the suppressor cells is removed). Therefore, generalized rather than specific autoimmune diseases should result, i.e. a panautoimmune disease affecting all the organ systems, circulating cells, and serum proteins. Since generalized autoimmune disease does not occur, the suppressor cell theory will have to be extensively modified before the suppressor cell can be seriously considered with any degree of credibility as a primary, rather than a coincidental, participant in the pathogenesis of immunologically mediated disease.

AUTOIMMUNE DISEASES

Up to this point, the main thrust of the discussion was to impart the status of legitimacy to autoimmune diseases and to elucidate the mechanism underlying the induction of autoimmune disease. It would now be appropriate to define and characterize autoimmune diseases in terms of their clinical manifestations and to present a functional classification of these diseases.

It is first necessary to clarify the distinction between autoimmunity and autoimmune disease. Up to this point, the terms autoimmunity and autoimmune disease have been used synonymously. This practice is inappropriate. Autoimmunity is an immunologic term used to designate a state characterized by the presence of circulating autoantibodies and/or sensitized cells. It does not necessarily imply autoimmune disease and pathology. On the other hand, autoimmune disease is a term used to designate a clinical syndrome frequently accompanied by circulating autoantibodies and/or specifically sensitized cells. However, these reactants need not be present in the circulation continually or at any one particular time. Failure to detect circulating autoantibodies or sensitized cells may be attributed to "mopping up" of these reactants by the target organ as quickly as they can be formed and released into the circulation.

The detection of circulating autoantibodies is often an incidental finding in the laboratory investigation of a patient and does not imply concurrent autoimmune disease. Many individuals possess circulating autoantibodies to smooth muscle without any symptoms of myositis. Individuals with autoimmune Hashimoto thyroiditis invariably possess circulating autoantibodies to thyroglobulin and other thyroid follicle-specific antigens. Their off-

Table 12.1
A Classification of Autoimmune Diseases

Autoimmune Disease		Reactants Implicated		Antigens
		Autoantibodies	Sensitized Cells	
I.	Hemolytic anemia	Yes	No	Erythrocyte
	Leukopenia	Yes	No	Leukocyte
	Thrombocytopenia	Yes	No	Platelet
	Rheumatoid arthritis	Yes	No	IgG
II.	Systemic lupus erythematosus	Yes	No	DNA
	Glomerulonephritis (Goodpasture)	Yes	No	Basement membrane
III.	Diabetes	Yes	?	Insulin, islet cell
	Pernicious anemia	Yes	No	Intrinsic factor, parietal cell
IV.	Thyrotoxicosis (Graves' disease)	Yes	No	Follicle membrane
V.	Thyroiditis (lymphocytic)	No?	Yes	Thyroglobulin, thyroid follicle
	Encephalomyelitis	No	Yes	Grey matter
	Aspermatogenesis	No	Yes	Spermatozoa
	Peripheral neuropathy	No	Yes	Myelin sheath
	Myasthenia gravis	No	Yes	Myoneural junction
VI.	Polyarteritis nodosa	?	?	?
	Scleroderma	?	?	?
	Dermatomyositis	?	?	?

spring often have circulating autoantibodies; however, they do not develop autoimmune thyroiditis nor any other thyroid dysfunction. Another example is the presence of rheumatoid factor in the circulation of normal children of parents afflicted with rheumatoid arthritis. Although a pathogenetic role is generally attributed to rheumatoid factor, its presence often in high concentration in unaffected individuals detracts from its role as the primary or necessary etiologic agent.

It has been stated above that individuals with autoimmune diseases usually possess circulating autoantibodies and specifically sensitized cells. However, autoantibodies bear a causal relationship with only certain select autoimmune diseases, while sensitized cells and not autoantibodies are directly implicated in other autoimmune diseases. Table 12.1 serves to clarify this point.

It will be noted that group I diseases which involve the circulating constituents—red blood cells, white blood cells, platelets, and IgG—are mediated exclusively by autoantibodies. In sharp contrast, group V diseases are organ specific and are mediated almost exclusively by sensitized cells. Autoantibodies do not appear to participate in the initiation of the lesion, although they may have an incidental or supportive role.

It is instructive to note that autoimmune diseases involving the circulating cells or proteins (group I diseases) have not been successfully induced in the experimental animal. In contradistinction, autoimmune diseases involving specific organs have been induced in the experimental animal with almost embarrassing ease (group V diseases). Almost without exception, the former are mediated by autoantibodies while the latter are mediated by sensitized cells. One interpretation of these results is that Burnet's proposed mechanism concerning the pathogenesis of autoimmune disease—that is, the eradication of autodirected immunocompetent cells in utero—may be correct only with respect to the potential autoantigens present on the circulating cells and serum proteins. In other words, immunocompetent cells formed during embryogenesis capable of interacting with and responding to the circulating elements may indeed be obliterated in utero prior to birth, and they may only reappear as "forbidden clones" postnatally as a pathologic condition. On the other hand, immunocompetent cells capable of interacting with organ-specific autoantigens would not be expected, during embryogenesis, to be exposed to organ-specific antigens which are normally sequestered within the specific organs. These cells would, therefore, be permitted to survive and proliferate and to attain immunologic maturity in the postnatal period, at which time they would respond immunologically if confronted with organ-specific autoantigens. This duel theory of the ontogeny of autoimmune disease provides an explanation for the consistent failure to induce, experimentally, autoimmune disease toward the circulating elements, as contrasted with the ease with which autoimmune diseases can be induced toward parenchymally and anatomically distinct organs.

To recapitulate, it is necessary to consider two different mechanisms to account for the spontaneous appearance of autoimmune disease. These are:

1. The pathologic emergence of neo or mutated ("forbidden") clones of immunocompetent cells directed toward the circulating cells and proteins. Autoreactive clones of cells, if they exist during embryogenesis, must be eliminated early during fetal life if the individual is to survive. It may be speculated that at some period

during the evolution of the species individuals may have been born with immunocompetent cells possessing receptor sites directed toward circulating autoantigens. However, such individuals would surely have succumbed at an early age and would not have been able to propagate and perpetuate the species.

2. The existence, normally, of immunocompetent cells capable of interacting with organ-specific (sequestered) autoantigens normally not present in the circulation. These cells are stimulated following the introduction of these antigens into the circulation.

Immunocompetent cells capable of responding to stimulation with organ-specific autoantigens can be tolerated and are, in fact, innocuous, as long as organ systems do not release potential autoantigens into the circulation. As long as the presence of these autoantigen-directed cells does not interfere with the reproduction of the species, the cells may be permitted to survive. Once the individual becomes expendable from the evolutionary point of view, and his demise no longer poses a threat to the perpetuation of the species, the activation of the ever present immunocompetent cells directed toward autoantigens may be countenanced. Since the autodirected immunocompetent cells are exposed to and activated by specific autoantigens with an increasing frequency in the individual as he ages as a consequence of degenerative changes, repeated insult, trauma, bacterial- and viral-induced damage, or simply normal wear and tear, autoimmune disease, with notable exceptions, increases markedly in frequency and severity with advancing years. It is a disease of the aged, not of the young. In fact, evolution might even have dictated that these cells be sustained as a means of limiting the life-span of the individual and thus preventing overpopulation which could threaten the survival of the young, sexually immature members of the species.

The explanation presented above begs the question why autoimmune diseases are not observed more frequently than they are. Certainly, if unchecked, one would expect the appearance of new clones of immunocompetent cells directed toward circulating autoantigens and the existing clones of cells directed toward organ-sequestered antigens to pose a serious threat to the survival of the individual and, therefore, the species. One would, therefore, anticipate, in strict adherence to the Darwinian theory of evolution, the development of a mechanism to annul this threat. Nature's answer appears to be the provision of clonally selected suppressor cells capable of inhibiting immune responses toward specific autoantigens.

Experimentally, an autoimmune disease affecting a specific

organ can be consistently induced in the animal only if the antigen is administered as an emulsion with complete Freund's adjuvant, which consists of killed *Mycobacterium tuberculosis*, a water-soluble fat, and an emulsifying agent. This mode of immunization is generally the method of choice to induce a cell-mediated immune response. A feature of this immunization procedure is the formation of a subcutaneous antigen depot surrounded by layers of mononuclear cells, mainly macrophage-like foam cells, some of which may appear to be binucleate and epithelioid. Mitotic figures can also be seen. Small and medium-sized lymphocytes are interspersed among the phagocytes (see Chapter 4).

If one extrapolates from the experimentally induced autoimmune disease to that which appears spontaneously in humans, it would be necessary to presume that a similar autoimmunization takes place. The necessary events, in their chronologic order of occurrence, would be: (a) trauma to a specific organ, followed by (b) a localized inflammatory response characterized by the infiltration of mononuclear, especially phagocytic, cells. The lesion would then assume a chronic state, with specific sensitization of the circulating lymphocytes (preordained or precommitted to transform into or generate sensitized cells) occurring at the site of the accessible antigen depot and not within the lymphoid organs where the humoral immune response is normally initiated. The sensitized cells would be liberated into the circulation, where they would then be detected by conventional immunologic assay.

Important

1. The results of numerous investigations have suggested that circulating autoantibodies often appear to prevent the induction of organ-specific autoimmune disease, whereas sensitized cells predispose to it. This is due not to suppression of the immune system by the circulating autoantibodies but to the competition of both the autoantibodies and the sensitized cells for the same antigenic determinants. The autoantibodies are generally not complement fixing and are, therefore, innocuous. Their sole function, it would appear, is to prevent the autoantigen from interacting with the sensitized cell and thus prevent the destructive sequelae of this reaction.

2. The autoantibodies detected following the induction of autoimmune diseases affecting particular organs are generally non-complement fixing, whereas the autoantibodies directed toward the circulating constituents are generally complement fixing and capable of inducing pathology and disease. Nature, therefore,

appears to provide the host with antibodies capable of protecting tissues and organs from reacting with specifically sensitized cells while not harming these tissues themselves due to their inability to activate complement. On the other hand, the immune system may not have anticipated the "spontaneous" emergence of forbidden clones of autoantibody-forming cells and has not yet, in an evolutionary sense, established mechanisms to prevent the highly destructive effects following the interaction of complement-fixing autoantibodies with the circulating elements (serum proteins and white blood cells).

The above scheme of the mechanism of induction of autoimmune disease is consistent with current knowledge concerning the distribution of the immediate precursors of the committed immunocompetent cells. The virgin cells which participate in the primary antibody response, the ARC and the uncommitted pre-AFC, reside in the parenchymal lymphoid organs and not in the circulation. The AFC only transiently invade the circulation at the peak of the immune response. On the other hand, the precursors of the sensitized cells in the cell-mediated immune response are present in the circulation in larger numbers, proportionately, than they are in the parenchymal lymphoid organs. These cells (a) respond with blastogenesis and mitosis upon stimulation with allogeneic cells (the MLR) or the plant mitogens phytohemagglutinin, pokeweed, or concanavalin-A; (b) constitute the cellular infiltrate in the delayed hypersensitivity skin reaction; and (c) generate or transform into cytotoxic cells in vitro. All of these diverse responses and activities are not considered to be the properties of a single pluripotent immunocompetent cell. Rather, they are properties which characterize a number of functional classes or subsets of lymphocytes, all of which participate in the cell-mediated immune response in one form or another.

CHAPTER 13

Nutrition and Immunity: The Role of Prostaglandins

A factor which is usually overlooked in the quest to understand the etiology and pathogenesis of noninfectious diseases, especially those attributed to a defective or deficient immune system, is the nutritional state of the affected individual. This is probably because good nutrition is taken for granted, especially in the Western world. We assume that the majority of people, intentionally or by chance, invariably consume a diet which provides for optimum or near optimum nutrition. Many consider it unthinkable that in North America or Europe it is possible to avoid splendidly balanced diets in view of the wide variety of easily available foods produced by the world's most efficient and productive agricultural industry. Unfortunately, the vast array of foods available to us at the supermarket is quite often highly caloric but not nutritious. Therefore, as paradoxical as it may seem, many people are in fact malnourished or undernourished, sometimes nutritionally deficient.

It is customary to consider a diet nutritious as long as the protein/calorie intake is adequate to maintain a positive nitrogen balance. The carbohydrate content is usually not stressed "as long as there is some." Only cursory attention is paid to the vitamin content of the diet, and scant or no attention is paid to the fatty acid and trace metal content.

The role which sound nutrition plays in maintaining and preserving good health has been demonstrated so unequivocally that its credibility cannot be questioned today. The role which good nutrition—which implies an adequate intake of protein, fats (essential fatty acids), vitamins, and trace metals—plays to reverse a disease state back to a healthy state is currently being investigated. Although all the evidence is not yet in, results of current investigations strongly indicate that chemotherapy may be overstressed and scientifically based nutrition undervalued and underemphasized in the treatment of a not insignificant number of diseases.

Prior to the 1970s, the practice of medicine, in the Western world at least, was totally committed to the utilization of synthetic or biologically derived drugs produced by the pharmaceutical houses to treat diseases and to reinstate a condition of good health. The role of nutrition and specific nutrients (vitamins, trace metals, fatty acids) in the treatment of conditions other than the obvious vitamin deficiency diseases was only considered in an anecdotal and cursory manner. In the late 1960s and early 1970s, it was demonstrated that certain forms of diabetes mellitus could be controlled, regulated, and stabilized without insulin or other chemotherapy by prescribing a high-fiber diet which includes large quantities of whole bran. Gastrointestinal disorders such as the "lazy gut syndrome," which may be experienced secondary to gallbladder insufficiency or for long periods following surgery, can be successfully treated and normal bowel movement restored by prescribing a diet with a high fiber content. The beneficial effects of parenteral hyperalimentation have been observed in patients with mycotic infections resistant to conventional chemotherapy. Such patients would normally succumb to the systemic mycotic infections were it not for the infusion of proteins, fatty acids, vitamins, and trace metals. Gold has long constituted a primary treatment in the attempt to relieve the pain and disfigurement of rheumatoid arthritis. The oldest specific chemotherapeutic agent, salvarsan, developed and synthesized by Ehrlich for the treatment of syphilis almost a century ago, is dependent for its effectiveness as an antibacterial agent on its content of arsenic, a trace metal.

The results of current investigations consistently indicate that proper nutrition is invaluable in the treatment of cancer. It is well known that patients who are permitted to follow their normal diets tend to lose weight as a result of diminished food intake due to lack of appetite (the result of a depressed mental state and the nausea and malaise induced by the chemotherapeutic drugs). Such patients do not tolerate the cytotoxic drugs very well, and the incidence of complications and morbidity is high. On the other hand, it has been repeatedly demonstrated recently that patients whose diets are supplemented with essential fatty acids, vitamins, and trace metals and who are subjected to intravenous hyperalimentation when necessary to achieve a positive nitrogen balance and to maintain body weight, tolerate the drugs to a much better degree and suffer fewer complications. Their general state of health is better and their mental outlook is superior as compared to patients in the control group.

It has been repeatedly observed that hospitalized patients on long-term intravenous therapy develop iatrogenic diseases due to malnutrition, especially diseases due to a deficiency of the essential fatty acids which are not usually administered intravenously with the other fluids. These diseases vary from the relatively innocuous but debilitating forms of contact dermatitis to the more serious exfoliative or bullous-type dermatitis to life-threatening leukopenia, thrombocytopenia, and anemia. The latter display many features of autoimmune thrombocytopenia and autoimmune hemolytic anemia. This syndrome, precipitated by a deficiency of the essential fatty acids, is similar to that which develops in weanling or immature rats placed on a fat-free diet. The rats grow poorly, lose hair (alopecia), lose weight, and develop splenomegaly, lymphadenopathy, and hepatomegaly. They also tend to develop an eczema-like scaly skin which can progress to frank exfoliative dermatitis. Death is usually preceded by severe leukopenia and/or anemia. A variety of autoantibodies may be detected in the circulation. This syndrome is considered to be the consequence of a panautoimmune disease due to the lack of T suppressor cells resulting from a functional thymectomy induced by a deficiency in essential fatty acids. Provided the condition has not been permitted to deteriorate too far, it can be successfully treated and permanent remission established by incorporating essential fatty acids into the daily diet.

It has been demonstrated that NZB/W F_1 hybrid mice spontaneously develop an autoimmune syndrome similar to that of patients with systemic lupus erythematosus (SLE), an autoimmune disease characterized by the presence of autoantibodies to native DNA. This disease in the mouse invariably progresses to an acute immune complex glomerulonephritis followed by renal failure, uremia, and death. There are also defects in cell-mediated immunity expressed by the affected NZB/W F_1 hybrid mice since they fail to reject allografts and transplantable tumors and their circulating lymphoid cells respond poorly to stimulation with mitogens and allogeneic cells (the MLR). There is also marked loss of cells from the T cell-dependent areas in the lymphoid tissues. The autoimmune response in these mice can be explained as a consequence of generalized loss of suppressor cells; however, the marked deficiency in the expression of the cell-mediated immune response cannot be similarly explained. At least one form of treatment of the autoimmune disease in the NZB/W mice involves the administration of prostaglandin E_1 (PGE_1).* Mice so treated exhibit a restoration of the immunologic

* The prostaglandins are a family of fatty acid derivatives numbering as many as 14 to 18 related compounds. They were called prostaglandins by von Euler in the

imbalance to normalcy and reestablishment of normal immunocompetence. Thus, the symptoms of the SLE-like syndrome abate, especially the glomerulonephritis. The mice regain the ability to respond with a cell-mediated immune response following appropriate immunization, and the circulating T cells respond to mitogen stimulation. There is also reconstitution of normal architecture in the T cell compartments of the lymph nodes and spleen and in the cortex of the thymus. Since normally the cortex houses the more immature T cells, it has been postulated that there is a maturation block of the thymic T cells in the mice which develop the SLE-like syndrome which is corrected by the administered prostaglandins.

When linoleic acid is added to the diet of NZB/W mice, especially at the age when they are most susceptible to the spontaneous emergence of the SLE-like syndrome, the animals grow normally and remain normal. Thus, the addition of an essential fatty acid to the diet of SLE-prone NZB/W mice prevents the symptoms and the disease. The substitution of nonessential saturated and monounsaturated fatty acids for linoleic acid does not result in protection of the animals to the occurrence of the disease. The explanation for this finding is that linoleic acid serves as the precursor of the prostaglandins and their immediate precursor, arachidonic acid. It is the prostaglandins and not the linoleic acid which are the active therapeutic agents in this disease. The prostaglandins can also control or ameliorate the autoimmune disease in adjuvant-induced arthritis in rats, probably via the same mechanism as they reverse the SLE-like syndrome in the NZB/W mice.

These results in the rodent indicate that immunologically mediated (autoimmune) diseases may be due to failure of prostaglandin synthesis secondary to a nutritional deficiency of essen-

---

1930s on the mistaken belief that these compounds were localized to the prostate gland and seminal fluid. Today, the prostaglandins are viewed as ubiquitous compounds found in all organs of the body, especially the pancreas, lungs, and liver.

The prostaglandins can be synthesized in vivo from the polyunsaturated essential fatty acids linoleic, linolenic, and arachidonic acid but not from the saturated and monounsaturated nonessential fatty acids. Mammals can synthesize the nonessential fatty acids from precursors but not the essential fatty acids—linoleic ($C18{:}2^{\Delta 9,\ 12}$) acid, linolenic ($C18{:}3^{\Delta 6,\ 9,\ 12}$) acid, and arachidonic ($C20{:}4^{\Delta 5,\ 8,\ 11,\ 14}$) acid. The latter is partly derived from linoleic acid in vivo (Fig. 13.1). Linoleic and linolenic acid are obtained primarily from plant sources, and arachidonic acid is obtained chiefly from meat. These fatty acids and the prostaglandin derivatives are characterized by a five-member cyclopentane ring (C8 to C12) (Fig. 13.1). The differences between the prostaglandins are due to the different constituents attached to the cyclopentane ring.

tial fatty acids. Nevertheless, until very recently, a diagnosis of nutritional deficiency was rarely entertained as the underlying cause of immunologically mediated or immunodeficiency diseases, although individuals suffering from moderate to severe malnutrition generally present with defective antibody and cell-mediated immune responses and exhibit mild to marked lymphopenia. Analysis of the lymphocytes in terms of T, B, and null cells usually reveals a severe T cell lymphopenia, normal numbers of B cells, and a null cell lymphocytosis. Furthermore, among the T cells in malnourished individuals, the proportion of cells with receptors for Fc(IgM) (T_M cells) is decreased, whereas the proportion of cells with receptors for Fc(IgG) (T_G cells) is increased. Since T_M cells have been shown to constitute the helper cells in the antibody immune response and T_G cells the suppressor cells, the shift in favor of T_G cells in the malnourished individual may explain the decrease in immune responsiveness of such individuals. It also helps to explain the greater deleterious effect of malnutrition on the primary, rather than the secondary, antibody immune response. The primary immune response, especially to T-dependent antigens, requires a T helper (or T_M) cell in addition to the B cell to facilitate antibody synthesis. Since there is a marked reduction in the T_M cells in severe malnutrition, these cells may not be present in adequate numbers to promote antibody formation. Furthermore, the increased number of T_G suppressor cells may inhibit the T_M helper cells from carrying out their functions. The suppressor cells act on the helper cells and not on the B antibody-forming cells in suppressing antibody formation (see Chapter 8). On the other hand, the secondary immune response is T cell-independent, as it does not require the mediation of T_M helper cells. It is strictly a memory B cell response. Even with an intact immune response system, a severely malnourished individual may still develop signs of clinical immunodeficiency with respect to invading pathogenic bacteria due to deficiencies in the various components of the complement system which are necessary to effect immune cytolysis of the microorganism.

The altered state of the immune system in the malnourished individual is not so much affected by the general state of malnutrition as it is by the deficiency of one or more specific nutrients. Thus, the antibody immune response is especially depressed if there is a deficiency of zinc, magnesium, ascorbic acid (vitamin C), and pyridoxine (vitamin B_6). Zinc deficiency results in a syndrome with symptoms of immunodeficiency disease. Normal immunity is restored with the oral administration of zinc (in the form of zinc sulphate). Acrodermatitis enteropathica, a systemic disease with characteristic dermatologic manifestations and a generalized immunodeficiency state, was invariably fatal due to the absence of specific therapy. However, this disease can now be totally controlled, if not cured, by the administration of the trace metal zinc, suggesting that the underlying cause of this disease is a zinc deficiency and/or a failure to store zinc. Zinc deficiency also results in progressive thymic involution and the indiscriminate loss of T cells of all classes, thus accounting for the marked defect in cell-mediated immunity. It is probably more than just a coincidence that prostaglandin synthesis from linoleic acid is also dependent upon adequate concentrations of zinc, magnesium, ascorbic acid, and pyridoxine and that the prostaglandins can correct the imbalance of T_M to T_G cells and restore normal T cell numbers and function.

Aside from specific effects which the prostaglandins may have in activating T suppressor cells and restoring the T_M and T_G cells to their normal proportions and states of activity, the prostaglandins may also influence the progression of autoimmune lesions through their effects on the inflammatory response. It will be recalled that autoimmune lesions are characterized by massive infiltration of phagocytic cells and lymphocytes. The prostaglandins of the E_1 series (PGE_1) exert antiinflammatory activity, similar to that exhibited by steroids, aspirin, and other nonsteroid anti-inflammatory agents. There is evidence that these chemotherapeutic agents act by stimulating the synthesis of the PGE_1 prostaglandins. On the other hand, the prostaglandins of the E_2 series (PGE_2) actively promote inflammation. There normally exists a feedback stimulation and inhibition interrelationship between the PGE_1 and PGE_2 prostaglandins. The PGE_1 prostaglandins are synthesized in vivo from linoleic acid, and the PGE_2 prostaglandins are synthesized in vivo from arachidonic acid in the presence of adequate levels of ascorbic acid, magnesium, zinc, and pyridoxine (Fig. 13.1). The PGE_1 prostaglandins inhibit the synthesis of the PGE_2 prostaglandins, and the PGE_2 prostaglandins stimulate the synthesis of the PGE_1 prostaglandins. However, in the absence of or a deficiency in the PGE_1 prostaglandins which may result from an inadequate intake of linoleic acid and/or excessive intake of arachidonic acid, excessive quantities of the PGE_2 prostaglandins will be synthesized. Since the PGE_2 prostaglandins actively promote inflammation, such an individual is susceptible to the development of inflammatory lesions to minimum (autoantigenic?) stimuli which can progress (or degenerate) pathologically to autoimmune lesions and clinically to autoim-

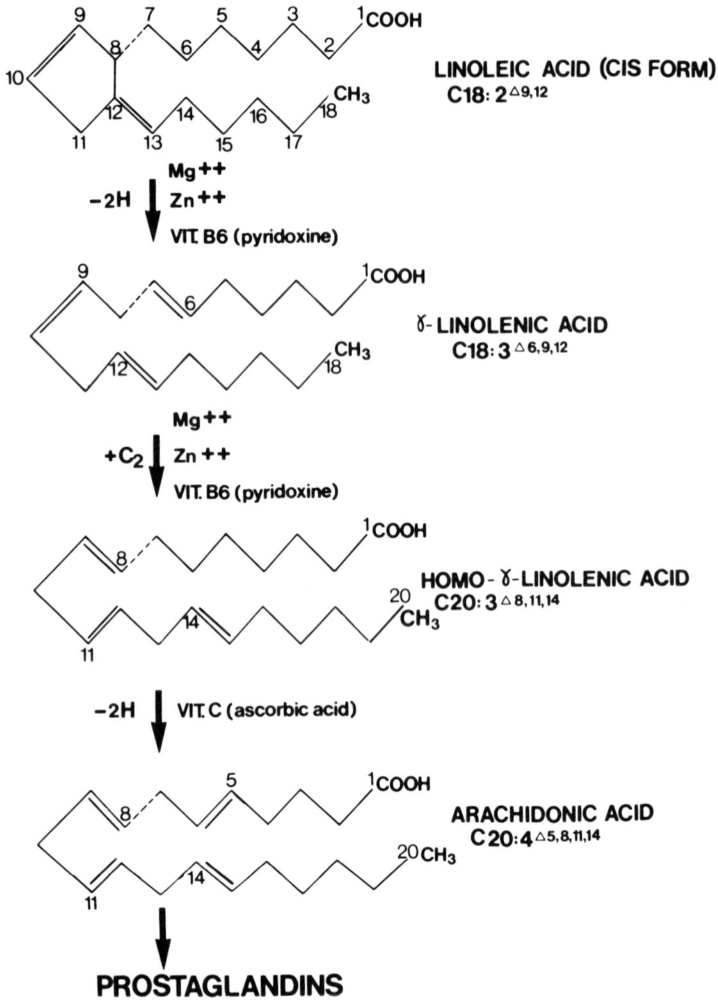

Figure 13.1 *The role of the essential fatty acids, vitamins, and trace metals in the in vivo synthesis of the prostaglandins.*

mune disease. It is, therefore, essential to ensure an adequate intake of the essential fatty acids—especially linoleic acid—in their proper proportions, ascorbic acid, zinc, magnesium, and pyridoxine in order to facilitate normal synthesis of the regulatory PGE_1 and the PGE_2 prostaglandins.

The field of nutritional immunology is a relatively new area of investigation. It is rapidly attaining respectability and credibility.

Undoubtedly, nutritionally dependent mediators or pathways for the expression of immunity remain to be discovered. It is this for the emergence of nutrition as a major vehicle in the treatment of many diseases, especially those with an immunologic etiology and pathogenesis.

CHAPTER 14

Immunopathology

The subdiscipline of immunopathology is concerned with those diseases the etiology and pathogenesis of which may be directly attributed to immune reactions (antibody or cell-mediated) or mediators released following the immune reactions. Immune reactions may lead to pathologic sequelae when the antigen is a constituent of a parenchymal cell (i.e. thyroid follicle cell, gastric parietal cell, spermatozoa), a circulating cell (i.e. erythrocyte, neutrophil, platelet), a hormone (i.e. insulin, growth hormone), a serum protein (i.e. gamma globulin), or connective tissue (i.e. collagen). Immune complexes formed as a result of the interaction between the antibody and the antigen are deposited onto the basement membranes of small blood vessels (postcapillary venules) and glomeruli. These complexes fix complement, resulting in the activation of anaphylatoxins and neutrophil chemotactic factors. Tissue damage occurs as a result of the release, locally, of histamine and highly destructive enzymes from the neutrophils chemotactically attracted to the sites of immune complex deposition. The cell-mediated immune reaction is not by itself destructive, but mediators released from the sensitized cells following interaction with the sensitizing antigen facilitate the tissue-destructive reactions.

Important

It must be emphasized again that the primary union of antigen with antibody or sensitized cell does not in itself induce pathology. Rather, it is the activation of complement and the production and release of pharmacologically active mediators which induce tissue damage.

The immune reactions which result in pathologic sequelae have been classified as Types I, II, III, and IV by Coombs and Gell, and Roitt. Types V, VI, and VII reactions have only recently been described (Table 14.1). A more detailed description of the diseases resulting from the immune reactions in vivo is presented in Table 14.2.

Table 14.1
A Classification of Immune Reactions with Potential Pathologic Sequelae

Reaction or Response	Pathologic Immunity (Immunopathology) ←	Immune Response	→ Normal Immunity (Resistance)
Type I—Clinical allergy IgE mediated Immediate skin reaction	Hay fever, asthma, food allergy, urticaria, angioedema, insect bite allergy, drug allergy, anaphylaxis	Humoral immunity (antibody mediated)	Resistance to most bacteria Resistance to some viruses Toxin-neutralizing activity
Type II—Autoimmune disease IgG mediated	Autoimmune hemolytic anemia, idiopathic thrombocytopenic purpura, pernicious anemia, thyroiditis		
Type III—Immune complex disease Arthus skin reaction	Glomerulonephritis, serum sickness, extrinsic allergic alveolitis, intrinsic bronchopulmonary aspergillosis		
Type V—Hyperreactive state IgG mediated	Hyperthyroidism		
Type VI—Antibody-dependent cell cytotoxicity (ADCC)	Rejection of allograft, autoimmune disease		
Type IV—Cell-mediated reactions Delayed hypersensitivity (skin) reaction	Rejection of allograft; cavitation and caseation of lung in tuberculosis; autoimmune diseases (orchitis, thyroiditis, ulcerative colitis, encephalomyelitis); contact dermatitis; graft versus host reaction	Cellular immunity (mononuclear cell mediated)	Cancer immunity Resistance to some bacteria (*M. tuberculosis*) Resistance to most viruses Resistance to fungi Resistance to parasites
Type VI—Antibody-dependent cell cytotoxicity (ADCC)	Rejection of allograft, autoimmune disease		
Type VII—Naturally occurring, antibody-independent cell cytotoxicity (NOCC)			Cancer immunity (to mutant cells) (immunologic surveillance)

Table 14.2
Some Properties Characteristic of Immune Reactions Initiating Pathologic Sequelae*

Type of Reaction	Pseudonym	Primary Mediators	Secondary Mediators	Characteristic Features	Diseases Mediated by or a Consequence of the Reaction
Type I	Allergy	IgE antibodies	histamine serotonin SRS-A+ ECF++	1. Non-complement-fixing reaction 2. Mast cell degranulation consequent to interaction of allergen with mast cell-IgE antibody complex, resulting in the release of histamine, serotonin, acetylcholine, heparin, SRS-A, ECF	Clinical allergy: hay fever, asthma, anaphylactic reactions to drugs
Type II(A)	Autoimmune disease	IgG antibodies	complement	1. IgG cytotoxic antibodies directed toward autologous cell membrane antigens 2. Complement-fixing reaction	Autoimmune diseases: SLE, AIHA, ITP
Type II(B)	Autoimmune disease	IgG antibodies		IgG antibodies directed toward non-cell surface antigens, i.e. hormones, DNA, gamma globulin, connective tissue	Autoimmune diseases: SLE, rheumatoid arthritis, diabetes mellitus, pernicious anemia, myasthenia gravis
Type III	Immune complex disease	IgG antibodies	complement neutrophils	1. Circulating complexes composed of IgG antibody and antigen 2. Immune complexes are deposited along or in intima of vessel wall and glomerular basement membrane. Complement is fixed resulting in release of neutrophil chemotactic factor. Infiltration of neutrophils results in release of proteolytic enzymes which induce a marked inflammatory response.	Immune complex disease: serum sickness, poststreptococcal glomerulonephritis, "Masugi-type" glomerulonephritis
Type IV	Cell-mediated immunity—"delayed hypersensitivity"	Sensitized lymphocytes	lymphokines	"Sensitized" lymphocytes are formed as a result of contact with specific antigen (autoantigen or microorganism). These cells interact directly with antigen, resulting in the release of lymphokines	Autoimmune disease: Hashimoto thyroiditis, postvaccinal encephalomyelitis Allograft rejection

				which mediate the reaction. Antibodies are not involved.	
Type V	Stimulatory immune reactions	IgG antibodies		Interactions between non-complement-fixing antibodies and cell surface antigens induces transformation and mitosis of cells and increased metabolism. If target is thyroid follicle, result is hyperplasia of thyroid follicle cells and increased secretion of thyroxin. Antibody has mistakenly been referred to as "LATS" (long acting thyroid stimulator).	Endocrinopathy: hyperthyroidism, Cushing's disease?, hyperpituitary syndromes?
Type VI	Antibody-dependent cellular cytotoxic reactions (ADCC)	Fc receptor-bearing lymphocyte		Normally circulating lymphocyte (not induced) capable of inducing cytolysis of target cell subsequent to interaction of target cell with specific antibody. Cytotoxic lymphocyte interacts with the Fc region of "cell-fixed" antibody via its Fc receptor, triggering changes in cell membrane and culminating in osmotic lysis.	Autoimmune diseases: thyroiditis Allograft rejection
Type VII	Naturally occurring antibody-independent cellular cytotoxic reactions (NOCC)	Undesignated lymphocyte		Normally circulating lymphocyte (not induced) capable of inducing cytolysis of target cells without the mediation of detectable antibodies. Target cells may be mutant (premalignant?) cells or overt malignant cells.	Prevention of primary malignancy and/or metastases

* SRS-A, slow reacting substance of anaphylaxis; ECF, eosinophil chemotactic factor; SLE, systemic lupus erythematosus; AIHA, autoimmune hemolytic anemia; ITP, idiopathic thrombocytopenic purpura.

TYPE I REACTIONS: IgE-MEDIATED ALLERGIC REACTIONS (DISEASES MEDIATED BY IgE ANTIBODIES)

Type I reactions constitute those immune reactions which are initiated by IgE antibodies and mediated by mast cell degranulation products (histamine, serotonin, slow reacting substance of anaphylaxis (SRS-A), and eosinophil chemotactic factor (ECF)). The clinical conditions which present include hay fever, asthma, urticaria, dust allergy, insect bite allergy, food allergy, drug allergy, photo or light allergy, and allergy to heat and cold. Type I reactions have been recorded toward (a) many foods (especially eggs, chocolate, shellfish, oysters, shrimp, nuts); (b) contaminants in the air; (c) products used to cleanse or beautify our bodies (aerosols, detergents, cosmetics); (d) constituents of common house dust (mites), pets (dog and cat dander, bird droppings); (e) insect stings (bees, yellow-jackets, hornets, wasps, red ants, black flies, mosquitos); (f) flower, tree, and weed pollen; and (g) drugs. The latter include the antibiotics, antifungal and antiprotozoal agents, sedatives, hypnotics, tranquilizers, anticonvulsants, central nervous system stimulants (analeptics, convulsants), antidepressants, psychotropics, narcotics, antihypertensives, anesthetics (local and systemic), radiocontrast solutions, and hormones. Even the common aspirin (acetylsalicylic acid) is capable of provoking an allergic response (aspirin-induced allergic rhinitis and asthma).

The majority of Type I reactions, although alarming and often frightening to the patient, do not constitute life-threatening situations and resolve without ontoward sequelae when treated in the appropriate manner. A minority of Type I reactions may become life threatening as a result of (a) systemic anaphylaxis resulting in cardiovascular collapse and shock (circulatory failure); or (b) localized anaphylaxis in the respiratory tract, resulting in acute asthma which may lead to status asthmaticus and death due to asphyxiation (respiratory failure).

All Type I reactions result in the illnesses classified under the heading of "clinical allergy." These illnesses are also referred to collectively as atopic diseases (from the Greek atopus—strange or out of place). The systems or organs affected include the upper and lower respiratory tract (rhinitis, hay fever, and asthma), the gastrointestinal tract (food allergy), the skin (allergic skin rashes which are often dermatologic manifestations of underlying drug allergy), and the cardiovascular system (systemic anaphylaxis). However, it should be stressed that not all allergies are caused by a Type I reaction. For example, contact dermatitis is caused by a Type IV reaction (see below).

The most common allergy in North America is hay fever, especially ragweed hay fever. About 5 to 10% of the population develop this condition following exposure to ragweed pollen. However, the term "hay fever" is a misnomer, as it implies a fever induced by hay. The initial description of hay fever is credited to Blackley in England in 1865. However, he was probably referring to farmer's lung, one of a large number of diseases classified under the category "extrinsic allergic alveolitis," rather than what is currently referred to as "hay fever" which is characterized by rhinitis, conjunctivitis, and recurrent bouts of sneezing. Extrinsic allergic alveolitis (EAA) is mediated by immune complexes and not by IgE antibodies (see Type III reactions). It is induced by the immune response (IgG antibodies) to fungal spores in moldy **hay**, animal and plant dust particles, industrial dust particles, etc. Farmer's lung, observed primarily in farmers, and considered to be an occupational disease, is a specific type of EAA characterized by respiratory distress following continuous intense exposure to moldy hay. Symptoms generally tend to occur 2 to 8 hours following exposure and include cough (sometimes very intense), chills, malaise, muscle pains, anorexia, weight loss, progressive dyspnea, and **fever**. Hence the term **hay fever**.

The inciting agent, in discussing the allergic state, is referred to as the **allergen** (in contradistinction to the term antigen), and the IgE antibody formed in response to it has been referred to in the past as **reagin, skin-sensitizing antibody**, or **homocytotropic** (affinity for cells) **antibody**. This antibody has a marked affinity for mast cells and basophils. Subsequent interaction of this cell-fixed antibody with the specific allergen (Fig. 14.1) results in the liberation of vasoactive amines (histamine, serotonin) (see below) which induce local vasodilatation and increased capillary permeability. Intradermal challenge with the allergen induces an **im-**

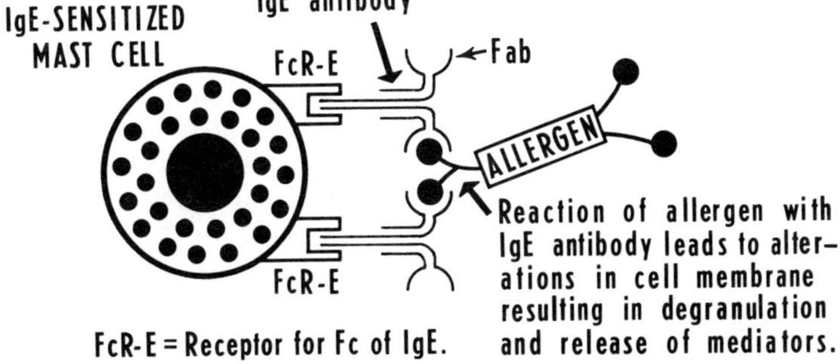

Figure 14.1 *The IgE antibody-allergen reaction on the mast cell surface and the consequence of this interaction.*

mediate skin reaction which is characterized by pruritis. A "wheal" (a white, raised, circumscribed swelling, a localized urticaria characterized by a transudate) is formed within minutes, and it is quickly surrounded by an erythema, referred to as a "flare" (localized hyperemia due to arteriolar dilatation). The reaction reaches its peak within 10 to 20 minutes accompanied by constant pruritis, and subsides to the normal state within 1 to 2 hours. There is no residual tissue damage. This reaction can be duplicated exactly by the intradermal injection of histamine. (The reader is referred to Chapter 7 for a discussion of the different skin reactions.)

Although the immediate skin reaction, following scratch or intradermal challenge with the allergen, has been utilized since the 1870s in the diagnosis of the allergic state, it was not until the mid-1920s that it was demonstrated by Prausnitz and Kustner that reagin circulates in the blood. These two investigators demonstrated that the serum of an allergic individual can sensitize the skin of a normal individual. Challenge of the "sensitized" skin site with the allergen to which the donor is sensitive results in an immediate skin reaction identical to that induced in the skin of the allergic individual. This test is referred to as the passive transfer or P-K (Prausnitz-Kustner) test.

The allergic state is a consequence of the formation of IgE antibodies to a host of innocuous, noninvasive, nonreplicating, and nontoxic substances or allergens which are either inhaled (grass, tree and plant pollen, fungal spores, dried animal fecal matter), ingested (parasites, foods), or injected (drugs, antibiotics). Only a small proportion of the population exposed to these substances will form IgE antibodies to them. The rest of the population (90 to 95%) will not respond at all. The individuals constituting the responding population are considered to be genetically disposed, to have a predisposition, to respond with the formation of IgE antibodies toward these agents. Obviously, initial contact with the allergen is required in order to trigger this IgE response.

The IgE antibodies secreted into the circulation by the stimulated lymphoblasts (or plasmablasts) adhere predominantly to the surfaces of mast cells and basophils. This adherence of the IgE antibodies to these cells is facilitated by the presence of Fc receptors on the surfaces of these cells specific for the Fc region of the IgE molecule. The cell-bound IgE antibody molecules are only slowly metabolized and can be found "stuck" to the mast cells months to a year after their synthesis. The mast cells are considered to be "sensitized" as a result of their being coated with the IgE antibodies (which, it must be remembered, are not directed to antigens on the mast cell surface but toward extrinsic antigens). If the individual is then exposed to the original sensitizing allergen, i.e. ragweed pollen, inhalation of the pollen will be quickly followed by absorption of solubilized components of the pollen, the allergens, through the mucous membrane of the respiratory tract where they will confront the mast cells coated with the specific IgE antibodies. These cells are packed with metachromatically staining granules containing highly potent vasoactive amines (histamine, serotonin), heparin, eosinophil chemotactic factor (ECF-A), etc. Interaction of the allergens with the Fab sites on these IgE antibodies results in reversible alterations of the mast cell membrane with the formation of intramembranous lesions or "holes" which may culminate in osmotic lysis of these cells. Irrespective of whether the mast cell is reversibly or irreversibly damaged, the granules will be disrupted and their contents released into the microenvironment of the cells, as well as in the secretions, and induce (a) contraction of smooth muscle; (b) increased capillary dilatation, resulting in hyperemia and engorgement with blood; (c) increased capillary permeability, causing transudation of fluid resulting in edema of the mucous membrane; (d) increased secretion of mucus by the mucus-secreting goblet cells; and (e) massive infiltration of eosinophils.

In addition to the mediators enumerated above, other mediators are also released from mast cell granules or activated from circulating precursor proteins. These are slow reacting substance of anaphylaxis (SRS-A) (from mast cells or adjacent cells), anaphylatoxin, and bradykinin (from precursor serum proteins or peptides).

All of the symptoms one sees in the allergic patient can be deduced from the actions of these mediators. The severity of the allergic reaction is governed by (a) the concentration of IgE antibodies coating the mast cells; (b) the susceptibility of the sensitized mast cells to degranulation; (c) the sensitivity of the target cells to the mediators released; and (d) the concentration of circulating enzymes capable of inactivating or neutralizing the mediators.

The eosinophilia which infiltrates the allergic reaction site secrete enzymes which degrade SRS-A, histamine, and kinins. The cells therefore appear to have a protective, and not pathologic, role—to localize the allergic reaction by preventing systemic spread of the mediators.

Important

1. The reaction between the allergen and the specific IgE antibody does not involve complement.

2. For degranulation of the sensitized mast cell to occur, the allergen must bridge *two* adjacent IgE antibodies via their Fab

sites. Otherwise, degranulation will not occur. In other words, the mast cell requires two simultaneous signals, and not a single signal, to initiate the degranulation reaction (see Fig. 14.1).

The reader may question why the triggering mechanism should require the bridging to two adjacent IgE antibody molecules by the allergen and not simply the interaction of a single IgE antibody molecule with the allergen. The interpretation which appears to have gained most acceptance is that the requirement for two signals constitutes a safety feature in the absence of which the mediators would be constantly secreted by the mast cells due to the myriad of different nonspecific stimuli to which the cells would be constantly subjected. The two-signal response ensures that nonspecific, unintentional, or inadvertent stimuli will not trigger the mast cells to secrete their content of the powerful pharmacologically active mediators.

Lest the reader consider that this two-signal, rather than the one-signal, response is one which has evolved only in the higher vertebrates, it should be pointed out that plants also utilize the two-signal mechanism very effectively. The venus fly-trap, a carniverous plant but a plant nonetheless, will snap shut over an unsuspecting fly or insect only after two of its internal sensitive hairs are stimulated simultaneously by the invader. Stimulation of only a single hair will produce no response. This ensures that the repeated "innocent" stimulation of a single hair, which can be effected by wind alone, will not send the plant into repetitive, exhausting convulsions.

We should, therefore, humbly conclude that the two-signal response mechanism evolved first among plants and was subsequently adopted by the animal kingdom.

Urticaria

The second most common manifestation of an allergic diathesis is urticaria or hives. Urticarial lesions may be localized or widespread. They are either induced by specific allergens—such as insect bites, cosmetics, foods, drugs, detergents, and simple chemicals (trace metals)—or they can be induced by nonspecific agents (intrinsic and extrinsic for which a cause-effect relationship is very difficult to establish). Urticaria due to a specific allergen is usually an acute, self-limiting condition and occurs only at the time of exposure to the allergen. It is a true allergic response and may be considered to constitute an anaphylactic reaction localized to the skin. The mediators involved in the induction of this reaction are identical to those which mediate hay fever and asthma. On the other hand, the urticarial reactions induced by nonspecific (nonimmunologic) agents are considered to be idiopathic, especially in instances when no etiologic agent can be identified, and the mechanism of the reaction and the mediators involved are obscure and speculative.

A urticarial lesion is a localized, red, warm, clearly demarcated raised area of the skin, resembling a large wheal. The fluid beneath the elevated epidermis is a sterile transudate facilitated by a marked increase in vascular permeability. It is basically a cell-free proteinaceous fluid. The reaction is invariably accompanied by intense pruritis. The lesion(s) may last for several hours to several days and resolve by resorption of the transudate.

The most common cause of allergic urticaria is food allergy, with drug allergy becoming more and more frequent as a primary cause. Urticaria may be produced irrespective of whether exposure to the offending allergen is via the mouth, the nose, or the skin. Urticarial eruptions are frequently encountered following repeated bites by common insects such as mosquitoes, lice, bedbugs, bees, wasps, hornets, and yellow jackets. In some individuals, infection with certain bacteria, viruses, and parasites is accompanied by hives.

Urticaria may also be induced by nonimmunologic causes such as heat and cold applied locally, pressure, and direct exposure to the sun. The mechanism whereby these agents induce the urticaria is not known. This form of urticaria can often be transferred with serum from sensitive individuals. It is, therefore, obvious that in the affected individual, the mast cell-bound nonantibody IgE immunoglobulins respond to the physical agents in much the same way as the mast cell-bound antibody IgE immunoglobulins respond in the presence of the specific allergen. The result is that degranulation occurs accompanied by release of histamine, serotonin, ECF, and SRS-A.

Another form of urticaria quite distinct from that induced by specific allergens or physical agents is that induced by emotional stress, a warm bath, or intense exercise. The urticaria in these individuals takes the shape of very small macular or papular wheals. Since challenge of these individuals with either mecholyl or acetylcholine invariably induces a similar lesion, this form of urticaria is often referred to as cholinergic urticaria. This urticaria, also referred to as generalized heat urticaria, may be related to the exercise (exertion)-induced anaphylactic syndrome. An anaphylactic-like shock may occur in individuals following intense exercise such as jogging, rowing, swimming, or tennis. Aside from the urticarial rash, the symptoms may include systemic manifestations such as abdominal pain, wheezing due to bronchial obstruction, and syncope due to vascular collapse. Treatment of the attack is identical to that for allergen-induced anaphylactic shock. Epinephrine should be administered intramuscularly if the hypotension persists for any period of time along with the appropriate fluids and oxygen. Life-threatening laryngeal edema requires emergency tracheotomy. The urticaria can be successfully treated with conventional antihistamines. It may be necessary to administer corticosteroids via the intravenous fluids should the response to these emergency measures be considered inadequate or sluggish. It is most important that the individual limit his exercise program to avoid these life-threatening anaphylactic episodes.

Important

1. Urticaria should not be confused with angioneurotic edema which is characterized by painless, nonpruritic swellings in the subcutaneous tissues. These lesions usually occur around the eyes, lips, and tongue, although they may occur with lesser or greater severity throughout the body. The hereditary form of angioedema is associated with a severe deficiency in circulating C′1-esterase inhibitor. This results in the uncontrolled and unpredictable activation of the complement system with the ensuing activation of kinins and anaphylatoxin from circulating protein precursors. Anaphylatoxin can induce the release of histamine from mast cells. These agents, therefore, act in a manner similar to histamine, causing smooth muscle contraction, generalized vasodilatation, and increased capillary permeability. Laryngeal edema may be life threatening unless treated promptly and aggressively.

2. Urticaria is often associated with systemic diseases of a nonallergic nature. These include neoplastic diseases such as Hodgkin's disease and lymphomas and immune-complex diseases such as systemic lupus erythematosus. The occurrence of cold urticaria suggests multiple myeloma, cryoglobulinemia, macroglobulinemia, and syphilis.

Animal Models

Are there prototypes or models for the allergic state in humans? Yes, but it is not anaphylaxis in the guinea pig which has mistakenly been considered to be *the* model for human clinical allergy (asthma). Generally overlooked is a condition in the horse called heaves which resembles human upper respiratory allergy in terms of etiology and pathogenesis better than does anaphylactic shock in the guinea pig. A relationship between guinea pig anaphylaxis and human asthma does exist on superficial analysis. However, on the basis of recent findings (1960–1976) concerning the etiology and pathogenesis of asthma, anaphylaxis in the guinea pig must be discarded as a working model for the human disease (see below).

What is the history of anaphylaxis and how was it discovered? Portier and Richet, two eminent French scientists (and immunologists) conducted a study, in the mid-1890s, of the toxic properties of jellyfish and sea anemones in the Mediterranean Sea off the south of France, the area which includes Nice and the Riviera and adjacent Monaco. The investigation was initiated during a cruise on the yacht of Prince Albert of Monaco. What inspired this investigation is not clear, although there are indications that the French government was very concerned about reports of sudden death among bathers along the seacoast and was very apprehensive of the adverse effects such news would have on the tourist industry if the causes for these deaths were not resolved. A more mundane explanation may be that the sea-bathing activities of the Prince of Monaco were hampered by these sea creatures. In any event, Portier and Richet prepared extracts from the tentacles of sea anemones and injected them into dogs, expecting the animals to die and thus demonstrate the toxic properties of anemones.

However, they were surprised when the dogs did not die even after massive injections with the anemone extract. In fact, many of the dogs did not even become ill. Less astute investigators might have given up right then and there. But Portier and Richet maintained the dogs for several weeks and decided, for reasons which are not obvious from the historical accounts of their work, to reinject the same dogs with the extract. All the dogs now became severely ill and most died within hours of the injection. Furthermore, the administration of even minute amounts of the extract was now capable of causing death in these dogs, whereas the injection of much larger amounts into fresh dogs was essentially innocuous and was not accompanied by immediate or delayed morbidity. Portier and Richet correctly concluded that the deaths could not be attributed to any toxic components of the extract but rather to an abnormal response of the host to the extract which manifests itself only upon the second or challenge injection of the material. They, therefore, coined this reaction **anaphylaxis** (ana—counter to; phylaxis—protection). The student should realize that there was no precedent for this reaction in the literature at the time, and this was indeed a major discovery for which a Nobel Prize was subsequently awarded.

Why did the dogs not die after the first injection of a large quantity of the extract, whereas they uniformly died within hours after a second administration of minute quantities of the extract 2 to 3 weeks after the first injection? The explanation appears to be as follows. The dog responds with antibody formation to the antigens in the extract within 1 to 2 weeks following its initial administration, just as it does to any other antigen. These antibodies circulate for several weeks and, if the animal is challenged with the original antigen intravenously during this period, the intravascular antigen-antibody reaction will result in the generation of vasoactive amines capable of causing smooth muscle constriction and increased capillary permeability. In the dog, the organ which appears to be the primary target for these mediators is the hepatic vein. Constriction of the smooth muscle in the wall of the hepatic vein causes engorgement of blood in the liver. Venous diastolic pressure increases, hepatic circulation diminishes markedly, and hypoxia results followed by massive hepatic necrosis with focal hemorrhagic areas. The dog dies as a result of massive internal bleeding.

It is interesting to note that Portier and Richet discovered anaphylaxis using the dog, an animal in which it is normally very difficult to induce this condition. They were very fortunate to have had at their disposal a strain of dogs which was susceptible to the induction of anaphylaxis. It should be recognized by the reader that the induction of fatal anaphylaxis in the dog is the result of a planned, contrived laboratory experiment. Normally, a dog would not be exposed to the same antigen within 2 weeks, and certainly the second exposure to the antigen would not normally be via the intravascular route. Subsequent to its discovery by Portier and Richet, other investigators reproduced anaphylaxis in other animal species, notably the guinea pig, which exhibits an exquisite susceptibility to the induction of anaphylaxis. Like the dog, the guinea pig displays no discomfort following the initial or **sensitizing injection** of the antigen. However, following the second or **challenge injection** of the identical antigen, given intravenously, the guinea pig immediately exhibits signs of apprehension and distress, the respiratory rate increases dramatically, and the breathing becomes more and more shallow and labored. Inspiration is much more difficult than expiration. Rhonchi and stridor become evident. The animal will retreat to a corner, become visibly cyanotic, scratch itself all over due to intense pruritis, defecate and urinate uncontrollably, begin to gasp, and die as a result of respiratory failure. This will all occur within 1 to 5 minutes following the challenge injection. At necropsy, the lungs are hyperinflated and float on water. On microscopic analysis, there is destruction of alveolar septa and morphologic evidence of pathologic emphysema.

The anaphylactic reaction in the guinea pig has fascinated immunologists since its description at the turn of the 20th century. It has been unequivocally demonstrated that it is not due to the interaction of antigen with circulating antibodies but that it is the consequence of the interaction between the antigen and cell-bound antibodies located on mast cells within the respiratory epithelium. Like in humans, this interaction results in degranulation of the mast cells and release of histamine, serotonin, etc., which cause bronchostriction and a clinical picture which certainly resembles human asthma. There the similarity ends. The antibody involved in the guinea pig is an IgG-2, not an IgE. The guinea pig can only be subjected to anaphylactic shock if challenged with the antigen over a specified period of time following sensitization—about 2 to 4 weeks. Challenge of the guinea pig prior to 7 days or more than 35 days postsensitization will result in few or no signs of anaphylactic shock. Furthermore, all soluble antigens can induce anaphylaxis in the guinea pig, whereas this does not appear to be true in the human. *All* guinea pigs exposed to the antigen in the manner described above will display symptoms of anaphylaxis, whereas *only a small percentage* of humans exposed to the allergen will develop an allergic diathesis, i.e. hay fever or asthma. The reaction in the guinea pig is an acute reaction, while that in the human is more chronic and protracted in its development.

Within several years following the description of anaphylaxis, it was observed that the guinea pig could be **desensitized** to anaphylactic shock if given small nonshocking doses of the antigen at 2- to 4-hour intervals beginning 24 to 36 hours prior to administration of the shocking dose (the challenge injection). The effect of the repeated injections of small quantities of the antigen is to neutralize the mast cell-bound antibodies in an incremental fashion, resulting in the release of insufficient histamine at any one time to shock the animal. After four to six of these desensitizing injections, most of the cell-bound antibodies are neutralized and there are insufficient cell-bound antibodies to interact with the antigen when it is administered in a large shocking dose which normally ensures the release of the mediators in pharmacologically active quantities. Since the desensitization procedure does not inhibit antibody formation to the antigen but only facilitates antibody neutralization in an orderly, controlled, graded manner, the animal becomes exquisitely sensitized to anaphylactic shock once more after the desensitization protocol is terminated. Nevertheless, the similarity of the clinical pictures of guinea pig anaphylaxis and human asthma prompted Noon, a British allergist, in 1911 to prescribe desensitization as a treatment for asthma and hay fever.

TREATMENT OF ALLERGIC DISEASE

Desensitization Treatment and Its Mechanism of Action

Desensitization consisted of frequent injections of the allergen in small doses during the few months preceding the allergy season. Dramatic claims of a positive, beneficial nature were initially made on behalf of the desensitization procedure in terms of its efficacy in the alleviation and eradication of allergic symptoms, and this mode of treatment rapidly gained credibility and acceptance by allergists. The claims were accepted at face value and were not scientifically validated. Today, approximately 70 years after its introduction, desensitization is still the method of choice in the treatment of the common IgE-mediated allergies. What is the scientific basis for the faithful adherence to this mode of therapy, and what are the alternative modes of treatment?

In point of fact, there were initially few objective in vitro or in vivo criteria with which to evaluate the benefits of the desensitization treatment since no one understood even remotely the nature of the allergic reaction. There was little advance in our knowledge between 1875, when Blackley demonstrated a relationship between allergy and skin reactivity, and 1923, when Prausnitz and Kustner demonstrated the presence of a skin-sensitizing factor (reagin) in the circulation of allergic, but not normal, individuals.

By the mid-1930s, it was assumed that the symptomatology characterizing the allergic state is inextricably related to the presence and activity of reagin in the circulation and that desensitization results in a lowering of the concentration of reagin in the circulation. However, when investigators finally attempted to relate reagin concentration with the clinical state following desensitization treatment, it was observed that, contrary to expectations, the reagin titer did *not* go down immediately following desensitization treatment; in most cases it increased in concentration and in some it remained stable. In only a small minority of cases did reagin concentration decrease. Thus, the rational basis for the desensitization treatment appeared to be in jeopardy.

At this time (1925–1940) the major research in allergy was conducted at the Roosevelt Hospital, New York City, first under the direction of the late Dr. Robert Cooke, and later the late Dr. William Sherman. These investigators discovered the presence of a second factor in addition to reagin specific to the circulation of the allergic individuals which they named **blocking factor**. This factor was shown to be capable of competing with reagin for the same site on the allergen in the conventional passive transfer test in the skin. However, the result of its interaction with the allergen did not result in a skin reaction in the host and did not lead to the release of histamine, serotonin, etc. It appeared to block the reaction between reagin and the allergen. The beneficial results of desensitization treatment were attributed to the induced synthesis of the blocking factor which was not detected in the circulation of normal individuals or in the circulation of allergic nondesensitized individuals; it could only be detected in the blood of desensitized allergic patients. Studies were carried out in the 1940s to determine the role of blocking factor. It was demonstrated that a definite link existed between desensitization and improvement of clinical symptoms, on the one hand, and the appearance of blocking factor, on the other. This reliance on blocking factor as the justification for desensitization treatment lasted until the 1950s, when it was demonstrated, in double-blind studies, that no relationship exists between the concentration of blocking factor, on the one hand, and any subjective improvement of the patient following desensitization therapy, on the other. It was found that approximately 33% of the patients improved, 33% reported a worsening in their allergic state, and 33% reported neither a worsening nor improvement in their condition following desensitization treatment, irrespective of what the accepted indicators, such as reagin and blocking factor concentrations, might suggest. It was also demonstrated that the blocking factor is an IgG antibody, like other protective antibodies formed in response to antigenic stimulation. The blocking factor was therefore renamed **blocking antibody.** Another finding was the existence of yet a third factor in the blood of the treated or untreated allergic individual which could agglutinate red blood cells coated with the identified offending allergen. This factor is also an IgG antibody, distinct from reagin and blocking antibody, and is referred to as **hemagglutinating antibody**. However, here again, no relationship has been demonstrated between the circulating concentration of hemagglutinating antibody and the subjective assessment of clinical symptoms following desensitization treatment.

The most recent and most revealing findings as to the nature of reagin were made by K. and T. Ishizaka in the late 1960s. They discovered that reagin is also an antibody but of the IgE type and that IgE antibodies tend to adhere, via receptors, to the surface of the mast cell. Following its interaction with the allergen, structural changes are induced in the mast cell membrane resulting in transmembraneous lesions or holes, alteration of the sodium-potassium pump and degranulation of the cell, resulting in the release of histamine, serotonin, ECF-A etc. These pharmacologic agents, as discussed above, induce the symptoms so characteristic of hay fever, asthma, and systemic anaphylaxis.

Thus, it might appear that we have come full circle with respect to our understanding of the immunologic mechanisms involved in the induction and expression of the allergic state. However, the goal of achieving a truly clinical withdrawal of allergic symptoms has proven to be a very elusive one. Desensitization therapy, hardly changed from that introduced by Noon in 1911, is still considered appropriate due more to the failure of chemotherapy to eradicate the allergic state than to the anticipated benefits obtained from this form of treatment.

Lest the reader feel that I have been excessively critical of the desensitization treatment and have condemned it to oblivion, let him take heart. Recent findings have shown that although the IgE antibody concentration does indeed rise during the first few years of desensitization, it drops dramatically after 6 to 8 years of this treatment. The clinical condition of the patient is also usually markedly improved after this time. The current interpretation for these findings is that the IgE antibodies are produced by selective clones of lymphoid cells and that these clones are exhausted and depleted following intensive continuous stimulation for 6 to 8 years. Thus, the prospect of long-term benefit may yet provide the raison d'etre for the desensitization therapy.

Desensitization treatment is the only treatment currently practiced which can justifiably be referred to as **immunotherapy**, since the individual is injected with antigens (or allergens) in order to effect a change in his immunologic responsiveness to these antigens. The term immunotherapy is incorrectly used by many oncologists who subject their patients to adjuvants in order to enchance or augment the cell-mediated immune response. This form of therapy should be designated as **adjuvant therapy** (see Chapter 16).

It is essential that the reader recognize that the term desensitization has a different operational meaning when it is applied to the treatment of hay fever or asthma as compared to when it is applied to the treatment of allergy to drugs, i.e. penicillin. In the former instance, desensitization is a long, drawn-out procedure aimed at diminishing the patient's sensitivity to the allergen after several years of treatment. In the case of drug allergy, desensitization is a short-term procedure, aimed at eliminating the patient's sensitivity to the particular drug within a time frame of only 1 to 2 days. A patient with subacute bacterial endocarditis or rheumatic heart disease requires intermittent prophylactic treatment with penicillin. The probability of such a patient developing an IgE-mediated allergy to penicillin is markedly greater than in the population at large. Should such a patient develop an IgE-mediated allergy to penicillin, he must be rapidly desensitized to it before further administration of penicillin is attempted. Desensitization treatment takes the form of a continuous intravenous drip of penicillin in isotonic saline. The concentration of the penicillin is initially very low, but it is gradually increased in an incremental fashion every 2 to 3 hours, providing all vital signs are stable, especially the blood pressure. By 24 to 36 hours, the concentration of the penicillin can usually be adjusted to be therapeutically effective. From this point on, the patient may take the penicillin three or four times daily, as directed, for as long as is required. However, it is essential that he take it according to a rigorously controlled schedule and that the penicillin be taken at least twice per day.

During the infusion (desensitization) period, the attending physician must continually monitor the vital signs, especially the blood pressure, in the event that a systemic anaphylactic shock is iatrogenically induced as a consequence of too rapid infusion of the penicillin. One must be prepared to intervene at any time to allay or prevent vascular collapse and shock by administering epinephrine intramuscularly every 15 to 20 minutes until the blood pressure is stabilized.

The effect of the desensitization is to neutralize the mast cell-bound IgE antibodies directed to penicillin as rapidly as possible without causing a systemic allergic reaction. Usually, the patient will be able to tolerate high doses of penicillin within 48 hours of initiation of the desensitization procedure.

A similar form of desensitization procedure can be instituted with respect to any drug which must be administered to a patient who is suspected of being allergic to it.

Drug Treatment in Allergic Disease

Most drugs used in the treatment of allergic disease in the nonacute or non-life-threatening stage (the drug indicated in the treatment of systemic anaphylaxis and the acute protracted asthmatic attack is adrenalin injected intramuscularly) fall into the broad categories of steroids (cortisone, prednisone, prednisolone, dexamethasone), antihistamines (Pyribenzamine, Benedryl, Phenergan, Actifed, Chlortripolon), xanthines (theophylline, aminophylline), sympathomimetic (adrenergic) drugs (isoproterenol, isoprenaline, adrenaline), and competitive inhibitors of adrenaline-inactivating enzymes, such as ephedrine. Newer classes of drugs include those which are primarily beta-2 adrenergic agonists, such as salbutamol, metaproterenol, and terbutaline. A number of topical corticosteroid derivatives such as beclomethesone, are given as an aerosol (for asthma) or by insufflation (for allergic rhinitis). These have minimal side effects because they are not absorbed to any great extent. However, there is some uncertainty as to the effects of the propellant in the aerosol when utilized on a long-term basis.

Intal (or sodium cromoglycate or cromolyn sodium) is apparently capable of preventing the degranulation of mast cells and the release of histamine and other mediators. This drug must, however, be given prophylactically because it does not inhibit or counteract the effects of histamine once it is released into the circulation or locally; nor does it relieve the symptoms of asthma once they have appeared. Since this drug has no apparent adverse action on cardiac smooth muscle, it is indicated, at least on a trial basis, for all patients with perennial asthma or allergic rhinitis and especially for those asthmatics with cardiac problems.

The drugs listed above, taken individually or in combination, usually stabilize the patient by ameliorating or controlling the symptoms of acute respiratory distress and reestablishing normal pulmonary function. However, they do not get to the root cause of the problem, which is the prevention of the allergic state. Only one of the drugs referred to above, Intal, can effectively prevent the allergic reaction, providing it is administered before the challenge.

Assays for IgE Antibodies

Using the passive transfer or P-K test to assay for IgE antibodies, one can obtain a relative, if not a semiquantitative, estimate of the IgE antibody concentration by passively sensitizing the skin of a normal individual with the allergic serum diluted 2×, 5×, 10×, 50×, etc. The specific IgE antibody or reagin titer of the serum is the maximum dilution of the serum which can still transfer skin-sensitizing activity.

The passive transfer skin test is no longer carried out due to the potential danger of transmitting serum hepatitis virus. When determination of IgE antibodies is necessary, an in vitro radioimmunoassay is used. The technique is referred to as the RAST or radioallergosorbent test. The allergen is coupled to an insoluble matrix and interacted with the serum of the allergic individual. The specific IgE antibodies will adhere to the insolubilized allergen and can be quantitated by their subsequent interaction with radiolabeled (^{125}I) anti-IgE antibodies. It is relatively simple to establish the relationship between the cpm and anti-IgE concentration. The latter bears a stoichiometric relationship to the human IgE antibodies bound to the matrix.

The limitations of the RAST technique reside in the fact that very few allergens have been sufficiently identified and purified to be utilized in a radioimmunoassay. Furthermore, many allergic individuals possess IgG (blocking) antibodies directed toward the allergen which will compete with the IgE antibodies for the determinant site on the allergen. Such a situation results in a false low value for the IgE antibodies. The use of this technique should be limited to a confirmation of the diagnosis on the basis of a properly documented case history. The RAST test may also be utilized if skin testing of the patient must be avoided due to either a history of extreme sensitivity to the allergen(s) or the presence of dermographism, a condition in which the individual gives a wheal and flare reaction to almost any stimulus applied to the skin.

Important

1. Allergic reactions may occur in 1 to 3% of all patients injected with iodinated radiographic contrast media for intravenous pyelography to demonstrate the presence of kidney stones (nephrocalcinosis), and for angiography to detect disturbances in the vascular system. The allergic reactions include urticaria, rhinitis, bronchospasm, dyspnea, systemic hypotension which may progress to vascular collapse, abdominal cramps, and laryngeal edema. Death may occur in 1 of every 10,000 of these patients. If one considers that more than 5 million contrast studies are carried out in the United States every year, then up to 500 people suffer fatal reactions to the injected contrast medium every year. This high incidence of morbidity and mortality following such a routine diagnostic procedure dictates that precautionary measures be taken in the form of readily available intravenous kits, replacement fluids, and injectable adrenaline, hydrocortisone, and antihistamines to ensure the safety of this procedure to the patient.

The systemic life-threatening allergic reaction is referred to as an anaphylactoid reaction which is an anaphylaxis-like reaction induced by a substance to which no prior exposure is recorded and to which no antibodies have been formed or are detected. All substances which induce the anaphylactoid reaction are considered to be capable of activating the complement system via the alternate pathway. The mediators which are activated are identical to those which are activated in the classical complement fixation reaction and they include anaphylatoxin, slow reacting substance of anaphylaxis (SRS-A), and bradykinin.

2. There is one association of health professionals other than physicians which encourages its members to utilize large quantities of drugs, specifically the local anesthetics. These are the members of the dental profession. It is now commonplace for a dentist to anesthetize the gums, using local anesthetics such as Xylocaine, Novocaine, and their derivatives, for such minor operations as the filling of a cavity. There are numerous dentists who even go so far as to administer these local anesthetics for as trivial a procedure as a dental examination and cleansing. This practice should be vehemently discouraged because it is fraught with potential danger for the patient. The fact is that these local anesthetics may function as allergens and induce IgE antibody formation in a not insignificant proportion of the recipients of these drugs. Up to recent

times, individuals were subjected to these local anesthetic agents only on occasions when extraction of teeth or oral surgery was necessary. Exposure to these drugs was minimal and probably did not exceed three to four times over a lifetime. Today, however, the situation is quite different. Pediatric dentists invariably administer local anesthetics to their young patients two to three times a year, and by the time the individual approaches the age of 20 he will have been exposed to the allergenic anesthetic agent approximately 10 to 20 times. Since the incidence of IgE antibody production increases with increased exposure to these agents, the susceptibility of the individual to local or systemic anaphylactic shock upon reexposure to these drugs is markedly increased. The incidence of sudden death in the dental chair, attributable to anaphylactic shock caused by the local anesthetic, has reached alarming proportions which must cause concern to the dental profession. An average of 300 dental-related deaths in the United States and more than 20 dental-related deaths in Canada are recorded yearly, directly attributable to anaphylactic shock induced by the injected local anesthetic. Undoubtedly, many more individuals die or become ill as a result of experiencing delayed anaphylactic reactions after they leave the dental office. There is no doubt in the mind of this author that ontoward immunologically mediated allergic reactions, the most severe and life threatening of which is anaphylactic shock, will increase in incidence and in severity as people are more and more frequently exposed to these allergenic anesthetic agents.

TYPE II REACTIONS: DISEASES MEDIATED BY AUTOANTIBODIES

All reactions characterized by the interaction of antibodies with autologous cell surface antigens, initiating complement-mediated lysis of the target cells, were initially designated as Type II reactions. By definition, all Type II reactions are autoimmune reactions, the consequences of which may be the induction of overt autoimmune diseases. An autoimmune disease is usually accompanied by obvious pathology providing the target is a specific organ and not a circulating hormone (see below). The targets of the autoantibodies are as follows:

1. Surface structures normally present on circulating cells, i.e. red blood cells (autoimmune hemolytic anemia), platelets (idiopathic thrombocytopenia purpura (ITP)).
2. Hormones, the inactivation of which subsequent to interaction with autoantibodies results in an endocrinopathy, i.e.

insulin (insulin refractory diabetes), thyroglobulin (thyroid insufficiency), erythropoietin (iron refractory anemia).

3. Circulating and noncirculating nonhormonal regulatory factors, i.e. antihemophilic globulin (hemophilia), intrinsic factor (pernicious anemia).

4. Antigens on invasive organisms which cross-react with autologous proteins. For example, antibodies to certain strains of streptococci react with glomerular basement membrane antigens resulting in a glomerulonephritis (poststreptococcal glomerulonephritis), or with antigens on cardiac valves resulting in rheumatic heart disease.

5. A new (neo) antigen on the target cell formed following its interaction with a drug (a drug-target cell complex), i.e. anemia and/or thrombocytopenia and/or leukopenia following treatment with Sedormid, penicillin, quinidine, or alpha methyldopa.

6. Sequestered antigens, not normally accessible to the circulating immunocompetent cells. These may consist of parenchymal organ-specific antigens (i.e. kidney- and liver-specific antigens located on the glomerular endothelial cell and hepatocyte, respectively) or constituents of connective tissue which may acquire autoantigenic properties subsequent to alteration at a specific site (i.e. synovial membrane collagen). Some of the diseases which arise as a result of these reactions are Masugi nephritis (the antigen appears to be specific to the glomerular basement membrane), Goodpasture's syndrome (the antigen is common to both the glomerular and alveolar tissues), myasthenia gravis (the antigen appears to be the acetylcholine receptor at the myoneural junction), and rheumatoid arthritis (the antigen was originally thought to be a somewhat altered circulating IgG molecule present in the synovial fluid; recent findings suggest that the pathology is primarily the result of interaction of autoantibodies with antigens specific to the synovial basement membrane collagen, not normally accessible to the immunocompetent cells).

In the instance where the target for the antibody is a neoantigen or a drug-altered autoantigen on an autologous circulating cell or an apparently unaltered structure on the cell surface, the target cell-antibody immune complex is eliminated in one or more of the following ways:

1. Phagocytosis and intracellular lysis of the target cell-antibody (IgG) complex by phagocytic cells following interaction of the Fc of the cell-bound antibodies with the Fc receptors of the phagocytic cells. This reaction is a complement-independent reaction.

2. Lysis of the target cell-antibody (IgG) complex following the interaction of the Fc of the bound antibody molecules with the Fc receptors of certain lymphocytes (Fc receptor-bearing

lymphocytes) capable of effecting the antibody-dependent cellular cytotoxicity (ADCC) reaction. This is a complement-independent reaction.

3. Lysis of the target cell-antibody complex following activation of and interaction with the complement system (complement-mediated lysis).

In the instance where the autoantigen is a parenchymal cell or a normally sequestered antigen, interaction with autoantibody usually results in the fixation of complement locally (except in the case where the antibody is a non-complement-fixing antibody). Anaphylatoxins and neutrophil chemotactic factors which are activated induce local hyperemia and infiltration with polymorphonuclear leukocytes. The latter release proteolytic and lipolytic enzymes which further exacerbate the inflammatory reaction. Phagocytic cells appear later in the reaction as the tissue and cell debris accumulates. The organ or tissue gradually, sometimes insidiously, loses its original architecture and function, and the original parenchymal cells are replaced by fibrous tissue.

TYPE III REACTIONS: DISEASES MEDIATED BY IMMUNE COMPLEXES

The pathology of a not insignificant number of diseases (see below) is today attributed to the harmful effects of immune (antigen-antibody) complexes. The pathology and the ensuing clinical symptoms vary depending upon the organ(s) in which the immune complexes are formed and/or are localized.

The skin reaction induced by immune complexes localized to the walls of the small blood vessels in the skin is considered to be a prototype of a Type III immune complex reaction. It is referred to as the **Arthus reaction**, named after Maurice Arthus who first described it in 1903 (see Chapter 7).

The skin reaction can best be induced at a time when the concentration of precipitating antibodies in the circulation is at or near its peak—that is, 8 to 12 days and 12 to 20 days following immunization of a rabbit or a human, respectively, with a soluble protein antigen. Within 2 to 4 hours following the intracutaneous (challenge) injection of the immunizing antigen, a diffuse non-itching swelling develops at the challenge site characterized by hyperemia, erythema, and petechial hemorrhages. The reaction, which rarely induces tissue damage, usually attains its maximum intensity by 6 to 12 hours and then subsides. However, in the hyperimmunized animal or the individual with a high concentration of circulating precipitating antibodies, the reaction may progress to necrosis of the skin followed by fibrosis and scar formation.

Histologically, the most striking features are the extensive infiltration of polymorphonuclear leukocytes in various states of degeneration, collagen fibers in various stages of digestion, and edema. Investigation by immunofluorescence reveals antigen-antibody complexes, free in the lumina of the blood vessels and in the interstitial spaces, localized to the blood vessel wall (in the subendothelial space between the endothelial cells and the basement membrane), and within polymorphonuclear leukocytes. The reaction of the immune complexes with the endothelial cells is facilitated by the presence of Fc receptors on these cells.

The pathology is not simply a direct consequence of the interaction of circulating precipitating IgG antibodies with intradermally injected antigen and the deposition of immune complexes upon and/or within basement membranes of small blood vessels per se. The immune complexes, especially when they are in a state of antigen excess, fix complement, resulting in the activation of a number of mediators such as the anaphylatoxins (histamine-releasing factors) and neutrophil chemotactic factors. The pathology which ensues is attributed to the activity of these mediators. The anaphylatoxins liberate histamine from mast cells which induces vasodilatation, resulting in a sluggish blood flow which facilitates further interaction between the antigen and antibody molecules, the formation of immune complexes, and their aggregation and deposition. The massive infiltration of polymorphonuclear leukocytes induced by the chemotactic factors is followed by the liberation of highly proteolytic and lipolytic enzymes, especially collagenase and elastase. The tissue destruction mediated by these enzymes induces further infiltration of polymorphonuclear leukocytes. Platelets are attracted to the site of the reaction, and blood-clotting factors are activated locally, resulting in the deposition of fibrin. Platelet, fibrin, or mixed thrombi are formed, resulting in ischemia of the tissues distal to the affected vessel(s). Thus, the reaction which presents initially as an acute inflammation may advance to hemorrhagic necrosis, ulceration, fibrosis, and scar formation.

The conditions which must be fulfilled in order to initiate the Arthus reaction are (a) the antibody must be a precipitating antibody, (b) the antibody must be a complement-fixing antibody, (c) complement levels should be normal, and (d) neutrophil function should be normal. Animals temporarily depleted of complement or neutrophils are not able to mount an Arthus reaction.

Important

The relevance of this skin reaction to clinical medicine lies in its use as a criterion designed to assess circulating antibody levels,

Table 14.3
Etiologic Agents in Extrinsic Allergic Alveolitis

Antigen Source	Disease	Usual Mode of Exposure
Molds associated with hay	Farmer's lung	Farming
Sugar cane	Bagassosis	Sugar cane processing
Mushroom compost	Mushroom worker's lung	Mushroom growing
Oak bark, cork dust	Suberosis	Cork making
Maple bark	Bark stripper's lung	Paper making
Barley, malt dust	Malt worker's lung	Malt processing
Wood dust	Sequoiosis	Sawmills
Bird droppings, i.e. pigeons	Pigeon breeder's lung	Bird breeding
Fur dust	Furrier's lung	Sewing furs
Pituitary powder	Pituitary snuff taker's lung	Pituitary snuff taking (in diabetes insipidus)
Coffee bean dust		Coffee processing

i.e. antidiptheria toxin antibodies. An individual with a high level of circulating antitoxin antibodies will present with a severe Arthus reaction if challenged intracutaneously with diptheria toxoid (Schick test). The same reaction will occur in individuals with high levels of antipenicillin IgG antibodies challenged intradermally with penicillin in an attempt to elicit an IgE-mediated immediate skin reaction to determine whether the patient is allergic to the antibiotic.

A number of diseases are characterized by a systemic Arthus reaction, with evidence of generalized or focal intravascular precipitation and deposition of antigen-antibody complexes and complement. These are: polyarteritis nodosa; extrinsic allergic alveolitis or hypersensitivity pneumonitis (originally referred to as cryptogenic alveolitis), i.e. farmer's lung; intrinsic bronchopulmonary aspergillosis; poststreptococcal glomerulonephritis; anaphylactic shock as a result of generalized intravascular precipitation of immune complexes followed by complement fixation and activation of anaphylatoxin; serum sickness.

Extrinsic Allergic Alveolitis

Hypersensitivity pneumonitis or extrinsic allergic alveolitis (EAA) is a consequence of the interaction of foreign antigenic particles or proteins and antibodies in the alveoli. Fungal spores in moldy hay or grass, dust particles from animal and bird droppings, plant dust particles, industrial dust particles, etc., upon inhalation, are deposited along the alveolar lining where they interact with antibodies formed in the affected individual. **Farmer's lung** is one of the diseases classified under the category of EAA (Table 14.3). The affected individual (usually a farmer) forms antibodies to the fungal spores in moldy hay and the antibodies combine with the inhaled spores in the alveoli causing an immune complex disease in the lungs, primarily the peripheral lung tissue (alveolar walls, respiratory bronchioles).

Respiratory distress commences 4 to 8 hours following exposure to moldy hay. The symptoms include cough (sometimes very intense), chills, malaise, muscle pains, anorexia, weight loss, progressive dyspnea, and fever. The symptoms persist in varying degrees of severity for up to 24 hours, although they may abate after only 4 to 8 hours provided exposure to the fungal spores has been terminated. The symptoms can be reproduced by provocative inhalation tests. The clinical distress is often out of proportion to the physical findings. Diffuse nodular infiltrates are detected radiologically. Pulmonary function tests indicate a restrictive pulmonary defect, with decreased lung compliance and diminished gas exchange. Skin testing with the suspected antigen results in an Arthus-type skin reaction. Circulating precipitating

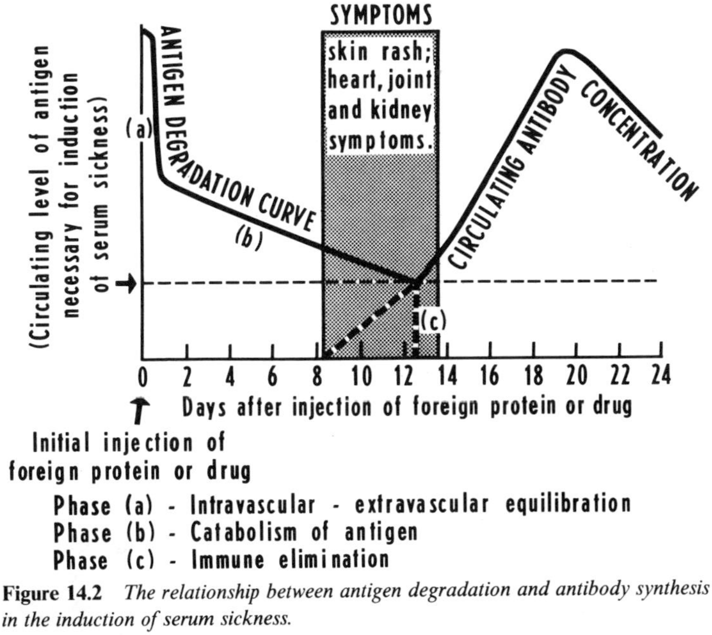

Figure 14.2 *The relationship between antigen degradation and antibody synthesis in the induction of serum sickness.*

antibodies to the suspected antigen can usually be identified by routine immunoassays, i.e. diffusion in gel.

The symptoms occur only following long-term intermittent or continuous exposure to moldy hay. The disease should, therefore, be considered to be an occupational disorder.

The danger is that the disease may develop insidiously, giving rise to obvious symptoms only late in its evolution. Permanent lung damage may ensue characterized by focal or diffuse fibrosis, leading inexorably to respiratory failure and death unless the individual is removed from the source of the provocative agent.

Important

If a patient presents with a history of recurrent severe bouts of coughing, occurring especially in the evening, accompanied by chills and/or fever, always inquire as to his/her vocation because it may be an occupational disease of the extrinsic allergic alveolitis type.

Serum Sickness

Serum sickness has been considered to be a model of an immune complex disease ever since its description by von Pirquet and Schick early in the 20th century. The term serum sickness was originally coined to denote an illness which occurs following administration of a xenogeneic antibacterial or antitoxin antiserum (i.e. horse antitetanus toxin antiserum (ATS)) used as a chemotherapeutic agent. The symptoms were initially attributed to toxic properties of the injected serum. However, in their classic book written in German entitled *Serum Krankheit*, von Pirquet and Schick demonstrated that serum sickness is not due to any toxic properties of the xenogeneic antiserum injected into the individual. It is, rather, an iatrogenic disease, the consequence of antibodies formed by the host toward proteins (antigens) in the xenogeneic antiserum. The coexistence of antibodies and the protein antigens in the circulation facilitates the formation of immune complexes in the circulation which induce what is referred to today as **immune complex disease** (Fig. 14.2). The symptoms of serum sickness are not observed until 10 to 20 days following administration of the xenogeneic antiserum, that is, at a time when the concentration of circulating antibodies directed toward the xenogeneic protein antigens will be at or near the maximum. The term "serum sickness," insofar as it implies an illness directly attributable to properties of the administered serum, is, therefore, a misnomer, but it has survived as a result of its being used synonymously with the term "immune complex disease."

The major clinical symptoms on physical examination are fever, malaise, lymphadenopathy, splenomegaly, rash (mild diffuse erythematous to gross urticarial), joint pains of a transient and fleeting character, and peripheral neuropathy (Guillain-Barré-like). Pericarditis may sometimes be detected as well as pleuritis. Wheezing may frequently be present. Laboratory investigation reveals an absolute leukocytosis with respect to neutrophils and a less but still obvious eosinophilia. The hemolytic complement titer may be half the normal level or lower. Examination of a skin biopsy will reveal diffuse, focal inflammatory lesions of small blood vessels in the dermis and hypodermis characterized by perivascular and intravascular infiltration of polymorphonuclear leukocytes, destruction of the blood vessel basement membrane with extravasation of blood, necrosis of adjacent collagen fibers and muscle bundles with invasion by phagocytic cells (multinucleate and foam cells), fibrinoid degeneration, and fibrosis. Urinalysis will reveal a proteinuria and usually a hematuria, suggesting acute glomerulonephritis. Renal biopsy will confirm the diagnosis of an inflammatory proliferative glomerulonephritis.

The clinical signs and symptoms generally reach maximum intensity 2 to 3 weeks after injection of the foreign proteins, following which the symptoms usually abate without complication or residual disease. It is not necessary for a patient to demonstrate all of the clinical signs and symptoms enumerated above. Some may present with only a rash, others a neuropathy, others with joint pains, others with malaise, edema, and proteinuria. Serum sickness can, therefore, mimic many diseases and may be mistaken for infectious arthritis, gout, acute glomerulonephritis, viral infections, pericarditis, pleurisy, peripheral neuropathy, etc.

The disease can occur not only following administration of a foreign serum protein but also following administration of antibiotics, especially penicillin (5 to 10% incidence), anesthetics, psychomimetic drugs, aspirin, etc. These drugs tend to autocouple to proteins and will thus behave as haptens. The antibodies formed toward these haptens will interact with the hapten-protein complex.

Why do only a small number (5 to 8%) of individuals present with symptoms of serum sickness following initial exposure to the antigen? The answer lies in the finding that only those individuals in whom the circulating antigen concentration is above a certain threshold level at the time when the antibody concentration attains an appropriate level develop signs and symptoms of serum sickness (Fig. 14.2). This condition will not be met in patients who metabolize the antigen at a very rapid rate (insufficient antigen in the circulation when antibody synthesis is normally underway) or who are delayed or poor antibody synthesizers (insufficient antigen in the circulation when antibodies are finally secreted into the circulation in sufficiently high concentration). On the other hand, some individuals synthesize and secrete antibodies so vigorously that a state of antigen excess will be very transient at best and will quickly be overtaken by a state of antibody excess. Since immune complexes formed in antigen excess fix complement to a much greater extent than do complexes formed at equivalence or antibody excess, patients in the latter category will rarely, if ever, present with serum sickness.

Following a second or third administration of the antigen, the antibody response is speeded up, with the result that the curves for antigen concentration and antibody concentration in the circulation intersect to the left in Figure 14.2, thus enhancing the opportunity to develop clinically overt serum sickness. Therefore, the incidence and severity of this disease increase with increased exposure to the antigen.

Immune complex disease may be superimposed upon an existing clinical condition and may, therefore, not be detected as such until late in the course of the disease, if at all. Often symptoms may be mistakenly considered to be complications of the primary condition (Table 14.4).

Table 14.4
Diseases Characterized by Superimposed Immune Complex Disease

Antigen	Disease
Bacteria	Symphilis
	Leprosy
	Poststreptococcal glomerulonephritis
Virus	Type-B hepatitis
	Infectious mononucleosis
Parasites	Malaria
	Leishmania
	Trypanosomiasis
	Schistosomiasis
Autoantigens	
DNA	Systemic lupus erythematosus
IgG	Rheumatoid arthritis
	Cryoglobulinemia
	Macroglobulinemia
Thyroid follicle	Chronic thyroiditis (Hashimoto)
Neoantigens on mutant cells	Cancer
Miscellaneous (unidentified antigens)	Benign monoclonal gammopathies
	Crohn's disease?
	Ulcerative colitis?

Important

1. Although the antibody response following initial administration of the antigen (drug or foreign protein) is invariably an IgG response, a minority of individuals synthesize IgE antibodies along with or in the absence of IgG antibodies. Such individuals may not present with serum sickness following initial injection of the antigen(s). However, they will present with life-threatening situations, usually systemic anaphylaxis, immediately following the second administration of the antigen(s) due to the interaction of the antigen(s) with cell-fixed IgE antibodies (Type I reaction). Therefore, individuals should be skin tested for IgE-mediated skin reactivity (immediate skin reaction) before a second administration of the drug or foreign protein (i.e., ATS).

2. Serum sickness is an iatrogenic disease, one of many diseases induced not by infectious agents or metabolic defects but by the drugs used to intervene on behalf of the patient. The overutilization of many drugs, such as the antibiotics (especially penicillin), cannot but result in an increased incidence of serum sickness. In the preantibiotic era, serum sickness could usually be attributed to the repeated administration of a xenogeneic antimicrobial antiserum. However, the majority of such antisera are now available following immunization of human volunteers. The administration of an allogeneic (human) antiserum does not normally result in any adverse reaction in the host, and serum sickness is not a consequence. Xenogeneic antisera should no longer be used except when the allogeneic antiserum is not available and passive immunization is indicated.

TYPE IV REACTIONS: DISEASES INCURRED AS SEQUELAE OF CELL-MEDIATED IMMUNE REACTIONS

As is discussed at length in Chapter 6, the immune response which nature dictates to many pathogens (some bacteria, most fungi, many viruses and parasites) is the cell-mediated (sensitized cells), and not the humoral (antibody), immune response. It may be detected by the delayed skin reaction following challenge with a soluble antigenic extract of the pathogen. This cell-mediated immune reaction is referred to as a Type IV reaction. This is also the immune system which is invariably activated following contact with poison ivy. Furthermore, autoantigens, transplantation antigens on allografted tissues, tumor antigens, and relatively simple chemical compounds (i.e. dinitrochlorobenzene or DNCB) also preferentially activate the cell-mediated immune system. The pathologic lesions are induced by sensitized cells only; antibodies, even if they are present, are not participants in or instrumental in the induction of these lesions. The disease states attributed to Type IV immune reactions are primarily autoimmune diseases. Allograft rejection, aside from the fact that an allogeneic rather than an autologous organ is affected, exhibits all the cardinal characteristics of an autoimmune disease. There are instances when the Type IV immune response to antigens other than infectious agents is obviously beneficial to the host, such as the immune response to tumor antigens.

Although the cellular immune reaction occurring either in the skin or within different organs always incurs some pathologic sequelae, it certainly facilitates the isolation and elimination of the invasive pathogen. When the intensity of the reaction is not too marked, the pathologic aspects are not obvious or disconcerting and the tissue damage is minimal and often reversible, and only the immune nature (i.e. resistance) of the reaction is seriously noted. However, at times the reaction can be explosive and the pathologic manifestations of the cell-mediated immune response can be just as life-threatening to the host as the infection itself.

Examples of disease and/or pathologic states, detrimental or beneficial to the host, which present as a consequence of complications or sequelae of what would otherwise be considered normal Type IV immune reactions are lung lesions in tuberculosis (Ghon tubercle; caseation, necrosis, and cavitation); autoimmune lesions, i.e. thyroiditis, adrenalitis, encephalomyelitis (including postvaccination), orchitis; rejection of an allograft; and rejection of transplantable and spontaneously occurring tumors.

The clinical diseases and/or pathologic lesions facilitated or induced by Type IV reactions are not due to a faulty immune system. The immune system is, in fact, operating very well. The fault lies with the inducers (the antigens) of the cell-mediated immune response. By and large, it is generally assumed that the immune system is normally incapable of recognizing autoantigens, or autoantigens are not normally secreted into the circulation and are, therefore, unable to stimulate the immunocompetent cells. However, situations may arise following trauma, surgery, or infection when antigens normally restricted or sequestered to a particular organ are permitted to invade the circulation. These organ-specific autoantigens may, under the appropriate circumstances, interact with immunocompetent cells, converting them to sensitized cells. These cells may then interact with the target tissue or organ (the source of the original sensitizing antigen), resulting in the release of powerful mediators (lymphokines) capable of inflicting extensive damage in the tissues culminating in curtailment or cessation of function, if not "rejection," of the autologous tissue or organ (please review Chapter 6). The pathologic lesions within the autologous tissues which characterize the cell-mediated autoimmune response cannot be distinguished morphologically from the lesions within grafted allogeneic tissues which characterize the allograft rejection reaction or the lesions which develop in the delayed (hypersensitivity) skin reactions. A constant and prominent feature of these lesions is the preponderance of mononuclear cells (monocytes in various stages of activity and degeneration, and lymphocytes of various sizes and shapes) which surround the small blood vessels (perivascular cuffs) and infiltrate the tissue proper.

The mononuclear cell infiltrate has been considered to be characteristic, if not pathognomonic, of the cell-mediated immune reaction. However, the discovery of the antibody-dependent cell-mediated cytotoxic (or ADCC) reaction in the late 1960s has greatly disturbed the tranquility in the transplantation sphere insofar as the underlying immune mechanism in the pathogenesis of allograft rejection is concerned. This is due to the difficulty in distinguishing between a mononuclear cell infiltrate carried out strictly by sensitized cells (a cell-mediated immune reaction) and a mononuclear cell infiltrate resulting from an ADCC-mediated immune reaction. The lymphocytes and monocytes involved in these two reactions are morphologically indistinguishable. However, upon elution of the mononuclear cells from the target tissue in vitro, it can be determined whether or not the cells possess receptors for Fc(IgG) [or Fc(G)]. If the vast majority of the cells do not, then it may be concluded that the infiltrate was inspired by the cell-mediated immune response. However, if a high proportion of the infiltrating cells are Fc(G) receptor-bearing cells, then an ADCC reaction in the target tissue cannot be ruled out. The absence of circulating antibodies does not rule out an ADCC reaction since the concentration of antibody molecules required to mediate the ADCC reaction is less than can be detected by even the most elegant and sophisticated antibody detection assays. Since Fc(G) receptor-bearing cells have, in fact, been isolated from rejected tissues, it would appear that the view generally adhered to—that allograft rejection is necessarily a consequence of a cell-mediated immune response—may not be valid.

Important

1. The cell-mediated immune response detected by the delayed skin reaction is the anticipated immune response to a large number of diverse antigens, such as all fungi, a large number of viruses, parasites, helminths, protozoa, and some bacteria. Failure to induce this form of reactivity implies an immunodeficient state.

2. Certain cell-mediated immune responses, such as poison ivy and tuberculin sensitivity, which have long been considered examples of allergic responses, are not allergic reactions but rather

the manifestations of cell-mediated immune responses anticipated and observed in all individuals exposed to the inciting agents.

3. As discussed above, Type IV reactions are not normally considered to be allergic reactions. However, there are individuals who indeed develop Type IV allergic reactivity toward highly reactive chemicals of low molecular weight capable of autocoupling to skin proteins and becoming haptens. These are referred to as contactants. The host response to a subsequent encounter with these agents takes the forms of a contact dermatitis, with the rash usually confined to the areas of contact. Examples are contact dermatitis to nickel, gold, platinum, detergents, lipstick, rouge, hair sprays, deodorants, soaps (especially those containing lanolin), "cleansing" solutions, nail polish, dyes, etc. Since only a small proportion of the population exposed to these agents ever display symptoms of a contact dermatitis, this response may be considered to be an allergic one, in accordance with the definition given for the allergic response.

TYPE V REACTIONS: ANTIBODY-INDUCED HYPERFUNCTION

Types V, VI, and VII reactions have only recently been introduced into the immunology lexicon. They are, therefore, still not well defined, possibly even suspect by many skeptics, but they have attracted an inordinately large number of investigators.

A Type V reaction appears to be at the basis of Graves' disease or thyrotoxicosis (Tables 14.1 and 14.2). Originally, a circulating factor referred to as the long acting thyroid stimulator (LATS) was blamed for this condition as it was shown capable of stimulating prolonged secretion of thyroxin from the thyroid. It has since been demonstrated that LATS is an IgG antibody molecule directed toward configurations on the thyroid follicle membrane, one of which is the receptor for the thyroid-stimulating hormone (TSH). The interaction of the antibody with this TSH receptor triggers off the synthesis and secretion of thyroxin. Unlike the synthesis of TSH, which is regulated by the concentration of circulating thyroxin, the synthesis of the LATS antibodies is under no such control and their continued presence in the circulation results in the constant stimulation of thyroxin synthesis and secretion.

Although endocrinologists may find it novel to attribute hyperfunction of the thyroid to antibodies, this form of antibody activity is not a precedent in the immunologic literature. As stated previously, non-complement-fixing antibodies directed toward cell surface antigens have a stimulating effect on the metabolism of the target cell, as do complement-fixing antibodies in the absence of complement in the artificial milieu of the test tube. For example, antilymphocyte antibodies and anti (lymphocyte-bearing) - immunoglobulin antibodies stimulate protein, RNA, and DNA synthesis in the target lymphocytes, with resultant blastogenesis and mitosis in vitro. It may, therefore, be anticipated that other endocrinopathies characterized by a hyperactive state may have an underlying immunologic etiology.

Evidence has recently been presented that certain features of malignant diseases of the lymphoreticular system may be attributed to an immune response by the host toward these malignant cells. Abdou and his colleagues have demonstrated that antibodies can be detected toward autologous plasmablasts and plasma cells in patients with multiple myeloma. It is conceivable that these antibodies, which must be non-complement-fixing (or else they would lyse the cells in vivo), directed toward plasma cell-specific antigen(s), are capable of stimulating blastogenesis of these cells on a continuous basis.

One may anticipate that other malignant diseases of the lymphoreticular system will be demonstrated to be the result of an "immune" response directed toward the malignant cells.

Important

The reader should be cautioned as to the terminology proposed for the antibodies implicated. They have been referred to as "stimulating" antibodies by endocrinologists investigating the pathogenesis of thyrotoxicosis. The reader should, however, realize that the antibodies, by themselves, are not stimulating; stimulation of cell metabolism and protein, RNA, and DNA synthesis is the result of the immune reaction occurring on the cell surface and has nothing to do with the properties of the antibody per se.

TYPES VI (ADCC) AND VII (NOCC) REACTIONS

These are the two most recently described reactions and they have not get gained uniform acceptance by the discipline as true immunologic reactions or as having a role to play in vivo (Tables 14.1 and 14.2). A number of recent investigations have revealed that Fc receptor-bearing cells, which mediate the ADCC reaction, infiltrate the lesions in experimentally induced autoimmune thyroiditis and malignant solid tumors. It has been postulated that these Fc receptor-bearing cells interact with the Fc regions of antibody molecules formed by the host toward thyroid follicle antigens and malignant cells, respectively. Once activated, these Fc receptor-bearing cells initiate the cytolysis of the antibody-sensitized target cells. Thus, the ADCC reaction may play a role in these two situations, in the former by inadvertently promoting even greater severity of the autoimmune disease and in the latter by facilitating the rejection of the tumor cells.

The role of the cells which mediate the NOCC reaction in vivo is even less understood than is that of the cells which mediate the

ADCC reaction. As stated previously (Chapter 7), mononuclear cells precommitted to interact with and lyse malignant cells without involving complement exist in the circulation of the experimental animal and humans in the absence of prior exposure to the targets. These NOCC effector cells do not appear to require antibodies on the target cells as a precondition for their interaction with these cells, in contrast with the ADCC effector cells. The NOCC effector cells, therefore, appear to possess receptors for surface structures intrinsic to the target malignant cells. Whether these surface structures are characteristic in a general sense of some or all malignant cells and whether the effector mononuclear cells constitute the elusive "immune surveillance" system whereby the normal individual suppresses the "spontaneous" emergence of malignant cells remain to be determined. Nevertheless, these effector cells provide food for thought for many investigators currently engaged in elucidating the mechanisms, assumed to exist in normal individuals, which provide resistance toward the emergence of malignant cells.

Important

1. Although the administration of almost any drug or foreign agent results in at least one of the reactions (Types I to VII) discussed above, a not insignificant number of drugs (e.g. antibiotics, local anesthetics, analgesics), insect bites, and xenogeneic antisera (such as antitetanus serum) administered prophylactically are, in fact, capable of inducing Types I, II, III, and IV reactions either sequentially or concurrently within the same individuals. For example, penicillin can function as (a) an allergen capable of eliciting the formation of IgE antibodies which will facilitate a Type I reaction upon challenge with penicillin; (b) an antigen (a hapten-protein conjugate to be precise) capable of stimulating the formation of IgG antibodies which will participate in a Type II and/or Type III reaction upon challenge with penicillin; and (c) an antigen capable of inducing sensitized cells which will evoke a cellular immune reaction (delayed hypersensitivity) upon challenge with penicillin. Furthermore, the cellular infiltrates in delayed hypersensitivity reactions attributed to sensitization to penicillin may be due to an ADCC reaction rather than, or superimposed upon, a purely (sensitized) cell-mediated reaction.

2. A drug which induces a Type I reaction in one individual may induce a Type II or Type III or Type IV reaction in another individual. In other words, different individuals may respond differently to the same drug. Since the treatments for the conditions characterized by the Types I to IV reactions are different, it is of practical, not just theoretical, importance for the physician to recognize the potentially harmful immunologically mediated complications of the commonly used drugs.

CHAPTER 15

The Humoral versus the Cell-mediated Immune Response: A Phylogenetic Approach toward an Understanding of the Mechanisms Which Trigger the Selection of the Particular Immune Response to a Specific Antigen

Thus far, the humoral immune (HI) and cell-mediated immune (CMI) responses have been discussed as separate and distinct entities, without stressing or alluding to their possible interaction or interdependence. A question which the student inevitably brings up is why some antigens evoke an antibody response and other antigens a cell-mediated response. Certainly, there is need to provide a rational explanation with scientific credibility for this apparent phenomenon, to define the factors which influence the immune system to select the humoral or cell-mediated immune response to a particular antigenic stimulus. The explanation probably depends as much on an understanding of the phylogeny (development of immunity during the evolution of the different species) and ontogeny (the development of the immune system in the embryo and fetus) of the immune response as it does on our knowledge of the immune systems in the adult animal.

It is generally accepted that the immune response evolved to safeguard and protect the host from the myriad of invasive pathogenic microorganisms present in his environment. Since the immune response has been retained by all animal species investigated and, conversely, since no animal species exists which does not exhibit an immune response, it must be assumed that the immune response has great survival value. However, how does one account for the existence of at least two distinct types of immune responses, the humoral and cell-mediated responses? In attempting to justify the need for two types of immune responses, the investigator should consider that he is analyzing the immune mechanism at a moment during its evolution and should assume that the species and/or the immune response system may still be evolving. In other words, the ultimate state in the evolution of the immune response need not yet have taken place. Nature may still be experimenting with a number of immune systems to provide the host with protection toward extrinsic invasive agents and may still be undecided which should be retained. The reader is reminded that the purely humoral and cell-mediated immune responses are not the only mechanisms available to the host to protect him from outside invaders. Fc receptor-bearing cells exist capable of lysing antibody-sensitized target cells in the absence of complement, and other cells exist capable of lysing target cells without the apparent need for antibodies.

In analyzing the phylogeny of the immune response, the cell-mediated immune response would appear to be the more primitive as there are indications of an inflammatory-type resistance having evolved in the lower animal species, such as the invertebrates, in the absence of circulating antibodies which generally characterize immunity in the vertebrates. Cell-mediated immunity appears to be the immunity of choice by the host with respect to the generally non-exotoxin-producing organisms of low pathogenicity, virulence, and infectivity, which also happen to be the most primitive—those which tend to localize on the skin or within a particular organ and which may, in fact, establish a symbiotic relation with the host. A classification of such microorganisms includes the fungi, rickettsia, some large viruses, protozoa, helminths, and some (primitive) bacteria. Since the theory of Darwinian evolution dictates that the response by the host be just sufficient to satisfy the need and must be economical, the host mobilizes specifically sensitized cells which are attracted to the focus of infection, to either liberate there an agent toxic toward the invading organism or physically interact with the latter and eventually wall off the infected area. On the other hand, a much larger number of specifically sensitized cells would be required to combat a disseminated or generalized bacterial infection, especially when it is also accompanied by the secretion of exotoxins, a property attributed to more highly evolved microorganisms. To combat this type of infection, the host developed a specific defense mechanism based on the secretion of relatively low moleclar weight antibody molecules which circulate and confront the organism and the low molecular weight toxin molecules anywhere in the body and there neutralize it. This type of immune mechanism permits a conservation of the cell population with a concomitant lower expenditure of energy by the host, since the energy expended to synthesize a large number of antibody molecules is several orders of magnitude lower than for the generation of an equal number of specifically sensitized cells. However, since immunity mediated by antibody is dependent upon complement in order to successfully induce the lysis of the invading microorganism, humoral immunity had to await the evolution of the complement system before it could become effective and displace cell-mediated immunity. It has been suggested that complement evolved among the lower vertebrates. It is, therefore, of more than academic interest to note that antibody synthesis also appears to have evolved among the lower vertebrates in unison with the evolution of the complement system.

To bridge the gap which exists with respect to our understanding of the types of cells which evolved to mediate humoral and cell-mediated immunity, it is suggested that a receptor-bearing antigen-reactive cell constitutes the initial responder cell for both types of immune responses. With respect to the humoral immune response, this cell is not normally present in the circulation but appears to be confined to a particular lymphoid organ, such as the bone marrow (rabbit) or the thymus (mouse). The humoral immune response is generally directed toward antigens which invade the circulation, such as toxin molecules, and confront the antigen-reactive cell in the organ in which it is localized. This interaction provides the signal to an antibody-forming cell to synthesize and secrete antibodies (see Chapter 5). On the other hand, the antigen-reactive cell concerned with evoking cell-mediated immunity is normally present in the circulation since it must migrate to the areas of infection rather than vice versa. That these cells exist in the cirulation is demonstrated by the fact that the circulating leukocytes can participate in the mixed leukocyte culture reaction, a cell-mediated immune response. It is considered that these antigen-reactive cells transform to what are referred to as sensitized cells. The radiosensitive nature of the humoral, but the relative radioinsensitivity of the cell-mediated, immune response is attributed to a short life-span for the ARC cell involved in the humoral immune response and a long lifespan for the precursor of the sensitized cell effecting the cell-mediated immune response. A short-lived cell, because of its higher rate of metabolism and DNA turnover, would be expected to be more susceptible to the deleterious effects of irradiation than a long-lived cell.

To recapitulate, the primitive cell-mediated immune response, characterized by a long latent period, is recruited to counteract the primitive noninvasive, nonexotoxin releasing large microorganisms. The humoral immune response, characterized by a much shorter latent period, evolved to counter or neutralize the more highly pathogenic, exotoxin-secreting, highly virulent invasive small microorganisms. Thus, what is observed is strict adherence to the principles of Darwinian evolution, that is, the appropriate response to satisfy a particular need and no more.

The superimposition of Lamarckian evolution, or, as it should be called, adaptation, permitted refinements in the response or a dual response to the same antigen, humoral and cell-mediated, as sometimes occurs. It is known that the ability of a chemical contactant to evoke a cellular immune response, which manifests itself clinically as a contact dermatitis upon subsequent challenge with the specific contactant, is related to its ability to autocouple with proteins in the skin, i.e., collagen. However, if the contactant is artificially coupled to a serum protein and injected into the host, it will not evoke a cell-mediated immune response but rather a humoral immune response. It appears, therefore, that the carrier molecule to which that antigen is coupled, either naturally in vivo or artificially in vitro, is a determining factor in the selection of the type of immune response to be activated.

One other relationship exists which may provide some insight into the mechanism of selection of the immune response. The host response to all the microorganisms which activate a cell-mediated immune response is basically a mononuclear infiltration in the infected site consisting of lymphocytes and macrophages in their various functional and morphologic states (i.e. foam cells, binucleate cells, vacuolated cells, round cells, etc.), resulting in a granuloma. This mononuclear infiltration appears to be a common denominator with respect to all cell-mediated immune responses. It is, therefore, instructive to note that the injection of any antigen emulsified in Freund's complete adjuvant (which consists of *Mycobacterium tuberculosis*, an emulsifying agent and an oil) will evoke both a mononuclear cell infiltrate and a cell-mediated immune response. This is true even if the antigen normally stimulates only antibody formation following its administration without adjuvant into the host via the intravenous or subcutaneous route. One may, therefore, speculate that a mononuclear infiltrate about the antigen depot faciliates a cell-mediated immune response to the antigen.

A more precise and definitive understanding of the mechanisms which determine the selection of the appropriate immune response must await further investigation.

CHAPTER 16

Allograft Rejection, Pregnancy, Cancer, and the Immune Response*

The intention of the author is not to discuss in detail and attempt to resolve the many conflicting views concerning the role and the mechanism of expression of the immune response in allograft rejection and the control of malignant disease. One reason for this hesitancy is that many results of current investigations in each of these two areas are still very controversial, often insufficiently documented, and unconfirmed. Another reason is that these two areas of research, transplantation immunology and cancer immunology, are being flogged incessantly in almost every monthly journal and in myriads of yearly periodicals and symposia so that the addition of one more opinion or view at this time would not be very contributory. It is the aim of the author to establish the "causis belli" for the allograft rejection reaction and the apparent spontaneous appearance of a malignancy in terms of the phylogeny and ontogeny of the immune response per se. In this way, it is hoped that the reader will appreciate that both allograft rejection and malignant disease do, in fact, adhere to the basic framework of immunologic theory and the pathology which ensues should be viewed as no more conspicuous or out of place than that which accompanies many of the immunopathologic reactions discussed in Chapter 14.

---

* Several of the terms used in the text and their definition are as follows:

An isogeneic (or isologous) graft refers to a transplant of tissue from one area of the body to another on the same individual.

A syngeneic graft refers to a transplant of tissue from one individual to another genetically identical individual.

An allogeneic (or homologous) graft refers to a transplant of tissue from one individual to another genetically dissimilar individual of the same species.

A xenogeneic graft refers to a transplant of tissue from one individual to another of a different species.

THE IMMUNE RESPONSE AND ALLOGRAFT REJECTION

There is now overwhelming and seemingly indisputable evidence, based on more than 20 years of investigation, that the immune response is the primary mechanism involved in the allograft rejection reaction. The original experiments of Medawar, Brent, and Billingham in the post-World War II period laid the foundation for the discipline of transplantation immunology. They demonstrated that the graft rejection reaction occurs in accordance with established immunologic principles and that transplantation antigens are genetically inheritable. With the perfection of the surgical skills and techniques required for skin, kidney, and heart transplantation, it has been repeatedly shown that an allograft—that is, tissue transplanted between two unrelated individuals of the same species—is uniformly rejected within an established time frame. However, transplants between syngeneic animals—that is, animals of the same genetic inbred strain—are not rejected. The rejection of the allograft by the host has been attributed to the generation of sensitized lymphocytes by the host following sensitization to transplantation antigens of the allograft. Cell transfer experiments have unequivocally established that the capacity to reject an allograft can be conferred with lymphocytes but not with serum obtained from an animal which has already rejected an allograft.

A second allograft is rejected much more rapidly than is the first allograft from the same donor. This is referred to as an accelerated or second-set rejection, in contrast with a first-set rejection reaction. These reactions may be compared to the secondary and primary immune responses, respectively.

A third type of allograft rejection is referred to as the hyperacute or immediate rejection reaction. The lesions which characterize this host response to the allograft begin to develop within minutes and are usually marked within several hours of engraftment of a skin allograft or revascularization of a kidney allograft. The hyperacute rejection is initiated and is sustained as a consequence of the interaction of the allografted cells with preformed allograft-specific antibodies present in the circulation of the allograft recipient at the time of transplantation. This type of rejection will, therefore, take place under conditions where the donor and recipient are totally mismatched with respect to the ABO blood groups; in recipients who were multiply transfused on previous occasions with histoincompatible lymphoid cells and platelets; and in women who have given birth to a number of children. Individuals transfused with allogeneic lymphoid cells tend to synthesize antibodies to antigens on these allogeneic (foreign) cells, several of which cross-react with antigens on the allografted tissues. These antigens are referred to as transplantation antigens, histoincompatibility antigens, or HLA (human leukocyte antigens) antigens. Women who have borne a number of children invariably possess circulating antibodies directed toward paternally derived fetal (HLA) antigens. Allograft-specific antibodies may also be induced as a result of previous infection with microorganisms which cross-react with HLA antigens on the paternal cells.

The pathogenesis of, and the lesions which characterize, the primary or first-set rejection, the secondary or second-set rejection, and the hyperacute rejection reactions are quite distinct and pathognonomic.

The sequence of events which characterizes a hyperacute rejection of the allograft begins immediately following anastomosis of the blood vessels and reestablishment of blood flow. The IgG antibodies adhere to the endothelial cells (probably via the interaction of the IgG molecules with the Fc receptors on the endothelial cells). This is followed by complement fixation, aggregation of polymorphonuclear leukocytes and platelets and precipitation of fibrin, the coagulation of blood and the formation of pure platelet and/or mixed thrombi which may occlude the lumen, and endothelial injury which may progress to a necrotizing vasculitis. Focal necrosis of the allografted tissue, often avascular in nature, is well underway within the initial 2 to 4 hours following implantation. Massive ischemic necrosis is evident shortly thereafter (cortical necrosis in a kidney allograft). If the rejected allograft is not extirpated in an expeditious manner, gangrene may set in. Furthermore, the release into the circulation of highly potent intracellular proteolytic enzymes from the degenerating allografted cells may induce the release of potent pharmacologic mediators from the mast cells (histamine, serotonin) and from precursors in the blood (kinins) with resultant generalized increase in vascular permeability and vascular collapse (anaphylactic shock).

A primary rejection episode does not present with the suddeness of the hyperacute rejection. In most instances, the transplanted tissue or organ functions normally for a few days following revascularization. However, over the following week or so, function becomes progressively diminished and more strained. In the case of a kidney allograft, renal function is normal for the first week or so following implantation of the mismatched allogeneic kidney. The blood urea nitrogen (BUN) and creatinine levels are normal. However, within a week, the BUN begins to rise slowly and the telltale signs of renal insufficiency—oliguria, proteinuria, hematuria, edema, and later renal failure—make their appearance. The functional deterioration of the engrafted organ is accompanied by pathologic changes within the allograft. The hallmark feature of a primary rejection is the massive infiltration of mononuclear cells into the parenchyma of the tissue. These cells include lymphocytes (sensitized cells) and macrophages (probably transformed blood monocytes) in various stages of maturation and degeneration. The small blood vessels may become clogged with these cells attempting to penetrate the organ proper, and the cells surround the vessel after they emigrate through the basement membrane at the endothelial cell junctions. These cells are referred to as perivascular infiltrates or cuffs. The damage in a primary rejection is directed principally at the parenchymal cells of the allograft by the specifically sensitized lymphocytes in what appears to be a pure cell-mediated immune response.

The vascular damage at this stage is minimal, unlike that in the hyperacute rejection reaction, and would not by itself suggest the extent of destruction within the allograft proper. However, as the days progress, the invasion of the vessel wall by the mononuclear cells results in vacuolation and focal degenerative changes. There is a marked increase in vascular permeability with accumulation of fluid in the interstitial space, causing edema. This is followed by vasoconstriction of the small arteries and arterioles. Within a few days, blood flow ceases and necrotic changes set in. This reaction is not associated with antibodies or complement, and it does not, initially, involve accumulation of polymorphonuclear leukocytes or platelets. Polymorphonuclear leukocytes can be detected in large numbers within the parenchyma of the allograft after rejection has already occurred, and their role is a "mopping-up" operation. Antibodies to the HLA antigens of the allograft may also be detected following rejection of the allograft. The loss of function in a primary rejection may be so gradual and insiduous as to often initially disarm the investigator as to the true nature of the situation.

A secondary rejection episode is observed in a recipient who has already previously rejected an allograft from the same donor. It does not begin as innocently as a primary rejection reaction. This reaction is more rapid and violent in onset and obvious, as the clinical signs and symptoms of severe malfunction or severe restriction of function of the allograft, i.e. kidney, make their appearance in rapid order within 1 to 2 days following implantation of the allograft. In this instance, the pathologic lesions appear to be due to both humoral and cell-mediated immune responses. Thus, mononuclear cells infiltrate and invade the parenchyma while antibodies inflict their damage in the vasculature. The interaction of preformed circulating antibodies with the endothelial cells lining the small blood vessels initiates complement fixation, which results in neutrophil infiltration, platelet aggregation, and fibrin deposition. Occlusion of the small blood vessels leads to destruction of the arteries and arterioles and to hemmorhagic necrosis locally and ischemic necrosis of the tissue distal to the occluded blood vessels. Examination of the biopsy by immunofluorescence reveals IgG antibodies and complement bound to the vascular endothelium of the small vessels. In the case of a renal allograft, the cessation of blood flow due to obstruction and occlusion of the arteries and arterioles results in severe afferent vasoconstriction, which is followed by aggregation of erythrocytes and platelets in the glomerular capillaries, deposition of fibrin in glomerular capillaries and afferent arterioles, renal tubular cell necrosis, and finally cortical necrosis due to marked renal ischemia.

It might strike the reader as incongruous that the host should reject an allograft via an immunologic mechanism. After all, the immune response evolved to protect the host from exogenous, invasive, tissue-destroying microorganisms, to eliminate them as expeditiously as possible. Why then should this same mechanism be provoked by noninvasive, nontoxic, nonaggressive allografted cells? The answer probably lies in the fact that the allografted cells are foreign and the immune system, not being perfect and not being able to anticipate such an abnormal imposition as an allograft, responds to the allografted cells as it should to any foreign cells, by invoking an immune response toward them. The immune system is, therefore, behaving quite correctly with respect to the allograft. It is simply that we are expecting too much of it, imploring it not to recognize or to respond to antigens or foreign allografted cells intentionally implanted into the host, but to recognize and respond to antigens on all foreign invasive cells such as pathogenic microorganisms which have breached the host's outer defense mechanisms (i.e. the skin) by their own devices. Although the aim of a virulent pathogen is probably only to parasitize the host and thrive on its nutrients, the end result is often death of the host. The immune response personifies the evolutionary ascendancy over the microorganism. Without the immune response mechanism we could never have evolved beyond serving as living culture media for the proliferation of microorganisms. Instead, it is we who grow microorganisms in synthetic culture media.

Control of Allograft Rejection in Patients: Immunosuppressive Drugs

It is one thing to define the basic immunologic mechanism(s) operating in the allograft rejection reaction in the experimental animal. It is quite another to be able to intervene therapeutically to the unequivocal benefit of the human patient. Progress in the establishment of therapeutic regimes essentially free of deleterious side effects has not kept pace with the burgeoning knowledge of the mechanism of the allograft rejection reaction per se and still remains a distant but hoped-for attainable goal.

The allograft rejection reaction is today successfully circumvented or abrogated, in the majority of patients, primarily through the administration of immunosuppressive highly toxic drugs. This is not to say that there do not exist other means presently being considered to control or regulate the graft rejection capability of the host (Fig. 16.1). Although avenues such as the induction of tolerance to the transplantation antigens of the allograft or "enhancement" of the allograft by antibodies are currently being explored, work along these lines has so far not been sufficiently fruitful to displace immunosuppressive chemotherapy as the treatment of choice. The most popular drugs are (a) purine and pyrimidine analogues, such as 6-mercaptopurine and its derivative, azathioprine (Imuran); (b) certain antibiotics, such as actinomycin D; (c) steroids, such as dexamethasone and prednisone; and (d) ALG (antilymphocyte globulin) or ATG (antithymocyte globulin).

ATG is the gamma globulin fraction of horse (or cow or goat) antiserum obtained following immunization with human thymic or T lymphocytes. Absorption of this antiserum in the appropriate manner with human serum proteins, erythrocytes, platelets, and bone marrow (B) lymphocytes results in an antiserum which is remarkably specific in its cytotoxic activity for human T lymphocytes. This is the cell which has been most implicated as the harbinger of an impending allograft rejection and as the assassin directly involved in the killing of the allografted cells.

Along with these drugs, there are a large number of other agents which are continually being promoted as immunosuppressants on the basis of very limited supporting evidence. Unfortunately, like other initially promising approaches, immuno-

Factors Which Inhibit or Deter Rejection of The Allografted Cells

1. A weakly responsive immune system.
2. The presence of continually circulating transplantation antigens (?).
3. The presence of immune complexes in the circulation (—●—C) capable of competing with sensitized cells for the cell-bound transplantation antigens (?).
4. The synthesis of noncomplement fixing (protective?) antibodies by the host.
5. The induction of a state of immunologic tolerance toward the transplantation antigens.
6. Immunosuppressive drugs.

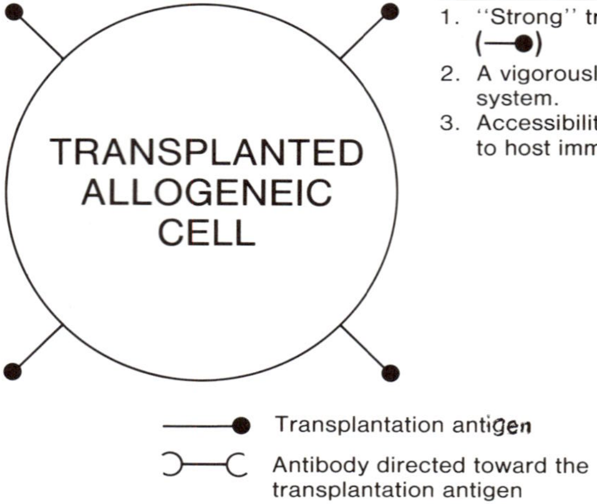

Factors Which Favor or Promote Rejection of The Allografted cells

1. "Strong" transplantation antigens (—●)
2. A vigorously responsive immune system.
3. Accessibility of the allografted cells to host immunocompetent cells.

Figure 16.1 *Factors affecting the acceptability of an allograft by the host.*

suppressant therapy as presently practiced will probably go the way of the dinosaur as a long-term approach to the prevention of allograft rejection. The reasons for anticipating the demise of currently practiced immunosuppressant chemotherapy are as follows: 1. The application of aggressive measures to prevent or quickly contain infections permits survival of the allograft without immunosuppressant therapy, even in the presence of an incompatible donor-host relationship.

2. The dosages of the immunosuppressive drugs administered, in the absence of a rejection crisis, are so low that their pharmacologic effects in vivo may be seriously questioned. Certainly the drugs exert little immunosuppression in the animal when administered at the same dosage per kilogram body weight as is utilized in the allografted patient. To be effective in the experimental animal, the dosage of each of the immunosuppressants must be increased 3- to 5-fold. Unfortunately, the incidence of death directly attributable to the toxic effects of the immunosuppressive agents administered also increases to a level which would be totally unacceptable in the human population treated with these drugs. Therefore, the dosage of the drugs administered to patients represents a compromise between a toxic (and most effective immunosuppressive) dose and a nontoxic (and much less effective immunosuppressive) dose.

3. The most effective of the drugs are immunosuppressive only in the broadest sense. They are, in fact, toxic to most cells, especially lymphocytes, granulocytes, platelets, erythrocytes and their precursors, gastrointestinal epithelial cells, endothelial cells, etc. There is, therefore, no specificity in their action. Several major complications following the administration of these drugs are hemorrhage, aplastic anemia, and immunodeficiency disease. The latter is attributed to the lymphocytotoxic properties of these drugs.

4. The drugs tend to act indiscriminately with respect to both the humoral and cell-mediated immune responses.

5. ALG, and more recently ATG, which many transplantation surgeons and immunologists anticipated would overcome all the obstacles in the way of a permanent graft take, have unfortunately been accompanied by unexpected serious complications. Even before these agents were used in human patients, experimental work in animals disclosed that the host could respond to the foreign proteins in the xenogeneic antiserum and form antibodies toward them. The circulating antigen-antibody complexes induce immune complex diseases, i.e. serum sickness, proliferative glo-

merulonephritis. The latter is a most serious occurrence if the allografted organ is the kidney, as it usually is. After a relatively short trial period, the use of ALG or ATG in patients has been markedly curtailed due to its dangerous side effects. Its use is primarily indicated during an acute rejection crisis.

The nonspecificity of these drugs with respect to the immune mechanisms affected makes their utilization hazardous at best, as it is now generally accepted that allograft rejection is primarily a function of the cell-mediated immune system. Furthermore, enhancement of graft survival is often accompanied by the formation of noncomplement-fixing antibodies which may protect the grafted cells from incipient or long-term damage by sensitized cells. It would seem advisable, therefore, to administer a drug which would temporarily suppress the cell-mediated, and not the humoral, immune response. This would also ensure the unhampered functioning, if not compensatory augmentation, of the antibody-forming system, thus minimizing the risk of bacterial and most viral infections, the immunity to which is provided primarily by circulating antibodies. Proper immunosuppressive therapy will, therefore, have to await the discovery, by chance or by design, of agents capable of specifically inhibiting or enhancing only one of the two major immune systems without simultaneously inflicting generalized tissue damage due to their innate toxicity. One drug which shows promise of fulfilling these conditions is cyclosporin-A, a fungal metabolite. In initial clinical trials, its immunosuppressive properties were not hampered or compromised by complications or side effects. Furthermore, cyclosporin-A can suppress the rejection reaction without the need to simultaneously administer steroids, Imuran, or ATG. Only time will tell whether cyclosporin-A is really the "wonder drug" which has been sought for in the treatment of the allografted patient.

If immunosuppressive drugs do not provide the answer to the total control of the allograft rejection reaction, what measures can we anticipate will emerge to facilitate the attainment of the objective? Future treatment must be far more specific and be noninjurious to the host (see Fig. 16.1). It should not affect the immune system in its capacity to form antibodies to pathogenic microorganisms. The treatment will probably take the form of an induced state of permanent immunologic tolerance toward the transplantation antigens of the allograft. Evidence has been presented, with increasing frequency in the past few years, that the administration of solubilized transplantation antigens into the experimental animal induces a state of tolerance toward them. Thus, it is probable that the human will respond in a similar fashion following the injection of the transplantation antigens in the appropriate physical state. It will be necessary to have a bank of the major and minor transplantation antigens in a tolerogenic form ready to be administered to the designated recipient following tissue typing of the allograft donor.

ALG (or ATG) may again be utilized but under circumstances which will ensure no immune response to it. It has been shown that a state of tolerance can be induced toward xenogeneic gamma globulin, provided the latter is injected in a nonaggregated form. Thus, the administration of nonaggregated equine gamma globulin will induce tolerance to it and the subsequent injection of equine ALG gamma globulin will be tolerated by the host without any ontoward reaction.

As stated above, the objective of this form of treatment is true immunotherapy and is mainly prophylactic, not chemotherapeutic. The immune system should not be affected insofar as its capacity to respond to pathogenic microorganisms is concerned. However, there should be no immune response toward the allografted cells because a state of tolerance toward the transplantation antigens of the allograft will have been induced.

Transplantation Antigens

Forgotten in the discussion related to the body's immune responses to implanted allogeneic cells is the need to define the raison d'etre for the response. Why do antigens exist on an allograft capable of evoking an immune response in the host? What are transplantation (or histoincompatibility or HLA) antigens, and why did they evolve in the first place? Since, under normal conditions, the immune system would never be exposed to these antigens, one must surmise that the ability of the immune system to respond to them implies the existence of preprogrammed or precommitted cells directed to interact with antigens which possess surface configurations identical to or cross-reactive with the transplantation antigens. The transplantation antigens, therefore, only serve as probes to detect and activate immunocompetent cells which evolved to react to quite different antigenic stimuli. Viewed in this light, the immunologically mediated rejection of an allograft results from the incidental activation of immunocompetent cells which exist for reasons other than to empower them to reject an allograft.

How and why have transplantation antigens been introduced into the genetic, and consequently antigenic, make-up of the cell? Why do cells possess transplantation antigens, and is their incorporation into the cell genome related to the evolution of the mammalian or other animal species? A consideration of the evolution of the transplantation antigens on a phylogenetic basis may help resolve this enigma.

Any proposed mechanism for the evolution of transplantation antigens should take into account the following considerations:

1. The transplantation antigens surely did not evolve in order

to permit an individual to reject an allograft, a most unnatural event. Therefore, their evolution must, in some way, be related to the preservation of the species and its protection from the environment. They must have survival value or they would have ceased to exist, in accordance with Darwinian concepts of evolution.

2. The transplantation antigens must have a raison d'etre as defined by natural phenomena or selection and should not be arbitrarily defined in terms of experimental findings in the laboratory. As recently stated by Burnet, we are dealing with Darwinian evolution at the level of cell surface antigens or recognition sites.

3. Animals and humans are not naturally inbred. Therefore, results of experiments with animals of highly inbred strains may not be relevant to, and might in fact detract from, the elucidation of the evolution of transplantation antigens.

4. Nature's primary preoccupation is to ensure survival of the individual up to the stage of sexual maturity and successful reproduction of the species. Once reproduction has occurred, the participants of the act of procreation become dispensible. Therefore, dysfunction and/or aberrant behavior of the immune system should be anticipated in the individual as he ages.

Let us confine the discussion of the evolution of transplantation antigens to the human being (Fig. 16.2). It is proposed that the transplantation antigens reflect the antigenicity of microorganisms which constituted the immediate environment to which the species was exposed during its evolution. Humans, by Darwinian evolution, probably evolved from lower animal species in a somewhat haphazard fashion on different parts of the globe. Let us assume that there originally existed two geographically isolated and distinct human populations, A and B. The (ARC) cells of some individuals in population A would, by chance, bear surface protein configurations (designated Ag-X) identical to the major antigen(s) characteristic of a particular virulent pathogen, arbitrarily designated pathogen X in Figure 16.2. Such individuals would, therefore, be immunologically tolerant with respect to this pathogen since surface structures or recognition sites on their (ARC) cells would be identical to those characteristic of this pathogen. These individuals would, therefore, succumb as a result of infection with this pathogen. Other individuals would be immunologically resistant to this pathogen as a result of their (ARC) lymphoid cells possessing receptor sites (RS-X) capable of cognizing (or recognizing) the major antigenic site on the surface of the pathogenic organism and of interacting with it, thus initiating the events which culminate in the immune re-

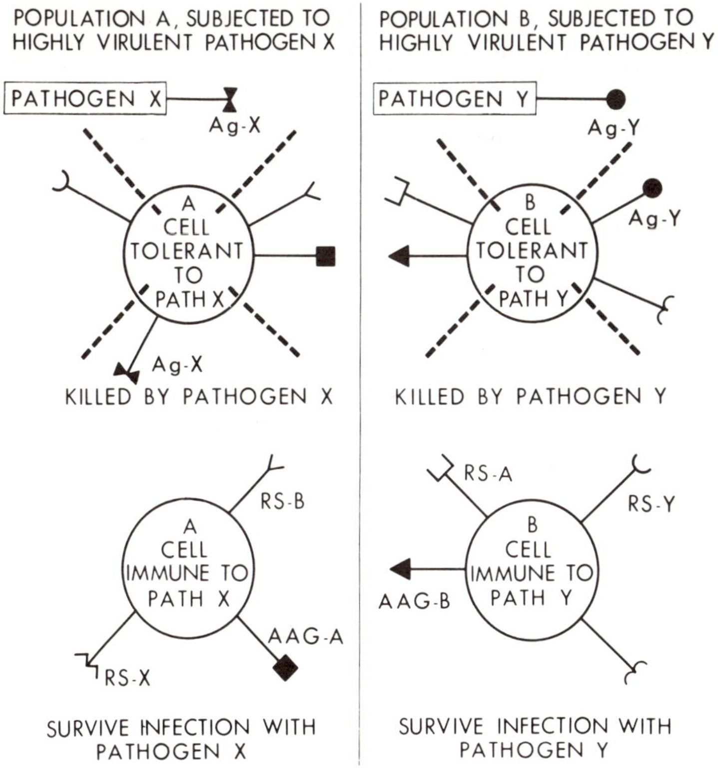

Figure 16.2 *The possible evolution of the transplantation antigens.*

sponse. A similar set of circumstances would govern the survival of individuals comprising population B with respect to pathogen Y, and their cells would possess the receptor sites (RS-Y) capable of interacting with the main antigen(s) characteristic of pathogen Y (Ag-Y). It is also proposed that the immunocompetent cells would possess surface structures identical to antigens characteristic of microorganisms of little or no virulence. Since such a state of affairs could not pose a threat to the survival of the individual, these cell surface constituents would be tolerated. Since these cell surface constituents would be transmitted from one generation to another in accordance with genetic laws governing inheritance, they exist today, although the organisms with which they originally cross-reacted may no longer exist or prove difficult to identify. It is proposed that these latter cell surface constituents, referred to as AAG-A and AAG-B in Figure 16.2, constitute what is referred to today as the transplantation or histoincompatibility antigens and that the allograft rejection reaction is the result of interaction of these antigens with receptors present on the cells of the allograft recipient.

To recapitulate, the concept proposed above is that the cell capable of responding immunologically to exogenous antigen X has a receptor RS-X capable of interacting with antigen X and has, therefore, lost the surface structure immunologically identical to exogenous antigen X. On the other hand, the cell capable of responding immunologically to exogenous antigen Y possesses a surface receptor RS-Y capable of interacting with antigen Y and has lost the surface structure immunologically identical to antigen Y. Implicit in this proposal is the mandatory deletion on the cell of sites which are configurationally complementary to receptors on the same and other autologous cells. If this condition were not to be realized or were it to be compromised, then obviously lymphoid cells would be able to interact with syngeneic lymphoid cells, thus initiating autoimmune disease and generalized immunodeficiency disease due to ablation of the thymoreticulolymphoid system. Such a state of affairs would constitute a lethal threat toward the survival of the species and would be quickly discarded by nature.

The cell surface antigens have been called the "differentiation antigens" by Boyse and Old. Presumably, they would be "recognized" by other molecules configurationally complementary to the differentiation antigens which have been referred to as "recognizers" by Bodmer. Bodmer postulated that any given cell may possess both differentiation antigens and recognizers providing the recognizers are not directed toward syngeneic cell surface antigens. In this context, the differentiation antigens and the recognizers are analogous to the transplantation antigens (AAG) and receptor sites (RS) for these AAG on allogeneic cells in the scheme proposed above to account for the evolution of transplantation antigens. This proposal is based upon phylogenetic and evolutionary considerations rather than on purely contemporary genetic considerations.

In support of the concept presented above, evidence has appeared suggesting an immunologic relationship between transplantation antigens and antigens present on some viruses and bacteria. Many investigators have observed cross-reactions between *D. pneumoniae, H. influenzae,* and streptococcal M proteins and human transplantation antigens. Recent findings in the guinea pig suggest that the genes controlling the immune response to antigens, the Ir genes, are closely linked to the genes controlling the major transplantation antigens. It has been suggested that the transplantation antigens may, in fact, be related to as yet unidentified exogenous antigens. Thus, it would appear that the capacity to respond to an antigenic stimulus with antibody formation or cell-mediated immunity is inextricably related to the presence or absence of the appropriate transplantation antigen.

Recent findings utilizing the MLR reaction also tend to support the proposal presented above. In the MLR composed of the allogeneic A and B cells, one may speculate that responder A cells react in at least two different ways to the stimulator B cells (Fig. 16.3). One may anticipate that the responder A cells undergo blastogenesis in the manner analogous to that of virgin antigen-recognizing cells (ARC) of the mouse or the rabbit confronted with an antigen for the first time. These lymphoblast A cells may release their recognition sites (transplantation antigens?) (Fig. 16.3, *left*) and transform into killer cells in vitro. Secondly, interaction of the responder A cells with the stimulator B cells, via interaction of the RS-B receptor on the A cell with the AAG-B antigen on the B cell, may result in the release from the A cells of the receptor sites which would behave functionally like antibodies (Fig. 16.3, *right*). A number of investigators have recently demonstrated the secretion of antibodies in the MLR. Since the MLR as described above is a two-way (or bidirectional) MLR and not a one-way (or unidirectional) MLR, the responder B cells would also simultaneously respond to the stimulator A cells in a similar fashion.

It has been demonstrated that the cell-free supernatant of an MLR, but not of a syngeneic cell culture, contains a blastogenic

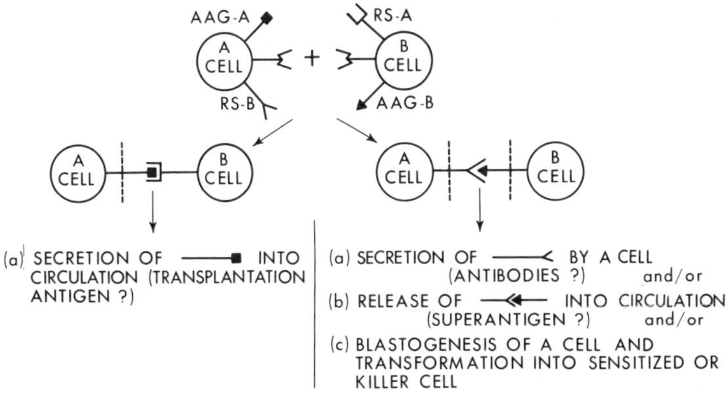

Figure 16.3 *The mixed leukocyte culture reaction (MLR): A proposal of the different cellular interactions and products released in this reaction.*

factor capable of inducing blastogenesis and mitosis of either of the cocultured lymphocytes as well as third-party cells. Since antiallotype and antilymphocyte antibodies also induce blastogenesis of human lymphocytes, and antibodies have been detected in the cell-free culture fluid of an MLR, it is probable that the blastogenic factor is an antibody secreted by the responder cells.

An understanding of the allograft rejection reaction greatly facilitates the appreciation and understanding of the autoimmune response. It is probably more than coincidence that the histopathologic characteristics of these two immune reactions are so similar as to suggest identical mechanisms. The effector phases of these two reactions display similar features, namely the infiltration of lymphoid cells, macrophages, pyroninophilic cells, and some plasma cells into a particular organ accompanied by inflammation and endothelial cell damage. This is followed by occlusion of the small blood vessels by platelet or platelet-fibrin thrombi, stasis, ischemia of the distal cells and tissues, necrosis often fibrinoid in character, and healing by fibrosis. The result may be total loss of function and failure of the organ affected. The pathogenesis of autoimmune disease as it affects a particular organ system dictates as one of the initiating events the emergence of new (forbidden) clones of immunocompetent effector cells, or the activation of normally dormant immunocompetent effector cells, capable of responding to stimulation by the autoantigens. In the transplant rejection reaction, it is considered that normal immunocompetent effector cells react to antigens present on the surface of the implanted allogeneic cells. The autoimmune reaction is, therefore, similar to that which occurs in the allograft rejection reaction.

THE IMMUNE RESPONSE AND PREGNANCY

A question often posed to the immunologist rather innocently by students, facetiously by residents and postgraduate students, and frequently antagonistically by physicians and investigators in other disciplines, is: "If you are so certain of a primary immunologic role in the allograft rejection reaction, then why does the female not reject her conceptus?" Since the cells of the embryo, even at the early trophoblast stage, possess surface antigens which are both maternally and paternally derived, one might anticipate that the maternal immune system would recognize these cells as foreign and mount an immune response to eliminate them. The normal individual is endowed with the capacity to reject all surgically allografted tissues genetically (and, therefore, antigenically) different from her own tissues. Then why does the pregnant female not reject her fetus, which in many respects may be considered to be an allograft? Of course, no such thing happens and the fetus is permitted to thrive in vivo until it is expelled at birth. The apparent lack of adherence by the immune system to the basic rules of transplantation immunity has been the subject of many monographs and books, but the explanation for this deviation from the anticipated response appears to have evaded us thus far.

As stated previously, one may seriously question whether the immune system evolved to provide the host with the capacity to reject an allograft. An allograft is, after all, a most unnatural event which would not occur under normal circumstances during the lifetime of the individual. The immune response provoked as a result of the well-intentioned surgical implantation of a lifesaving allograft may be nothing more than the normal response of the immune system to invasion by large numbers of foreign cells. Whether or not these foreign cells are pathogenic is irrelevant.

Our puzzlement concerning the lack of a response by the host to a foreign allogeneic fetal implant is probably the result of our having been conditioned to consider a heart or kidney allograft to be a natural or normal event and, paradoxically, the fetal allograft to be an unnatural or abnormal event, rather than vice versa. Investigators are constantly apologizing for the fact that the fetus appears to be the only allograft (semiallogeneic graft to be more precise) capable of surviving in the host and are constantly attempting to explain this within the framework of accepted immunologic principles and dogma governing the transplant rejection reaction. It is necessary that we realize that the fetus is not an allograft like all other allografts. The paramount importance of internalized pregnancy and gestation to the survival of the species should be obvious, and any explanation proposed to account for allograft rejection must take into account the normal maternal acceptance of the fetal allograft without the need to intervene with immunosuppressive drugs.

Furthermore, the fetus, certainly in the early stages of embryogenesis, behaves more like an uncontrolled malignant lesion than the precursor of a human being. Normal individuals are considered to possess natural immunity toward malignant cells, preventing the spontaneous occurrence of a tumor (see below). It is, therefore, necessary to conclude that, with regard to pregnancy and gestation, the immune system twice contravenes its own rules concerning the response of the pregnant female to her fetus since the latter may be considered to be both an allograft and a malignant process.

One theory which has been proposed to explain why the fetal

allograft is not rejected is that the uterus is an immunologically privileged site. Another theory is that the trophoblast cells are not antigenic. Both of these arguments have been refuted by investigations carried out in the experimental animal. A third theory is based on the finding that the cells in the outer layer of the trophoblast, the syncytiotrophoblast, possess only maternally derived antigens. This theory proposes that the syncytiotrophoblast functions as an "immunologic (placental) barrier" to protect the developing embryo from potential or actual maternally derived immunocompetent cells capable of interacting with fetal cells possessing paternally derived antigens on their surface. However, little evidence has been forthcoming to substantiate this theory. In fact, all evidence points to the inappropriateness of the term "barrier" because there are very few materials which cannot traverse the placenta. The placenta does appear to be impermeable to maternal cells, though, at least up to the time of parturition.

Another theory to account for fetal survival is based on the finding that antibodies are synthesized by the mother toward the fetal cells which protect the fetus and enhance fetal growth and development. These protective antibodies would have to be non-complement-fixing and would be similar to the allograft-"enhancing" or -"blocking" antibodies which are synthesized in allograft recipients toward cells of the allograft.

The most recent theory advanced to explain the failure of the mother to reject the fetal allograft is the suppressor theory. It is proposed that suppressor cells and/or circulating soluble suppressor factors can be activated and/or newly generated, capable of inhibiting the immune response and thus limit the capacity of the pregnant female to reject the fetal allograft. Suppressor cells have been detected in the fetal circulation capable of inhibiting maternal circulating lymphoytes from responding to the fetal and paternal cells in an MLR. Several placenta-derived hormones and alpha-fetoprotein, a glycoprotein secreted by fetal cells into the circulation, are capable of inhibiting reactions in vitro which are synonymous with immunocompetence. Their function in the maternal circulation may be to induce a transient immunosuppressed state in order to facilitate the induction of tolerance to the fetal transplantation antigens and thus ensure the survival of the fetus. However, this immunosuppressed state would have to be specific to fetal antigens since only the ability to reject the fetus is suppressed and not the immune response to all other antigens, especially pathogenic microorganisms. The incidence of serious infections is not significantly higher in pregnant women than it is in the general population. Despite its shortcomings, the suppressor theory as the explanation for the "phenomenon" of normal pregnancy and gestation is very attractive as it reflects contemporary immunologic thinking.

The author would like to propose one more mechanism to account for tolerance to the fetal allograft not alluded to above. The reader will recall from the discussion of immunologic tolerance (Chapter 11) that very small doses of an antigen are just as effective in inducing tolerance (low dose or low zone tolerance) as are massive doses of the antigen (high dose or high zone tolerance). It may not be irrelevant to point out that tolerance can be induced to an implanted tumor if the host is first injected with only a very few (10^2 or 10^3) tumor cells (the "sneaking-through" theory of tumorigenesis). On the other hand, pretreatment of the host with large numbers of cells (10^5 or 10^6) of the to-be-implanted tumor invariably provokes an immune response which will prevent the growth and result in death of the tumor once it is implanted. It may, therefore, be that the very minute quantity of paternal antigens presented to the maternal immune system in the initial stages of embryogenesis (morula and blastocyst stage) may invoke a state of low dose tolerance toward the embryo, which will last until either tolerance is prematurely broken (i.e. idiopathic abortion?) or the infant is born.

It may very well be, therefore, that low dose tolerance is the mechanism which permits tumor and fetal (allograft) survival in the normal individual. Cancer may be the penalty we pay in order to provide an internal milieu for pregnancy and gestation.

THE IMMUNE RESPONSE AND CANCER

The cornerstone of the proposed immunologic role in the control and eradication of malignant disease rests upon the presumed capacity of the immune system to recognize the malignant cells as foreign (Fig. 16.4), since no immune response can be mounted in the absence of a tumor-specific antigen(s). Antigenic differences between the normal cell and its malignant counterpart are usually demonstrated by injecting the experimental animal with malignant cells and observing that the antiserum, following absorption with normal cells, retains the capacity to react with the malignant cells. However, this does not necessarily indicate that the immunocompetent cells in the human patient from whom the tumor cells have been isolated can differentiate between normal and malignant cells and form antibodies to the malignant cells. It is important that the reader realize that the term "tumor-specific antigens" alludes to the capacity of cells of the immunized xenogeneic animals to recognize these antigens

Factors Favoring Inhibition of an Immune Response to Tumor Cells

1. Absence of tumor-specific antigens.
2. Immunosuppressor factors secreted by tumor cells.
3. Immunoincompetence induced by chemotherapeutic agents.
4. Formation of noncomplement fixing antibodies.
5. Presence of circulating antigen-antibody complexes. (→≻—≺)
6. Continued presence of excess antigen in the circulation (→), competing with cytotoxic antibodies and/or sensitized cells for cell-bound antigen.

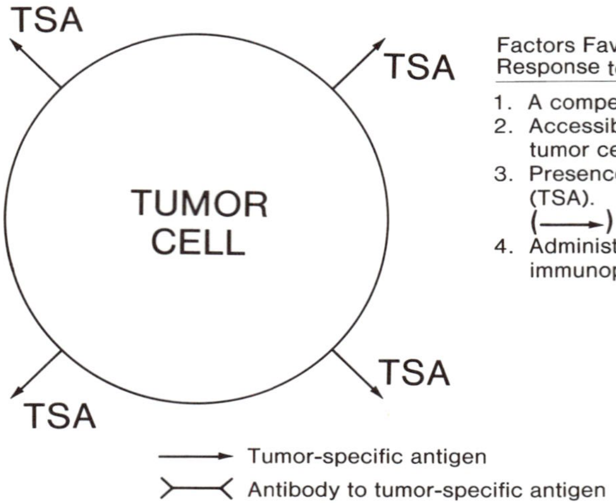

Factors Favoring an Immune Response to Tumor Cells

1. A competent immune system.
2. Accessibility of lymphocytes to the tumor cells.
3. Presence of tumor-specific antigen (TSA). (——→)
4. Administration of specific immunopotentiating agents.

Figure 16.4 *Factors favoring and inhibiting an immune response to tumor cells.*

and respond immunologically to them. When it was recognized that tumor antigens could sensitize the allogeneic host toward both tumor cells and normal cells from the donor, these tumor-specific antigens were referred to as **tumor-specific transplantation antigens** (TSTA).

The finding of TSTA on malignant cells encouraged speculation concerning immunologic mechanisms whereby malignant disease is suppressed in the normal individual, assuming that mutant, potentially malignant cells emerge continually in the host.

Theoretically, a finite number of malignant cells or their immediate (malignancy-committed) precursors are expected to arise spontaneously as a result of mutations within a small proportion of the cells which are normally rapidly dividing, i.e. the cells of the lymphothymoreticular system, the bone marrow, the gastrointestinal tract, and the urogenital system. If even less than 1 of every 100,000 mitoses results in a mutated cell endowed with unregulated proliferative capacity, each individual could possess more than 10,000 of these cells at any one time, a number which can induce malignant disease in the experimental animal. However, in reality, the incidence of malignant disease is many times lower than would be predicted, suggesting that the host possesses a mechanism to thwart the emergence of malignant cells. The concept of **immunologic surveillance** as a normal protective mechanism was proposed in the 1960s, and it ascribed "search and destroy" activity to a class of circulating T lymphocytes. This proposal was based on the fact that, with a few exceptions, the incidence of malignant disease increases with aging coincidentally with involution of the thymus and its diminishing ability to generate new T cells. Although the concept of immunologic surveillance was initially greeted with enthusiasm by the discipline, its credibility was seriously eroded a few years later in the face of documented evidence that the incidence of malignant disease in neonatally thymectomized T cell-deficient mice, or "nude" mice born euthymic or with a severely hypoplastic thymus, is not significantly greater than in the normal population. This is contrary to what would be anticipated if indeed the major protection from, and barrier to, the establishment of malignant disease is provided by the T cells. Furthermore, humans deficient in circulating T cells as a result of immunosuppressive chemotherapy present with an increased incidence of lymphoreticular malignancies but not with an increased incidence of other types of malignancies. These findings forced a reassessment and reevaluation of T cells in the provision of natural immunity to malignant disease in the early 1970s. Fortunately, there was another cell in the wings waiting to be assigned an anticancer role, the so-called natural killer or NK cell. This cell, first described by Richter in 1971, is a normally circulating cell capable of effecting antibody-independent lysis of selected target cells in vitro (see Chapter 7). Numerous malignant cell lines and nonmalignant, nonreplicating cells can function as target cells. However, the identity of this cell is uncertain due to the fact that T, B, and null lymphocytes, and even monocytes, exhibit NK cytotoxic activity depending upon the target cell selected in the in vitro assay. It is probable, therefore, that the circulating NK cells constitute a functional class of numerous unipotent cytotoxic cells with varying morphology rather than a single pluripotent or omnipotent cytotoxic cell.

That NK effector cells, in general, have an antitumor role to play in the host has gained support over the past several years. The circulating cells of cancer patients treated with interferon, Bacille Bilié de Calmette-Guérin (BCG), and *C. parvum*, all of which enhance anticancer immunity, exhibit enhanced NK activity. It has also been observed that mice with few and/or slowly responding circulating NK cells are susceptible to greater numbers of spontaneously arising tumors than are mice with large numbers of rapidly responding circulating NK cells. Furthermore, the transfer of cells with high NK cytotoxic activity to syngeneic animals possessing cells which exhibit low NK cytotoxic activity protects the latter from the emergence of tumors. It has been postulated that mutant cells with surface configurations recognized by NK cells are not normally given the opportunity to become overt tumors because they are susceptible to lysis by the NK cells and are thus eliminated.

A seemingly contradictory finding is the relative insensitivity of freshly explanted tumor cells to lysis by the patient's own NK cytotoxic cells. The explanation currently favored for this finding is that tumor cells are generated and proliferate due to the absence of specific NK cells capable of interacting with these malignant cells. Conversely, some mutant cells initially susceptible to lysis by NK cells may shed the surface configuration(s) which serves as the target for the NK cytotoxic cells, and these mutant cells may now become overtly malignant and evolve into a solitary tumor and/or present as metastatic disease.

In addition to the naturally occurring NK cytotoxic cells which may function in a prophylactic manner to deter the emergence of malignant cells, it is also necessary to acknowledge an antitumor role to the (antigen-responsive) immune system, especially the cell-mediated immune system, which is impressed with the role of eliminating the tumor cells following failure of the NK cells. It has been consistently demonstrated in the experimental animal that stimulation of cell-mediated immunity to a transplantable tumor prior to implantation of the tumor invariably results in rejection of the tumor rather than rapid growth and spread of the tumor which results in death of the animal. The resistance toward the generation and proliferation of malignant cells appears, therefore, to be provided by both naturally occurring NK cells which function independent of prior antigenic contact and the cell-mediated immune mechanism which requires activation by the antigen.

Important

1. Malignant cells are mutant cells or cells which have dedifferentiated antigenically to embryonic status. It is postulated that these cells have lost the gross surface features or specific surface configurations which are recognized by the naturally occurring cytotoxic cells and are, therefore, no longer susceptible to lysis by these cytotoxic cells. As a result, these cells are no longer regulated by the control mechanisms to which normal cells are subject.
2. For the acquired or adaptive immune mechanism to be recruited on behalf of the host, it is essential that the malignant cell possess surface configurations recognized as foreign by the host's immunocompetent cells, to which they can react with an immune response. These configurations are, therefore, not present in the normal counterpart cells.
3. The induced immune response consists of the formation of cytotoxic cells and/or complement-fixing (lytic) antibodies directed toward the malignant cells. Non-complement-fixing antibodies will tend to protect the malignant cells as a result of competition with the complement-fixing antibodies and sensitized cells for the identical antigenic sites.

Evidence that immunity plays a role in resistance to, or rejection of, cancer in humans is mainly anecdotal and circumstantial. No one factor listed in Figure 16.4 can be singled out as the primary inhibitor or stimulator of the immune response to the malignant cells. Each of these factors has been implicated in different patients and the experimental animal as instrumental in both inhibiting and augmenting an immune response. One reason for the apparent conflicting results is the adherence by investigators to the assumption that immune responses to all malignancies are identical. This may be a very invalid and ill-conceived assumption. More likely than not, different tumors may evoke different types of immune responses and some may not evoke any. Thus, it is imperative that each type of tumor be investigated as a specific disease process. Patients with leukemia should not be investigated as part of a group of patients where the other members may be suffering from such diverse malignancies as cancer of the bowel (carcinoma), bone (sarcoma), lymph gland (lymphoma), ovary (mucinous tumors), nervous system (neuroblastoma, glioma), etc. An evaluation of the immune responses of the individuals in such a heterogeneous group of patients can only confuse the investigator, because specific, consistent immune responses of one type to any of these tumors may be masked by the lack of responses or different responses to the other tumors. Statistical analysis of the combined data obtained from such a heterogeneous sample is, therefore, a most inappropriate and often misleading way to evaluate the immune response to tumors.

Nevertheless, results of investigations in the experimental animal, mainly the inbred mouse, subjected to transplantable virus-induced and chemical carcinogen-induced tumors, strongly indicate that the immune response to the tumor antigens, when it occurs, is a cell-mediated one and that antibodies tend to protect the tumor cells from lysis by the sensitized cells. Results of investigations in humans afflicted with various types of malignant diseases generally confirm this view. From an immunologic point of view, it would seem appropriate to treat the patient with drugs which stimulate the cell-mediated immune system and suppress an antibody response to the tumor antigens. A number of substances, including Freund's complete adjuvant, levamisole, *C. parvum*, and endotoxins, have been promoted as possessing the capacity to preferentially enhance the cell-mediated immune response. These agents are capable of nonspecifically stimulating the reticuloendothelial system and thus enhancing the phagocytic capabilities of the phagocytic cells (the angry macrophage). They also function as adjuvants since they can augment or enhance an immune response to an antigen (see Chapter 4). **Immunotherapy** in the treatment of cancer consists of the administration of the tumor-specific antigens along with an adjuvant in order to induce a significant immune response to these antigens. When only a small quantity of the antigen is injected along with the adjuvant, the result is usually the induction of a cell-mediated, not a humoral, immune response. For this reason, these agents have been incorporated into chemotherapeutic regimens.

Important

If the antigen is injected in a subimmunogenic dose along with the adjuvant it will tend to preferentially stimulate a cell-mediated immune response. However, as the concentration of the antigen is increased to the level approaching the normal immunogenic dose, the humoral immune response is also markedly augmented by the adjuvant. The investigator or chemotherapist must be assiduously cognizant of this dual role of Freund's adjuvant, *C. parvum,* levamisole, endotoxin, and other agents which function to selectively enhance the cell-mediated immune response provided the dose of antigen administered is in a concentration below that which normally provokes an antibody response. Otherwise, both cell-mediated and humoral immune responses are enhanced, thus neutralizing the anticipated beneficial effect of the adjuvant.

As was discussed above, tumor cells must possess tumor-specific surface configurations capable of being recognized as antigens by the host's immunocompetent cells if a specific immune response to the tumor cells is to take place. Support for the existence of tumor-specific surface structures is derived from the findings that unique tumor-specific proteins, carcinoembryonic antigen (CEA), and alpha-fetoprotein (AFP), are detected in the circulation of patients afflicted with cancer of the gastrointestinal tract (primary adenocarcinoma) and the liver (primary hepatoma), respectively. It has furthermore been demonstrated that antibodies to CEA and AFP generated in the xenogeneic animal adhere to the surface membranes of the tumor cells which secrete these tumor-specific proteins as demonstrated by indirect immunofluorescence staining (see Chapter 7).

The detection of AFP in the serum, especially if its concentration is found to rise in a follow-up assay, is indicative of a primary tumor (carcinoma) of the liver (with the obvious exception of the pregnant woman in whom AFP is synthesized by the developing fetus), while a rise in the concentration of CEA is indicative of a primary malignancy in the gastrointestinal tract or possibly the gall bladder, pancreas, or breast. Of course false positives do arise, and these must be differentiated from patients with malignant disease. For example, excessive cigarette smoking has been shown to result in relatively high concentrations of circulating CEA; however, the concentration of CEA drops to normal when the individual ceases to smoke.

In view of the unavoidable occurrence of false positives and false negatives in the CEA and AFP assays, it would be inappropriate, if not hazardous, to screen all individuals in whom a diagnosis of malignant disease is entertained on the basis of intuition rather than corroborating clinical and/or laboratory and/or radiologic evidence. From a logistical point of view, it would not be feasible to attempt to utilize the CEA and AFP assays as routine screening tests for the entire population at large. Nevertheless, the immunoassays for CEA and AFP provide highly relevant, if not critical, data when carried out in follow-up studies on known cancer patients at intervals of time following initial treatment of the tumor (surgery and/or irradiation and/or chemotherapy) to monitor recurrence of the malignancy. A sharp drop in the concentration of the tumor-specific antigens in the immediate posttreatment period and their subsequent absence from the circulation are good prognostic signs, whereas failure of these antigens to decrease in concentration following treatment or a subsequent sharp rise in their concentration indicates metastatic disease and a bad prognosis. This type of monitoring for progression and/or recurrence of a malignant disease can now be carried out routinely with respect to malignancies of the gastrointestinal tract and the liver. Recurrence of a malignancy can be diagnosed early by a radioimmunoassay test, and treatment can be initiated before the disease has progressed and/or metastasized to any significant degree.

Efforts are currently underway to establish radioimmunoassay procedures for the detection of prostate and breast tumor-specific antigens, and success may be anticipated in the not too distant future.

What factors and conditions limit the application of immunologic tests to the diagnosis of cancer? Several of these are as follows:

1. Tumor-specific antigen(s) must be present in the circulation of the host in the presence of malignant disease and must be absent from the circulation in the absence of malignant disease. It must be emphasized once again that the term "tumor-specific antigen" used in its present context does not imply antigenicity in the host but antigenicity in a xenogeneic animal, such as the rabbit, horse, or goat.

2. The test must be such that it can be carried out using only the serum or plasma of the patient. The factor detected in the serum or plasma must be stable in vitro and should withstand freezing, thawing, and mild pH changes.

3. The test must be inexpensive, reproducible, relatively simple to perform, and, most important, highly specific for the malignancy in question. Not only must there be minimal numbers of false positives and false negatives, but the test must also be infallible with respect to the specific malignancy.

4. The specificity of an immunologic procedure in terms of its reliability to detect and quantitate circulating tumor-specific antigens depends entirely upon the purity of the immunizing antigen and its cross-reactivity with normal tissue proteins. The more pure the antigen, the more specific will be the antiserum following immunization of the xenogeneic animal. Conversely, the less pure the antigen, the more will the antiserum cross-react with normal body constituents, thus allowing for false positive reuslts.

5. Although the tumor-specific antigen(s) may be relatively pure, it does not necessarily follow that it will be identical in different individuals with the same type of tumor. For this test to be effective as a general screening or follow-up tool, it must be demonstrated that the antigen is tumor-specific and not individual-specific.

6. Even if the antigen isolated is tumor-specific, it does not necessarily follow that the xenogeneic antibodies generated toward the antigen will be identical in their specificity and avidity. Since the antisera are obtained from different outbred animals, they may be more or less specific depending on the individual response. It is, therefore, necessary to compare batches of different antisera before selecting the most appropriate one to be used in the radioimmunoassay.

The reader should not be intimidated or depressed by the above discussion. An understanding and appreciation of the relevant factors at play may limit freedom with respect to the utilization of the test procedure but will greatly enhance its predictive value.

It is necessary to ensure that patients are not unduly or inappropriately subjected to chemotherapy to the point where the immune system is compromised and is unable to provide immunity, not only toward the tumor cells but, even more importantly, toward pathogenic microorganisms in the environment. The attempt to manipulate the immune systems with crudely defined highly toxic drugs only exacerbates the already tenuous immunologic homeostatic balance in the patient by inducing an iatrogenic immunodeficiency state, thereby facilitating the imposition of a severe bacteremia and septicemia following exposure of the patient to even minimally pathogenic microorganisms from which the patient may not recover. The recognition that a major complication of chemotherapy is the induction of an immunodeficiency state, and that this and not the malignant disease is often responsible for the death of the patient, is attracting considerable attention.

The chemotherapeutic drugs induce an immunodeficiency state probably as a result of their lymphocytotoxic properties. They also exhibit psychodepressive properties, which diminish the appetite and contribute toward the loss in weight characteristic of many cancer patients frequently long before the terminal stage of the illness is reached. Recent findings indicate that, even in the absence of malignant disease, prolonged negative nitrogen balance preceded by severe weight loss due to markedly diminished intake of the appropriate nutrients results in an immunodeficiency state. However, immune responsiveness can be restored by intravenous hyperalimentation. Therefore, diminished food intake and/or an inadequate diet followed by a lengthy period of negative nitrogen balance should be considered contributory factors in the induction of an immunodeficiency state.

The different forms of treatment used, especially chemotherapy and irradiation, are not selective in their action and they tend to adversely affect multiple organ systems, especially the lymphoreticular (immune) system. It is, therefore, prudent, if not obligatory, to monitor the immune status of the patient on chemotherapy. The institution of reliable tests which monitor and help maintain an immunocompetent state would be expected to be accompanied by improvement in the prognosis of the cancer patient. The role of the immune response in cancer must be specifically defined before intervention can be instituted with drugs selective in their effects on the humoral and cell-mediated immune responses, capable of enhancing or augmenting one and suppressing the other to the benefit of the host. Unfortunately, the drugs presently utilized, the "immunotherapeutic drugs," do not come close to achieving this objective. The continued funding of "field trials" aimed at establishing in a very empirical manner a statistical validity for a particular drug cannot but hamper initiative to extend our basic knowledge of the metabolic and immunologic properties of malignant cells, a prerequisite for a rational and responsible approach to drug therapy. The proper therapeutic agents will only be found once we have established scientifically based criteria to be used in their evaluation.

CHAPTER 17

Immunity and the Aged

"The seas are strewn with the wreckage of unverified facts and abandoned theories." (M.A.R.)

A great deal is being written these days about the health and social needs of the aged, and the reason for it is self-evident. An inordinately high percentage of the North American population is presently in the 40 to 55 age group and getting older. It is estimated that, in Canada, the percentage of people in the postretirement age category (65 and over) will reach record proportions within 15 to 20 years, with this age group constituting approximately 18 to 22% of the population. This figure is probably valid for the United States as well. This should be contrasted with the fact that only 5 to 8% of the population constituted the "over 65" age category between 1950 and 1970, years when new institutions and social measures were enacted to cater to postretirement age people.

Old age may be a blessing to the person who experiences it, but society projects a very ambivalent attitude toward the aged in our population. On the one hand, industry and, therefore, the economy benefit from the existence of the elderly who are the primary consumers of specialized products and services designed to meet their needs. Construction of chronic care hospitals and nursing homes for the bedridden as well as lodges to house those who are in good health and mobile (ambulatory) is a booming industry, creating many job opportunities at a time when other sectors of the economy of North America are stagnant. Counterbalancing these positive economic benefits is the general financial burden society associates with old people since a not insignificant number of the elderly become senile and debilitated and require frequent hospitalization long before the terminal illness sets in.

Government demographers view with alarm the projected statistics for the late 1990s and the first decade of the 21st century, when one of every five individuals will belong to the post-65 age group. Furthermore, one of every three individuals in the post-18 age group, that is 33% of the adult population, will be in the post-65 age group. It is also estimated that the budget to finance the needs of the elderly will multiply 4- to 5-fold by the late 1990s. How, it may be asked, will our institutions be able to discharge their obligations to the aged, from both cost and manpower points of view, without causing excessive harm to our social structures and the other sectors of our economy? This is the dilemma facing government and society at large—the obligation to provide appropriate services to a large dependent aged population without placing excessive strain on existing institutions with responsibilities toward other segments of the population. We must ensure that our social and financial institutions will not be jeopardized by the heavy burden of caring for a large elderly population. Translated into simple terms, the question really posed is how can a contracted working population support an ever growing elderly population sufficiently to ensure that the latter will be properly fed, properly housed, and maintained in good health.?

It is a fact that as people age, especially when they enter the eighth decade of life, the incidence of morbidity rises sharply. Not only are illnesses more difficult to treat and cure, but they often become chronic and debilitating. This translates into a high financial cost to society.

Obligatory retirement at age 65 is most damaging to the individual in a psychologic sense and undoubtedly hastens his transformation from a responsible, independent, and active member of society to a dependent, depressed, and noncontributing member of society. Such an individual tends to suffer a loss of appetite and becomes malnourished within a short period of time. His state of health deteriorates and he becomes abnormally susceptible to infectious disease. Many of the health problems facing the elderly stem from the increased susceptibility to infection after exposure to even mildly pathogenic microorganisms. The infections are often severe and unresponsive to conventional antibiotic chemotherapy, and the individual requires lengthy hospitalization. Other diseases are also more prevalent in the elderly. In general, it can be stated that:

1. The incidence and severity of infection are markedly increased in the aged.
2. The incidence of autoimmune disease is markedly elevated in the aged.
3. The incidence of malignant disease is markedly elevated (10 to 100 times) in the aged.

The role of the immune system in the prevention of autoimmune disease and cancer has been discussed at length in previous chapters. Evidence has been presented strongly indicating that the presence of autoimmune or malignant disease is usually accompanied by one or more identifiable defects in the immune system. Therefore, on the assumption that the state of the immune response system plays a pivotal role in the control of morbidity and disease, these findings of increased morbidity in the aged due to infection, autoimmune disease, and cancer suggest a generally defective immune system in the aged. Is there any evidence which would support such an assessment? The answer would have to be a guarded yes. The evidence to date strongly suggests that aging is accompanied by a lessening ability to respond immunologically. Immunocompetence generally declines as the individual grows older—imperceptibly between the ages of 10 and 65 but with apparent suddenness between the ages of 65 and 75. The data are largely anecdotal, however, as very few in-depth systematic studies have been carried out. Nevertheless, evidence from numerous investigations conducted on both animals and humans indicates that:

1. The humoral or antibody response is less vigorous in the elderly as compared to that observed in individuals in the young and middle-aged groups. The onset of antibody synthesis is slower, and the peak antibody titer is generally lower. Often, no immune response is detected in the elderly following what would otherwise be considered appropriate immunization. The effect of aging is far greater on the primary immune response than on the secondary immune response.

2. The cell-mediated immune response is also diminished in the elderly and sometimes cannot be detected.

3. The ratio of nonspecific suppressor cells (T_G cells) to helper cells (T_M cells) is markedly altered and often inverted in the diseased elderly individual as compared to that in the normal individual. The absolute numbers of T_G cells may not be increased, reflecting a general decrease in the numbers of T_M cells. However, sufficient studies of this nature have not been carried out in the healthy aged population to warrant any conclusions at this time.

4. The number and/or activity of the naturally occurring killer (NK) cells appear to be decreased in the aged individual. If current concepts as to their role in the provision of innate antitumor immunity are correct, then these individuals would be more than normally susceptible to malignant disease.

Thus, the increase in incidence of disease in the elderly with its attendant morbidity and other sequalae can be attributed, at least in part, to a loss of immune responsiveness to invasive agents, an enhanced ability to respond to autoantigens, and a diminished ability to eradicate malignant cells.

Are there any changes in the tissues or organs of the immune system which correlate with this loss of effectiveness of the immune system? The answer again would appear to be yes, based on the following findings:

1. The thymus in terms of its size and cell content is but a vestigial remnant in the aged individual, in comparison to its size and lymphoid cell content in the young or mature individual.

2. The spleen and lymph nodes also undergo atrophic changes with the approach of old age. The lymph nodes shrink, the lymphoid follicles decrease in number and size, and the total number of lymphoid cells in the lymph nodes and spleen decreases. The percentage of T cells in the lymph nodes and spleen decreases markedly, while the percentage of B cells increases. The lymphoid follicles are replaced by fibrous elements.

3. The phagocytic capacity of the monocytes and neutrophils in the elderly also appears to be impaired. These cells do not respond normally to conventional chemotactic stimuli, and the opsonization index is usually lower in comparison to cells of young individuals.

The lack of vigor in the immune response is not apparently due to the absence of, or defects in, the B cells since B cells are detected in normal numbers in the circulation of the elderly. Furthermore, the immunoglobulin levels do not decrease appreciably, even well into old age (i.e. 80 to 90 years of age), indicating that the synthesis of immunoglobulins in general is not significantly impaired. The fault appears to lie with the thymus and the thymus-dependent cells. As stated previously, the thymus attains its maximum (relative) size at birth and begins to involute before puberty. From that point on, the thymus continues to shrink in size and in its cellular content, thus resulting in the diminished generation of the immunocompetent thymus-derived T cells. Investigators who have been concerned with these changes in the lymphoid organs in the person as he ages chronologically have suggested that the thymus functions as the biologic time clock, the pivotal organ balancing the see-saw of life and inevitable death. As they explain it, the thymus, as it involutes, generates and secretes lesser and lesser numbers of T cells, especially those immunocompetent T cells which participate in the induction of the antibody and cell-mediated immune responses. The secretion of the thymic hormones, such as thymosin and thymopoietin, also diminishes markedly. Furthermore, the thymus also ceases to generate the precursors of the suppressor cells, thus facilitating the autoimmune responses and autoimmune diseases. Thymus-derived NK cells diminish in number and/or activity in the circulation, enhancing the opportunity for mutant cells to survive and transform into malignant cells.

Thus, as the individual ages, he suffers irreplaceable losses of immunoresponsive T cells, immunoregulatory suppressor T cells, and the thymic hormones on which the transformation of stem cells into T cells depends and which sustain the T cells in the peripheral lymphoid tissues. The aged individual becomes more susceptible to infections with microorganisms to which he would previously have responded with a vigorous immune response, and he becomes susceptible to malignant disease due to loss of T NK cells which provide innate immunologic surveillance. The increase in incidence of autoimmune disease can be attributed to the generalized loss of suppressor cells. All in all, this is a neat picture providing one does not examine it too closely or approach it with a critical mind. Unfortunately, there are several flaws in the scheme described above which would tend to suggest that it is the investigator who is often incompetent rather than the immune system. These "flaws in the ointment" are as follows:

1. There is really no solidly based evidence that suppressor cells actually decrease in numbers and function as the individual ages. In fact, results of a number of investigations indicate that suppressor cell activity is alive and well in the aged individual. Therefore, the high incidence of autoimmune disease in the aged cannot presently be attributed specifically to a loss of suppressor cells. As stated previously, our concept of suppressor cells is very naive and is based on highly artificial (and suspect) in vitro assay systems. We may very well be identifying an artifact and assigning mystical powers to it; conversely, suppressor cells may truly exist in vivo which have not as yet been identified due to inadequacy of the assay systems.

2. Results of investigations in the experimental animal should not be extrapolated without qualification or reservation to the human. It is true that NZB/W F_1 hybrid mice tend to die at a young age (for the mouse) as a consequence of development of a panautoimmune syndrome with characteristics similar to the systemic lupus erythematosus syndrome in humans. Death in the affected NZB/W mouse is invariably preceded by loss of suppressor cells, autoantibody synthesis especially to circulating DNA, deposition of immune complexes in the renal glomeruli, acute (proliferative) glomerulonephritis which progresses to chronic glomerulonephritis, glomerulosclerosis, nephrotic syn-

drome, and uremia. However, it must be kept in mind that this disease picture occurs only in this highly inbred strain of mouse and it may represent the picture one observes in the individual suffering from progeria, but it is highly unlikely that it is representative of the disease which arises with increasing frequency in the normal aging population.

3. The incidence of malignant disease rises sharply with aging, and it occurs with alarming frequency in the elderly. However, this is not an across the board finding, as only certain malignant diseases fall into this category. It is important to stress that the majority of malignant diseases do not present with a greater incidence in the elderly.

4. The failure to detect a cell-mediated immune response may be more an illusion than reality. In the majority of instances, the diagnosis of cell-mediated immunodeficiency is made on the basis of a negative delayed skin reaction in response to the intradermal challenge with the sensitizing antigen. This is fine insofar as the normal young or middle-aged adult is concerned in whom it has been shown that the absence of skin reactivity is indicative of defective cell-mediated immunity. Unfortunately, this relationship does not hold true with respect to the elderly. It has been demonstrated that the skin in the elderly is incapable of serving as the stage for the delayed skin reaction, due to defects within the constituents of the skin and/or the cellular constituents. Thus, sensitized cells may be present in the circulation in the aged individual, but the delayed skin reaction will be negative.

5. Frequently, the terminal infection is not due to out of the ordinary normally nonpathogenic bacteria—i.e. *Serratia marcescens*, *Pseudomonas aeruginosa*, *Proteus vulgaris*, *Staphylococcus epidermidis*—but to bacteria which were previously encountered and which were eliminated via the normal antibody response—i.e. *Diplococcus pneumoniae*, *Haemophilus influenzae*, *Staphylococcus aureus*, *Streptococcus pyogenes*. Presumably, the individual would have generated long-lived memory cells directed toward these microorganisms as a consequence of prior encounter with them. It is possible that the memory cells in the aged individual may not survive well in the spleen, which may in itself become inhospitable to the immunocompetent cells; or it may be that the memory cells are, in fact, alive and well in the elderly, but that other factors which participate in the elimination of invasive pathogens via the specific immunologic route may be defective, i.e. the complement system and the phagocytic cells.

6. The results of a number of investigations support the NK nature of some T cells. However, the results of the majority of

investigations indicate that non-T lymphocytes, monocytes, and neutrophils also exhibit NK cytotoxic activity. Thus, the loss of T cells in the aged need not imply the loss of NK cytotoxic cells. Furthermore, as discussed elsewhere, only certain NK cells directed toward distinct malignant cells may be defective or absent.

The defects in the immune system in old age must be specifically identified if specific therapy to correct these defects is to evolve. The primary defects which appear to exist and which require correction may be summarized as follows:

1. Defect(s) in T cell maturation. It has been shown that the thymic hormones such as thymosin and thymopoietin secreted by the thymic epithelial cells are markedly decreased in concentration or are absent from the circulation in the elderly. These hormones function to drive the precursor T cells through the various maturation, transformation, and proliferative stages up to the mature T cell stage.

2. Defects in prostaglandin synthesis. This may be due to insufficient intake of the essential fatty acids (linoleic, linolenic, and arachidonic acid), vitamins, and trace metals. The administration of prostaglandins has been shown to reconstitute immunocompetence in otherwise immunoincompetent experimental animals.

3. Specific deficiency of trace metals. Trace metals may be required in the induction of the immune response. The injection of zinc can by itself reconstitute antibody synthesis following its administration to immunodeficient and zinc-deficient individuals.

4. Defects within or deficiency of naturally occurring killer (NK) cells. These cells respond to the administration of interferon.

Several forms of treatment of these defects not presently carried out are implied above and should be considered. These include:

1. The administration of thymus hormones which would promote the generation of T cells within the thymus and maintain the T cells in the peripheral lymphoid tissues.

2. A diet high in essential fatty acids, vitamins, and trace metals, administered periodically by intravenous hyperalimentation if necessary. This would ensure that the aged person is in a state of positive nitrogen balance and is not malnourished. It would also promote the synthesis of the prostaglandins which appear to exert a major beneficial influence on inflammation and the immune response.

3. The periodic administration of isologous T cells (T_M and/or T_G) generated in vitro following incubation with the T cell

mitogens phytohemagglutinin or concanavalin-A, to restore the normal balance of these cells.

4. The administration of interferon. Interferon appears to be capable of restoring normal function to incompetent NK cells and/or of inducing the generation of highly active NK cells.

It is, therefore, apparent to this author that the final chapter is yet to be written concerning the immune status of the aged. There is no question but that the immune system undergoes deterioration and/or degeneration with old age; however, the precise mechanism whereby the general reduction in immunity evolves and the specific defects remain to be defined. Once this information is forthcoming, it will be possible to contemplate intervention with specific drugs to correct specific defects and restore effective immunocompetence to the aged individual. The goal of clinical immunology is not to extend the normal life-span of the individual but rather to sustain him in good health as long as possible, obviating the need for depersonalized extended hospitalization and its attendant high financial cost.

CHAPTER 18

Nonspecific Mechanisms in Immunity

What is meant by the expression "nonspecific immunity"? A precise definition might be all the mechanisms which the body can call on in its battle with an invading pathogen other than that form of immunity characterized by specific antibodies or specifically sensitized cells. The latter constitute the specific immune mechanisms. Up to the mid-1960s, classical nonspecific immunity, also referred to as innate or intrinsic or natural immunity, was considered to consist primarily of (a) impermeable barriers such as the skin and all the epithelial surfaces with their lining of ciliated columnar or cuboidal cells and fatty acids, lactic acid, and mucin coating these surfaces; (b) secretions with their content of highly potent enzymes, i.e. lysozyme; (c) the phagocytic cells within the circulation (monocytes and neutrophils) and within tissues and organs (macrophages) which are the major participants in the inflammatory reaction; and (d) the complement system.

As a result of the discovery in the late 1960s and early 1970s of subclasses of normally circulating lymphocytes, monocytes, and neutrophils capable of mediating the antibody-dependent cell-mediated cytotoxic (or ADCC) reaction and the antibody-independent naturally occuring cell-mediated cytotoxic (or NOCC) reaction, one is today obliged to add a fifth nonspecific immune mechanism. This mechanism consists of the normally circulating ADCC and NOCC cytotoxic cells. Objection can be rationally raised to the inclusion of the ADCC cytotoxic cells since the effectiveness of these cells is dependent upon the presence of specific antibodies. However, the amount of specific antibodies required to mediate the ADCC reaction is so small that it may very well approximate that which has been referred to as naturally occuring antibodies (the opsonins).

Unquestionably, the acute inflammatory response constitutes the first line of defense, a major protective mechanism to invasion by pathogenic microorganisms. The basic objective of this response is to wall off the invader and to isolate it. A large proportion of the organisms are killed by the phagocytic cells; others are killed by the potent enzymes released from degenerating neutrophils which accumulate in large numbers at the site of inflammation. There can be no question but that many if not a majority of infections are aborted as a result of the acute inflammatory response long before specific antibodies are formed to the pathogen. The primary antibody response in humans is rather sluggish compared with that in the rodent or the rabbit. The latent period is about 10 to 14 days, and the peak antibody synthetic period may vary from 14 to 21 days postimmunization. Thus, the infected individual could be long dead or certainly moribund if the only defense to the pathogen were that provided by antibodies or sensitized cells. In the preimmunization era, it was not uncommon to record a 50 to 60% mortality rate following respiratory infections with *Corynebacterium diphtheriae*, *Diplococcus pneumoniae*, *Streptococcus pyogenes*, or *Haemophilus influenzae*. The objective of deliberate immunization is to induce an immune response at a time when it is not needed in order to establish the conditions whereby a secondary, and not a primary, response is initiated following infection at a later date. It will be recalled that a characteristic property of a secondary immune response is the much shorter latent period or the more rapid induction of antibody formation. Often, the latent period in a secondary immune response is less than half what it is for the primary immune response (i.e. 4 to 6 days instead of 10 to 14 days). This marked shortening of the time to respond with antibody formation toward the pathogen can literally spell the difference between life and death. Deliberate active immunization is, therefore, of great survival value to the individual. Infection with a virulent pathogenic bacteria in the absence of prior immunization today does not carry the fear of death it once did since it is invariably possible to intervene with at least one type of effective antibiotic during the early stage of the infection. Thus, the one-two punch of deliberate immunization prior to infection and antibiotic chemotherapy during the infection takes over when natural or acquired immune mechanisms may falter.

The complement system constitutes another nonspecific mechanism in the provision of resistance to pathogenic microorganisms. As was discussed in Chapter 7, antibodies by themselves do not kill the mircoorganisms to which they have been induced; rather, it is the activation of components of the complement system by the bacteria-antibody complex which guarantees the demise of the bacteria. However, as was also discussed in Chapter 7, the activation of the complement system by the antigen-antibody complex, referred to as the classical pathway, is not the only manner whereby complement can be activated. Many chemical compounds and constituents of bacterial cell membranes, especially gram-negative bacteria, are capable of activating the complement system in the absence of antibodies via a route referred to as the alternate pathway. Thus, the invading microorganism can frequently inadvertently activate the complement system, resulting in the generation of very potent bactericidal agents.

As we enter the decade of the 1980s, an uneasy, disquieting feeling pervades the discipline and occasionally surfaces among clinical immunologists involved in the treatment of infection, especially in the aged, the very young, and the immunologically compromised individuals treated with toxic chemotherapeutic drugs to eradicate a malignancy and immunosuppressive drugs to prevent an allograft rejection or exacerbation of an autoimmune disease. The euphoria engendered by the discovery of numerous highly effective nontoxic antibiotics in the 1950s and 1960s has been replaced in the late 1970s and early 1980s by a somber mood which can be described as guarded pessimism about our ability to continue to depend upon antibiotics in the ongoing battle against pathogenic microorganisms. The fact is that the pathogenic bacteria and viruses are mutating from antibiotic-sensitive to antibiotic-resistant states at a much faster rate than our ability to discover and develop new antibiotics to effectively combat these newly evolving strains. The newer antibiotics are, furthermore, less effective and often highly toxic; in other words, their chemotherapeutic indices are such as to discourage their utilization unless there are no other alternatives. Frequent, repeated immunization with numerous killed or attenuated microorganisms or refined toxins (5 to 10 times the number currently used in routine immunization schedules) may result in excessive stimulation of the immune system and result in an increase in the incidence of amyloidosis, a disease considered by many to be due to the continuous deposition of immune complexes and/or the activation of complement locally. Conversely, oft-repeated immunization may result in iatrogenically induced immunodeficiency disease due to clonal exhaustion or induction of nonspecific and/or specific suppressor cells.

It is the expectation of this author that the next major advance in our ability to cope with infectious agents will be the discovery of drugs capable of stimulating and activating the nonspecific immune mechanisms, especially the phagocytic cells (and possibly the ADCC and NK effector cells), converting these cells to "angry phagocytes" capable of selectively devouring and eliminating the invading pathogen even in the absence of a specific immune response. Drugs like interferon, BCG, and natural metabolites like the lymphokines (i.e. macrophage-activating factor), all capable of stimulating the phagocytic cells, may constitute the vanguard for a totally new group of antimicrobial chemotherapeutic agents capable of facilitating the elimination of the invading organism without damage to the host's tissues.

CHAPTER 19

The Clinical Immunology Laboratory

LABORATORY PROCEDURES APPROPRIATE FOR THE CONFIRMATION OF A DIAGNOSIS OF A DISEASE WITH SUSPECTED IMMUNOLOGIC ETIOLOGY AND/OR PATHOGENESIS

Clinical and Laboratory Procedures for the Diagnosis of Immunodeficiency Diseases

A. Physical examination
   1. Temperature (record if patient experienced fluctuations in temperature)
   2. Weight (record if child has gained expected weight)
   3. HEENT—otitis, sinusitis
   4. Respiratory system—cough, expectoration, blood, night sweats
      precussion—areas of consolidation
      auscultation—breath sounds
   5. Spleen—tenderness; increase in size by percussion
   6. Lymph nodes—tenderness, mobility, texture, change in size

B. Radiologic examination
   1. Anteroposterior and lateral of nasopharynx (Waldeyer's ring—tonsils and adenoid tissues)
   2. Anteroposterior and tomogram, when necessary, to detect thymic shadow
   3. Lung fields, for areas of consolidation.

C. Circulating cells
   1. Morphologic analysis
      a. Total and differential white blood cell count
      b. Monocyte count (stain for nonspecific esterase)
   2. Functional analysis.
      a. Monocyte and neutrophil chemotactic activity
      b. Monocyte and neutrophil phagocytic activity
      c. Lymphocyte blastogenic response to stimulation with
         (1.) Phytohemagglutinin (PHA), pokeweed (PWM), and concanavalin-A (Con-A) mitogens

(2.) Allogeneic cells in the mixed leukocyte reaction (MLR)
(3.) Specific antigens, where indicated

d. Synthesis of immunoglobulins in vitro by B cells following incubation of circulating T and B cells with pokeweed mitogen
e. Capacity of the circulating cells to mediate target cell lysis in the ADCC assay (polymorphs, monocytes, and lymphocytes)
f. Capacity of the circulating cells to mediate target cell lysis in the NOCC assay (polymorphs, monocytes and lymphocytes)
g. Capacity of the circulating cells to mediate target cell lysis in the MICC assay (polymorphs, monocytes and lymphocytes)
h. Capacity of the circulating cells of a sensitized individual to secrete lymphokines (MIF, transfer factor, MAF, mitogenic factor, lymphocytotoxic factor) in vitro upon incubation with the sensitizing antigen

3. Detection of suppressor cells
   a. Inhibition of PWM-driven immunoglobulin synthesis of normal B cells in vitro by circulating (T) cells of the patient suspected of harboring suppressor cells
   b. Inhibition of mitogen-induced blastogenesis of normal T cells in vitro by circulating (T) cells of the patient suspected of harboring suppressor cells
4. Analysis on the basis of surface receptors and markers:
   a. T cell—possesses receptor for sheep erythrocyte (E) and forms rosettes with E (E-rosette-forming cell)
      —possesses T cell-specific antigen, detected by immunofluorescence (horse anti-T cell-specific antiserum followed by FITC-conjugated anti-horse IgG)
   b. Null cell—possesses receptor for the Fc region of IgG antibody (A) adherent to the antigen. If the antigen is a sheep erythrocyte (E), the null cell will form rosettes with EA (EA-rosette-forming cell)
   c. B cell—possesses receptor for C′3 (C) complexed to antibody-sensitized ox erythrocytes (EAC), and forms rosettes with EAC (EAC-rosette-forming cell)
      —possesses receptor for mouse erythrocyte and forms rosettes with mouse erythrocyte (mouse erythrocyte rosette-forming cell)
      —possesses B cell-specific antigen, detected by immunofluorescence (horse anti-B cell-specific

antiserum, followed by FITC-conjugated anti-horse IgG)
—possesses surface immunoglobulins detected and semiquantitated by immunofluorescence (IgG, IgM, IgA, IgD, IgE)

D. Serum
   1. General
      a. Electrophoretic analysis of serum proteins
      b. Immunoelectrophoresis, where indicated
      c. Quantitation of immunoglobulins (IgG, IgM, IgA, IgD, and IgE) by radial immunodiffusion technique, where indicated
   2. Specific
      a. Hemolytic complement titer
      b. Circulating level of C′1 esterase inhibitor
      c. Circulating levels of C′3
      d. Circulating levels of C′1, C′2, and C′4
      e. Circulating levels of isohemagglutinins
      f. Circulating levels of antibodies following immunization with DPT, polio, mumps, pneumococcal polysaccharide, typhoid, paratyphoid A and B.

E. Biopsy examination
   1. Rectoanal (suction) biopsy—check for plasma cells
   2. Lymph node biopsy—check for T- and B-dependent areas:
      a. By normal histologic staining procedures (hematoxylin and eosin)
      b. By adherence of E and EAC to the T and B cells, respectively, on cryostat-fixed tissue specimens

The E and EAC may be considered as "vital stains" in this regard in view of their ability to bind specifically to T and B cells via cell surface receptors.

F. Skin tests
   1. Schick test—to detect the presence of circulating antibodies to diphtheria toxin.
   2. Dick test—to detect the presence of circulating antibodies to *Streptococcus pyogenes* toxin
   3. Delayed skin reactions—to detect presensitized cells to Koch's old tuberculin (O.T), histoplasmin, dermatophytin, mumps, Candida and to detect newly sensitized cells following intentional sensitization with DNCB or any of above agents to which the patient has not previously been sensitized.

Immunologic Tests and Immunologic-related Tests Recommended for the Differential Diagnosis of Specific Immunodeficiency Diseases

(The tests are listed in the sequence that they are used in the author's laboratory.)

A. History and clinical picture suggesting an immunodeficiency disease as a consequence of a diminished level or absence of circulating antibodies
   1. Electrophoresis—result presents a profile of the serum proteins and discloses the presence and concentration of the total gamma globulins.
   2. Quantitation of immunoglobulins—a "must" test as it provides immediate unequivocal and clear-cut indications of either hypo- or agammaglobulinemia with respect to any or all of the major immunoglobulin classes (IgG, IgM, IgA)
   3. Circulating levels of isohemagglutinins (IgM antibodies)
   4. Circulating antibodies to diphtheria and tetanus toxins, polio, *Salmonella typhosa*, and *Salmonella paratyphi* (IgG antibodies)
   5. X-ray of nasopharynx to detect the presence of tonsil and adenoid tissues
   6. Rosette formation of circulating lymphocytes with EAC—to disclose presence and numbers of B cells
   7. Immunofluorescence assay of circulating lymphocytes—to determine the number of cells bearing surface immunoglobulins (SIg)
   8. Intracellular adenosine deaminase activity
   9. Adherence of E (SRBC) and EAC to distinct areas in a frozen section of a lymph node biopsy to determine the presence and location (normal or pathologic) of the T and B cell-dependent areas, respectively
   10. The in vitro induction of plaque-forming (antibody-synthesizing) cells (PFCs) to sheep red blood cells (SRBC) from normal circulating lymphocytes. Cells normally present in the circulation can be induced to generate or transform into antibody-synthesizing cells. The cells must be subjected to two signals in vitro before they can transform into overt antibody-forming cells or AFC. One signal is provided by the antigen, the SRBC, and the other signal can be provided by any of a number of unrelated substances, one of which is the polyclonal

mitogen stimulant, pokeweed. One may rationally anticipate that evidence will shortly be forthcoming that these cells are lacking in the circulation of patients with diseases characterized by a deficiency of circulating antibodies; or that these cells are present and are capable of transforming to PFCs in vitro but not in vivo, suggesting that the non-antigen-specific second signal is not operating in vivo. This assay, once it is introduced as a routine test in the clinical immunology service, should be most useful in the differential diagnosis of the different subtypes of antibody immunodeficiency diseases.

B. History and clinical picture of humoral (antibody) immunodeficiency disease not corroborated by results of above tests. The physician should suspect a defect in the complement and/or phagocytic system. Determination of the following is recommended to help clarify the clinical picture:
   1. Hemolytic complement titer
   2. Circulating level of C′3
   3. Neutrophil chemotactic activity
   4. Neutrophil phagocytic activity
   5. Rosette formation of circulating lymphocytes with EA—to determine the presence and number of Fc receptor-bearing cells
   6. The ADCC cytotoxic activity of circulating neutrophils and mononuclear cells—to determine the functional activity of Fc receptor-bearing cells

C. History and clinical picture suggesting an immunodeficiency disease due to a defect in the cell-mediated immune system. The following tests are recommended:
   1. White blood cell differential—percentage and absolute number of circulating lymphocytes
   2. Rosette formation of circulating lymphocytes with E (SRBC)—to determine the presence and number of circulating T cells
   3. The blastogenic response of the circulating cells to stimulation with the plant mitogens PHA and Con-A. This response is given essentially by T cells and discloses the gross functional state of the T cells.
   4. The blastogenic response of the circulating cells to stimulation with allogeneic cells (the MLR reaction). This is a T cell response.
   5. Intracellular adenosine deaminase activity
   6. Anteroposterior x-ray and tomogram—to detect a thymic shadow.

7. Skin tests to O.T., histoplasmin, dermatophytin, mumps. If skin tests are negative, sensitize individual with these antigens and challenge 3 to 4 weeks later for delayed skin reactivity.

D. History and clinical picture of cell-mediated immunodeficiency disease not corroborated by results of above tests. The physician should suspect a defect in the phagocytic activity of the circulating cells, primarily the monocytes, and/or failure of the sensitized cells to secrete one or more of the identifiable lymphokines. Determination of the following is indicated:
   1. Monocyte and neutrophil chemotactic activity
   2. Monocyte and neutrophil phagocytic activity
   3. The ADCC cytotoxic activity of the circulating monocyte and neutrophil
   4. Assay of lymphokines secreted following in vitro stimulation of the circulating cells with the suspected infectious agent(s)

E. History and clinical picture of immunodeficiency disease not corroborated by results of any of the above tests. The physician should suspect specific clonal deletion (congenital) or clonal depletion (exhaustion of immunocompetent cells due to repeated or persistent stimulation) and/or excessive numbers of activated suppressor cells as the underlying cause. The following tests are indicated:
   1. Blastogenic response of the circulating cells to stimulation with the suspected or implicated microorganisms(s) or extracts thereof. The absence of a significant blastogenic response would suggest the absence of antigen-recognizing cells (clonal deletion or depletion).
   2. Electron microscopic analysis of cells which undergo blastogenesis following stimulation with PHA or Con-A. Look for defect or marked absence of endoplasmic reticulum and defects in Golgi apparatus in the blast cells.
   3. The NOCC cytotoxic activity of the circulating neutrophils and mononuclear cells
   4. The MICC cytotoxic activity of the circulating neutrophils and mononuclear cells

      Although the significance of these two latter tests is not known at the present time, they serve to identify populations of cells which may not be detected by any of the other assays.
   5. The analysis of the circulating cells for suppressor cells capable of inhibiting immunoglobulin synthesis and/or

cell-mediated immune responses and/or mitogen-induced blastogenesis by normal allogeneic cells
6. Analysis of lymphokines secreted in vitro by sensitized cells incubated with suspected infecting microorganisms or solubilized antigen
7. Capacity of affected individual to permit a delayed skin reaction by passively transferred normal allogeneic sensitized cells followed by challenge with the specific antigen

Clinical and Laboratory Procedures for the Diagnosis of Autoimmune Diseases and "Immune Complex" Diseases

A. History and physical examination
Complete physical examination, paying attention especially to the:
1. Skin: evidence of rash, discrete or confluent, macular or urticarial, accompanied by intense pruritis ("immune complex" disease); areas of nonpitting induration, not accompanied by pruritis (angioedema); "tightness" of the skin (scleroderma); excessive desquamation and flaking (eczema); dry scaling erythematous patches (psoriasis); crops of irregularly scattered bullae (pemphigus); hyperkeratosis, induration, papular rash (cell-mediated reaction, i.e. poison ivy), tendency to bruise easily, petechiae and/or echymotic and/or purpuric lesions (thrombocytopenia); pallor, especially mucous membrane (anemia)
2. Edocrine system
   a. Thyroid—hypothyroidism (autoimmune hypothyroidism or Hashimoto thyroiditis); hyperthyroidism (Graves' disease)
   b. Pancreas—insulin-refractory diabetes (antibodies to exogenous insulin); juvenile onset diabetes (autoantibodies to islet cells and/or autologous insulin)
3. HEENT: complaints of dryness of the eyes, tongue, and mouth (Sjögren's disease); conjunctivitis, rhinitis and recurrent bouts of sneezing (IgE-mediated hay fever); sympathetic ophthalmitis (cell-mediated autoimmune uveitis)
4. Lymph nodes and spleen: lymphadenopathy (axillary, inguinal, and popliteal lymph nodes) accompanied by tenderness, splenomegaly ("immune complex" disease)
5. Respiratory system: bronchial asthma (IgE-mediated or "immune complex"-mediated); recurrent severe episodes of nonproductive coughing, fever, malaise, related to season or occupation and symptoms abate dramatically

upon hospitalization ("immune complex"-mediated extrinsic allergic alveolitis, i.e. farmer's lung); bronchitis not related to obvious infection, i.e. intrinsic bronchopulmonary aspergillosis (immune reaction to mycotic agents—"immune complex"- and/or cell-mediated reaction)

6. Peripheral nervous system: paresthesia, hyperesthesia, dull ache, numbness, "pins and needles" ("immune complex" disease, i.e. Gullain-Barré syndrome, pernicious anemia)
7. Digestive system: dysphagia (scleroderma); melena, occult blood, recurrent episodes of diarrhea, abdominal pain and cramps (ulcerative colitis); recurrent episodes of pain localized to right lower quadrant (regional ileitis)
8. Kidneys: pain and tenderness on palpation (suspect "immune complex"-induced glomerulonephritis if tenderness is bilateral)
9. Circulatory system: nodules along blood vessels, tenderness (polyarteritis nodosa)
10. Musculoskeletal system: pain, swelling and tenderness of the joints (thrombocytopenia, rheumatoid arthritis, "immune complex" disease); lower back pain (ankylosing spondylitis or Marie-Strümpell disease); muscle tenderness and pain (dermatomyositis); general muscle weakness (myasthenia gravis)
11. Hematologic findings: thrombocytopenia ("idiopathic" thrombocytopenia purpura or ITP); persistent normochromic normocytic anemia and reticulocytosis (autoimmune hemolytic anemia or AIHA); megaloblastic anemia (pernicious anemia); absence or deficiency of C'1 esterase inhibitor (angioedema)

B. Circulating autoantibodies and other relevant serum constituents

Suspected Disease	*Detection Assay*
Autoimmune hemolytic anemia	Antierythrocyte antibodies (agglutination, hemolysis)
Idiopathic thrombocytopenia purpura	Antiplatelet antibodies (immunofluorescence)
Diseases of connective tissue (collagen disease)	
1. Scleroderma	Anticonnective tissue antibodies (immunofluorescence)
2. Dermatomyositis	a. Anti-muscle cell antibodies (im-

	munofluorescence)
	b. Perivascular infiltrates of mononuclear cells and degeneration and necrosis of adjacent muscle cells (biopsy)
3. Rheumatoid arthritis	Anti-IgG antibodies or rheumatoid factor [agglutination of IgG-coated latex particles or erythrocytes (Rose-Waller test)]
4. Polyarteritis nodosa	a. Anti-blood vessel wall antibodies (immunofluorescence)
	b. Perivascular infiltrates of mononuclear cells (biopsy)
5. Systemic lupus erythematosus	a. Anti-DNA antibodies (radioimmunoassay)
	b. Anti-RNA antibodies (radioimmunoassay)
	c. Antinuclear antibodies (immunofluorescence)
	d. Circulating immune complexes (inhibition of the ADCC cytotoxic reaction and C′1q binding)
	e. L-E cells
Diseases of the endocrine system	
1. Thyroid	a. Antithyroid antibodies (immunofluorescence)
	b. Antithyroglobulin antibodies (agglutination of thyroglobulin-coated latex particles or erythrocytes)
2. Diabetes	Antiinsulin antibodies (radioimmunoassay)
Glomerulonephritis	a. Antikidney (glomerular) antibodies (immunofluorescence)
	b. Deposits of immune complexes and complement (immunofluorescence)
Myasthenia gravis	Antimyoneural junction (acetylcholine receptor) antibodies (immunofluorescence)
Pernicious anemia	Antigastrointestinal (parietal cell) antibodies (immunofluorescence)

Pemphigus, psoriasis	Antiskin antibodies (immunofluorescence)
Infertility	Antisperm antibodies (immunofluorescence and/or agglutination and/or immoblization)
Hypersensitivity pneumonitis or EAA (immune complex disease)	Circulating precipitating antibodies to suspected bacterial and mycotic antigens and inhalable innocuous proteins (immune precipitation in gel)
Angioedema	C′1-esterase inhibitor (immune precipitation in gel)

Laboratory Procedures for the Detection of Circulating Tumor-specific Proteins or Glycoproteins

These are often referred to as "tumor-specific antigens" (see below and Chapter 16).

1. The concentration of carcinoembryonic antigen (CEA) in the circulation, to verify or suggest a diagnosis of a gastrointestinal carcinoma (and secondarily lung, pancreatic, breast, and ovarian carcinomas) and for follow-up to detect residual tumor and/or recurrence of the malignancy
2. The concentration of alpha-fetoprotein (AFP) in the circulation to verify or suggest a diagnosis of hepatic carcinoma or germ cell tumor and for follow-up to detect residual tumor and/or recurrence of the malignancy

A high concentration of alpha-fetoprotein in amniotic fluid and in maternal serum, especially during the second trimester of pregnancy, is considered to be indicative of neural tube defects, such as spina bifida. However, the use of this test in predicting congenital malformations will not be discussed here as it does not fall into the terms of reference of this book.

Laboratory Procedures to Predict (a) Histocompatibility Differences between the Prospective Allograft Donor and Recipient and (b) an Incipient or Imminent Rejection Crisis following Allografting

1. The one-way mixed leukocyte culture reaction (MLR) (see Chapter 7).
2. The lymphocytotoxicity assay. This procedure is used to determine the major and minor HLA antigens present on the lymphocytes of the prospective donor and recipient of an

allograft. It provides an assessment as to the histocompatibility relationship of the donor and the recipient.

In this assay, the lymphocytes are suspended in wells in microtiter plates, and antisera directed toward the different HLA (or transplantation) antigens are added along with complement. Lysis of the lymphocytes denotes the presence or the specific HLA antigen. Whereas the MLR demonstrates major HLA antigenic differences between the prospective donor and recipient (the minor HLA antigens do not appear to induce blastogenesis of the allogeneic lymphocytes, at least not in the normal 5-day culture), the lymphocytotoxicity assay demonstrates the major and minor histocompatibility differences. The lymphocytotoxicity test is the assay of choice when time is a factor and the allograft is not elective (i.e. kidney donated by a normal donor) since the MLR requires 4 to 5 days whereas the lymphocytotoxicity assay can be carried out in several hours.

3. The spontaneous blastogenic response of the circulating lymphocytes cultured for 3 to 5 days in the absence of any known mitogenic agent(s) (see below). A significant spontaneous blastogenic response is indicative of incipient allograft rejection.

INDICATIONS FOR AND INTERPRETATIONS OF THE ROUTINE IMMUNOASSAY PROCEDURES

The Appropriate Utilization of Electrophoresis, Immunoelectrophoresis, and Quantitation of Immunoglobulins in the Differential Diagnosis

It has been the experience of the author that very few physicians (and even fewer students and residents) have been sufficiently exposed to those now routine procedures in a manner which would permit them to properly interpret the results and relate them to the clinical state of the patient. Few physicians are able to properly analyze and evaluate the results obtained by these three techniques; nor do they have an appreciation of their shortcomings and limitations on the one hand, and advantages and usefulness on the other. A brief analysis of these basic methods and their application is, therefore, in order.

The electrophoretic analysis of a serum will disclose the concentration of the gamma globulins or total immunoglobulins, primarily the IgG, IgM, and IgA as these three classes of immunoglobulins constitute more than 99% of the gammaglobulins. Furthermore, the densitometer tracing of the electrophoretic pattern will also suggest whether any or one or more of the immunoglobulins is monoclonally derived or polyclonally derived, provided the proteins in the affected immunoglobulin class are present in relatively high concentration. The method is not sufficiently sensitive or discriminating to permit one to detect significant changes within any one immunoglobulin class if the total immunoglobulin concentration is within the normal range.

The advantages of the routine electrophoretic examination are that it is simple to carry out, requires very little time (several hours for the analysis of 12 to 18 sera), is inexpensive, and provides a reproducible absolute value with respect to the sum total of immunoglobulins present. It is usually carried out on cellulose acetate strips which provide an inert, uncharged surface upon which the serum proteins can migrate. A serious drawback inherent in this technique is the frequent failure to detect agammaglobulinemia or very severe hypogammaglobulinemia. Proteins tend to be irreversibly absorbed to varying degrees at the point of application on the cellulose acetate strip, and the absorbed proteins will remain at this point while the bulk of the proteins migrate in the electric field. Furthermore, the albumins, α and β globulins leave a "trail" of proteins as they migrate. Unfortunately, the gamma globulins or immunoglobulins do not migrate to any great extent electrophoretically (the reader should recall that the isoelectric point of the gamma globulins is closer to the pH of the buffer used in the electrophoretic analysis than are the other serum proteins) and remain around the point of application. A very low concentration of circulating immunoglobulins will, therefore, be recorded as a much higher concentration due to the contribution of the nonspecifically absorbed and trailing serum proteins. Therefore, agammaglobulinemia, even if it is present (25 mg% or less), will normally be recorded as a hypogammaglobulinemia. Hypergammaglobulinemia (greater than 2.5 g%) and hypogammaglobulinemia (less than 400 mg%) will invariably be detected.

Immunoelectrophoretic analysis provides a qualitative, not quantitative, assessment of the immunoglobulins. Its usefulness lies in the fact that it permits the identification of immunoglobulins as either monoclonal (heavy and narrow precipitin arc) or polyclonal (diffuse and broad precipitin arc).

The quantitation of immunoglobulins by precipitation in gel (immunodiffusion) is a sufficiently sensitive and specific technique to provide the precise concentrations of the immunoglobulin classes. However, one cannot determine whether the immunoglobulins are monoclonally or polyclonally derived by this method.

In summary, it is essential that the reader recognize the advantages of the different immunoglobulin assay procedures and not ascribe to them interpretations which are not valid. Immunoelectrophoresis tends to be overused or inappropriately used due to the invalid assumption that it permits a quantitative assessment of the immunoglobulins, which it does not. Similarly, immunodiffusion in gel only permits a quantitative determination of the immunoglobulin classes and not an analysis as to the homogeneous (monclonal) or heterogeneous (polyclonal) nature of the molecules within each immunoglobulin class.

Thus, if a patient is suspected to have an immunodeficiency with respect to circulating antibodies, electrophoresis followed by quantitation of the immunoglobulins would be the initial assays requested, not immunoelectrophoresis. On the other hand, if the patient is suspected of having lymphoproliferative disease, especially that characterized by a monoclonal plasma cell dycrasia such as multiple myeloma, macroglobulinemia, or cryoglobulinemia, then electrophoresis followed by immunoelectrophoresis would be the initial assays of choice, not quantitation of the immunoglobulins.

Significance of Receptor and Immunoglobulin-bearing Cells

The techniques available for the detection of these cells may now be considered as routine procedures and fall into the "available on request" category in any modern clinical immunology laboratory.

They can be classified into a number of categories.

A. Tests which identify surface markers

These markers include surface immunoglobulins (SIg) and the receptors for SRBC(E), the Fc region on the antigen-fixed IgG antibody molecule (EA) and C′3 adherent to the antibody-antigen complex (EAC) (please review section concerning rosettes, Chapter 7). Cells possessing these markers are identified and visualized by the utilization of the immunofluorescence assay (to demonstrate the presence of SIg) and by their ability to form rosettes with E, EA, and EAC (to demonstrate the presence of cell surface receptors).

B. Tests which indicate the state of functional activity of the receptor-bearing cells

The ADCC (antibody-dependent cell-mediated cytotoxic) activity is generally attributed to Fc receptor-bearing cells. Thus, this assay indicates the functional state of the cells which form rosettes with EA.

Important

It must be stressed that the presence of an Fc receptor on the surface of a cell does not necessarily endow that cell with the capacity to mediate the ADCC cytotoxic reaction. In point of fact, evidence has been presented which suggests that less than 5% of the Fc receptor-bearing cells capable of forming rosettes with EA can actually carry out the ADCC reaction. The rosetting technique provides a quantitative index as to the number of the Fc receptor-bearing cells and not an indication as to their functional state. On the other hand, the ADCC assay provides direct evidence for the presence in the circulation of cytotoxic Fc receptor-bearing cells but does not permit the estimation of the number of these cells. Therefore, at the present time, it is essential to determine both the rosetting capacity of the circulating cells and their ability to mediate the ADCC cytotoxic reaction.

Significance of the ADCC, NOCC, and MICC Cytotoxic Reactions

The ADCC and NOCC reactions in vitro may both be considered to represent reactions which may take place in vivo under the appropriate circumstances. As stated previously, the ADCC reaction is primarily attributed to an Fc receptor-bearing cell, capable of interacting with the Fc of IgG antibody molecules following their reaction with the antigen and, as a consequence, lysing the antigen should it be an erythrocyte or a bacterium. Thus, the Fc receptor-bearing cell should be considered as a cell which participates in the eradication of invasive organisms, capable of killing them in the presence of minimal quantities of IgG antibodies.

Similarly, the cell which mediates the NOCC reaction is considered to provide the "innate resistance," also referred to as "immunologic surveillance," toward the emerging of malignant cells in vivo. Although the cytotoxic activity of these cells has thus far not been shown to be dependent upon the presence of identifiable receptors, one may anticipate that this is probably not the final word on this matter.

Since the cells which carry out the ADCC and NOCC reactions are distinct cells, these two cytotoxic reactions in vitro serve to identify two potentially important immunocompetent cells not detectable by other conventional assays.

As far as the MICC cytotoxic reaction is concerned, it must presently be regarded as a means (or probe) to identify the existence of a cell type different from those which mediate the ADCC and NOCC relations. However, the immunologic significance of the MICC reaction remains to be determined. One would be safe to assume that a role for the MICC cell will be defined in the not too distant future.

Significance of Cell Surface Immunoglobulins

The circulating lymphocytes can be segregated into two categories—cells with receptors for immunoglobulins which facilitate the reversible absorption of immunoglobulins onto the surface membrane and cells with immunoglobulins which actually constitute an integral part of the cell surface. The immunoglobulins on the former cells can be eluted from the cells by incubation at 37°C for 1 to 2 hours. These immunoglobulins are referred to as cytophilic immunoglobulins and are usually IgG. The immunoglobulins on the latter cells cannot be eluted in this manner and are primarily IgM, at least in terms of the antigenicity of the heavy chain.

There is general agreement that the immunoglobulin-synthesizing B cells and the precursors of and actual antibody-forming cells are surface immunoglobulin (SIg)-bearing cells. However, one must be wary to ascribe excessive significance to the number of SIg-bearing cells. It has been documented that immunodeficiency disease of the Bruton type exists in the presence of normal numbers of SIg-bearing cells. On the other hand, normal individuals with normal levels of circulating immunoglobulins may possess few SIg-bearing cells. At best, therefore, the presence of a normal number of SIg-bearing cells serves as an indication of the potentially normal immunocompetent state, whereas the total absence of these cells would strongly indicate potential or actual immunoincompetence.

Significance of the Blastogenic Response of Cells in Vitro

The agents used to stimulate the blastogenic transformation of the circulating cells fall into two categories—nonspecific agents and specific agents. The former (category I) includes the plant-derived mitogens—phytohemagglutinin (PHA), pokeweed (PWM), and concanavalin-A (Con-A)—as well as allogeneic cells bearing transplantation antigens. The latter (category II) consists of antigens which have been used in routine immunization procedures, such as diphtheria and tetanus toxins, pneumococcal polysaccharides, typhoid and paratyphoid microorganisms, old tuberculin (OT), salmonella flagellin, endotoxins derived from gram-negative microorganisms, polio, rubella and rubeola viruses, and fungal antigens such as histoplasmin and dermatophytin, to name but a few.

It is generally agreed that the cells which respond to the stimulating agents listed in category I are T cells. The mitogen PWM is still considered by many investigators to be a B cell stimulant, although evidence is mounting that the blastogenic response to PWM requires the active participation of T cells and that, in fact, T cell proliferation exceeds B cell proliferation. Monocytes are definitely required for the proliferative response of the circulating lymphocytes, especially if low concentrations of the mitogens are used. It also appears that T cell proliferation is potentiated in the presence of B cells and that B cell proliferation is enhanced in the presence of T cells. The original views concerning the specificity of mitogen action should be reconsidered to take into account cellular interdependency.

The antigens listed in category II which normally induce a humoral (antibody) response, such as the bacteria and bacteria-derived antigens, stimulate the circulating B memory cells of the specifically immunized individual to undergo blastogenesis and mitosis in vitro. Those antigens which normally induce a cell-mediated immune response, the viruses and fungi, stimulate the circulating T memory cells of the immunized individual to undergo mitosis in vitro.

Important

1. The plant-derived mitogens—PHA, Con-A, and PWM—are very potent but nonspecific in their action. A blastogenic response to these agents by the circulating lymphocytes of immunologically mature individuals is, at best, a crude indicator of potential or actual immunocompetence. A blastogenic response does not, however, necessarily rule out a defect in the immune system. This cautious approach to the interpretation of the blastogenic response is due to the fact that the plant mitogens are polyclonal stimulants, capable of inducing blastogenesis of both immunocompetent lymphocytes and "bystander" lymphocytes not normally involved in the immune response. These latter cells have functions other than the provision of immune responsiveness and constitute the majority of the circulating lymphocytes. It is, therefore, possible to obtain a marked blastogenic response in the absence of virgin and/or committed immunocompetent cells. Such a situation is encountered in investigations with fetal and neonatal cells. Both give good blastogenic responses in culture upon stimulation with PHA, Con-A, and PWM; however, neither the fetus nor the neonate is normally capable of generating a significant immune response. On the other hand, the absence of a blastogenic response is a definite indication of a major defect in the immune response mechanism of the individual.

2. A normal mitogen-induced or antigen-induced blastogenic response is indicative of the presence of not only normal T and B cells, respectively, but also normal monocytes. In the absence of

normally functioning monocytes, the blastogenic responses of the T and B cells are drastically reduced, wrongly suggesting defects within the T and B cells. In actual fact the T and B cells may be perfectly normal, but they will not undergo blastogenesis and mitosis in the absence of normally functioning monocytes. Since the cells being analyzed are often deficient in monocytes, as they often are in patients with lymphoreticular proliferative diseases on immunotherapy, or may contain defective monocytes, the status of the circulating monocytes must be taken into account in the evaluation of T and B cell function.

3. Specific defects in the immune system which preclude a normal immune response, such as congenital specific clonal (ARC cell) deletion (as may be suspected in the case of recurrent infections to a single pathogenic organism commencing at 6 to 8 months of age), or acquired specific clonal (ARC cell) deletion (as may be suspected in the case of recurrent infections to a single pathogenic organism commencing insidiously in adulthood and increasing in severity with each passing episode), or exhaustion of the specific immunocompetent B cells, cannot be detected or surmised from the blastogenic responses of the circulating cells to stimulation with the plant mitogens for reasons stated above.

Significance of Circulating Autoantibodies and Autosensitized Cells

As discussed at length in Chapter 12, a pathogenetic or disease-inducing role is ascribed to sensitized cells and antibodies directed to autoantigens, especially autoantibodies directed toward the circulating erythrocytes, leukocytes, and platelets. However, neither autoantibodies nor specifically sensitized cells may be detected in the circulation at the time of investigation as they may be "mopped up" by the target tissue as quickly as they are released into the circulation. Examples of instances where autoantibodies are synthesized but not detected are autoimmune hemolytic anemia, autoimmune thrombocytopenia, and autoimmune glomerulonephritis. In the latter case, it can be demonstrated that the autoantibody titer rises sharply following bilateral nephrectomy (as has been done in the experimental animal). Therefore, the failure to detect either autoantibodies or sensitized cells is not necessarily indicative of the absence of an autoimmune disease. Furthermore, it is more than likely that the failure to demonstrate autoantibodies may be due to the failure to identify the appropriate autoantigen(s).

On the other hand, the demonstration of circulating autoantibodies or autosensitized cells supports the clinical suspicion of an autoimmune disease. However, it does not necessarily follow that they are implicated, in a cause-effect relationship, in the etiology and pathogenesis of the condition. Autoantibodies may be formed as a consequence of the initial insult, or they may be secondary, possibly irrelevant, concomitants of the clinical condition. Autoantibodies and sensitized cells can induce pathology only if the antigens which they are directed against are present on the surface of the target cell or tissue and are accessible to interaction with the antibody and/or sensitized cell.

The finding of autoantibodies in the circulation toward normally noncirculating constituents may simply reflect the fact that autologous proteins, normally inaccessible to the immunocompetent cells as they are restricted to specific organs, have been released into the circulation as a result of infection, inflammation, trauma, irradiation, malignancy, or surgery. The result is that the immunocompetent cells, recognizing those molecules as "foreign," respond with antibody formation and/or sensitization. In other words, the autoantibodies and sensitized cells may not make an appearance before the damage has been committed but subsequent to the pathologic event.

The physician is, therefore, advised not to be content at having identified circulating autoantibodies and/or autosensitized cells, and not to attribute the induction of the disease to them unless they corroborate the history, physical examination, and clinical findings. Laboratory data should only be used to reinforce the diagnosis already made and should not initiate a witchhunt for a diagnosis not suggested by the clinical picture.

Significance of Circulating Proteins Characteristic of and Specific to the Malignant State

Great stress is currently being placed upon the need to diagnose a malignant condition early, thus ensuring surgical and/or chemotherapeutic and/or radiologic intervention at a time when the malignancy is still very small and may not as yet have metastasized. The search is, therefore, on to characterize cancer-specific antigens (these are constituents which are antigenic in another animal, not necessarily in the affected individual) which, it is assumed, are liberated into the circulation by the proliferating malignant cells and can be detected by a radioimmunoassay technique. A very extensive and systematic investigation on gastrointestinal adenocarcinoma-specific "antigen" was initiated by Gold and Freedman at McGill University in the early 1960s which culminated with the demonstration that malignancies of the gastrointestinal tract and possibly other entodermally derived malignancies shed a rather complex constituent(s) into the circulation early in the oncogenic process. This constituent(s) has been called carcinoembryonic antigen (CEA), as it is a product of a dedifferentiated malignant cell which can also be detected during embryogenesis. CEA is antigenic in the rabbit, and thus rabbit antibodies can be utilized in a radioimmunoassay for the detection and quantitation of CEA.

As discussed in Chapter 16, the repeated finding of an abnormally high concentration of CEA in the circulation of a patient who does not smoke or drink to excess strongly suggests the presence of a malignancy in the gastrointestinal tract, pancreas, or gallbladder. Recent evidence indicates that even breast and ovarian carcinomas may be diagnosed at their early stages of oncogenesis by the detection of CEA in the circulation.

Nevertheless, it is universally recognized that one cannot screen the entire population for the malignancies referred to above, as good intentions cannot negate the tremendous cost which such an undertaking would entail, especially as it would have to be carried out at closely spaced defined intervals of time to be effective. A more plausible indication for the CEA assay is in follow-up studies of patients who have been treated for the specific malignancy of the gastrointestinal tract, i.e. adenocarcinoma, and are in a state of remission. It has been demonstrated that the recurrence of a malignancy and/or metastases can be detected much earlier via the CEA assay than by subjective and clinical criteria (nausea, dyspepsia, loss of appetite and weight, melena, recurrence and metastases detected radiologically), thus permitting early chemotherapeutic, radiologic, or surgical intervention which should be accompanied by a decrease in the incidence of tumor-related morbidity and death.

A second malignancy-specific constituent which can also be detected in the blood is referred to as alpha-fetoprotein (AFP), and its presence in the circulation is highly suggestive of a primary hepatic carcinoma or a germ cell tumor. It, like CEA, can be detected and quantified by a radioimmunoassay.

One may anticipate that more tumor-specific circulating "antigens" will be identified in the not too distant future, especially those specific to breast, lung, pancreatic, prostatic, and cervical tumors. These, along with gastrointestinal tumors, account for the majority of deaths due to malignant disease.

Significance of Circulating Precipitating Antibodies in Individuals with Suspected Extrinsic Allergic Alveolitis

The diseases referred to under the umbrella term "extrinsic allergic alveolitis" (EAA) have been discussed in Chapter 14.

They are invariably mediated by immune complexes formed between the solubilized constituent (usually protein) of the inhaled material and antibodies circulating in the capillaries in the alveolar walls, thus simulating an Arthus reaction. The demonstration of a precipitin band formed in a gel between the serum of the patient and the suspected antigen will usually suffice to nail down a diagnosis of EAA. However, a negative result, that is, the absence of a precipitin band, does not serve to rule out EAA. As is true with the majority of specific but relatively insensitive immunoassays, a positive reaction carries considerably more weight than a negative reaction. In the case of EAA, antibodies of a precipitating type must be present in the circulation in relatively high concentration in order to precipitate with the antigen. Therefore, the failure to detect an immune precipitin band does not rule out the presence of circulating precipitating antibodies. In fact, they may be present in the circulation in a concentration sufficient to facilitate a pathologic reaction in the lung upon contact with the specific antigen but below that necessary to give a visible precipitation reaction with the antigen in vitro.

Interpretation and Prognostic Value of the MLR and Lymphocytotoxicity Assays in Transplantation

Both of these assays are routinely used to help predict whether an allograft from a potential donor will be rejected by the prospective recipient. Unfortunately, neither of these tests can predict the outcome of an allograft with any degree of certainty. In fact, recent investigations have disclosed that a mismatched allograft has an almost equal chance of being accepted by the host as a matched (by MLR and lymphocytotoxicity assays) allograft. The management of the patient and the prevention of infection appear to be as important as the actual histocompatibility relations of the allograft and the recipient. Nevertheless, it is the accepted position that the less the antigenic disparity between the allograft donor and the recipient, the greater the probability of a "take" without the need to treat the recipient with immunosuppressive drugs.

The MLR is the result of a blastogenic response of the designated recipients' cells (responder cells) stimulated in culture with mitomycin-C-treated cells of the potential allograft donor (stimulator cells). Only strong histocompatibility (transplantation or HLA) antigens on the donor cells will provoke the blastogenic response in the recipients' cells. Furthermore, this reaction is permitted to proceed for only 5 days; therefore, any HLA antigens which cannot provoke a response within the accepted time frame of 5 days will not be detected. The MLR may, therefore, be able to predict acute and subacute rejection but not chronic rejection, which probably involves the host's response to minor antigens not detected in the MLR. The antigens on the stimulator cells responsible for the blastogenic response by the responder cells are referred to as "lymphocyte-determined" or LD antigens.

On the other hand, the lymphocytotoxicity assay utilizes antisera directed to both the major and minor histocompatibility antigens. Lymphocytes of the donor and recipient are compared for their susceptibility to lysis by various anti-HLA antisera and complement. Identical susceptibility to the different antisera (there are now more than 90 antisera, each of which is considered to detect a single HLA antigen) would suggest that the donor and recipient are well matched. On the other hand, markedly different susceptibility to lysis by the different antisera would suggest that the donor and recipient are mismatched and an allograft should not be attempted.

Unfortunately, this method also has limitations insofar as it can predict the performance of an allograft. In contrast to the MLR, the lymphocytotoxicity assay detects a much larger number of antigens (referred to as SD or serologically determined), some of which may not even be antigenic in the host. In other words, the allograft may very well take, although the donor and recipient may be mismatched with respect to a number of minor or even major HLA antigens.

It is, therefore, necessary to use prudence in the assessment of results of the MLR and lymphocytotoxicity assays insofar as their predictive value is concerned regarding the fate of the proposed allograft.

The Spontaneous Blastogenic Response as an Indication of Impending Allograft Rejection

Lymphocytes placed in culture will undergo some blastogenesis and mitosis even in the absence of a stimulating agent. This response is referred to as the spontaneous or baseline or control blastogenic response and is rarely more than 1% of the response given by the cells in the presence of mitogens (i.e. PHA) or allogeneic cell. However, in retrospective studies of allograft rejection, it has been observed that the circulating cells of allograft recipients undergo a much greater degree of spontaneous blastogenesis prior to a rejection crisis. The spontaneous blastogenic response will be found to be quite marked 1 to 2 weeks before clinical and other laboratory signs appear to indicate that the host is rejecting the allograft. Thus, the spontaneous blastogenic response of the cells, if determined at varying intervals of time postallografting, will alert the physician to an impending crisis and permit the institution of immunosuppressive chemotherapy more as a prophylactic (and, therefore, less agressive and toxic) measure than as a treatment for an ongoing rejection episode.

The interpretation for the dramatic rise in the spontaneous blastogenic response of the cells of the allografted patient a few days prior to the acute rejection crisis is that sensitization of the patient to the allograft has alrady been induced and that sensitized cells are present in the circulation at various stages of maturation. Some of these cells (less than 1%) are probably pyroninophilic blast cells and they are capable of continuing their blastogenic and proliferative response in vitro. These cells, and/or their progeny, are presumably the cells which infiltrate the allograft and initiate the rejection reaction.

CHAPTER 20

Future Expectations

"The only ideas worth exploring are those which do not disintegrate on impact with the critical mind." (M.A.R.)

The relationship of immunology with the other disciplines in medicine could for many years be compared to the skeleton and the interest engendered in it by anatomists only interested in physical characteristics of particular bones, but not in the whole. Experts concerned only with the study of the bones themselves could not possibly envisage or anticipate that the bones are connected to other bony structures by muscles, sinews, and tendons, which impart to the bones a function of locomotion. As recently as the 1940s, immunology was still considered to be an esoteric "basic" science. Its only accepted role in the field of medicine was the application of serology for the identification of infecting microorganisms and verification of the immune responses to them. By the late 1940s, immunology was composed of a number of subspecialties aside from serology concerned with (a) the composition of antigens, (b) the composition of antibodies, (c) the function and composition of complement, (d) the in vivo manifestation of the immune response, and (e) the delayed hypersensitivity reaction. However, there was little interaction between investigators in these different areas and investigators in the other disciplines (i.e. biochemistry, pharmacology, histology). When the era of antibiotics dawned in the late 1940s, those immunologists who recognized the long-term implications of the event must have despaired as the only apparent link of immunology to medicine, that of serology, was threatened with extinction, to be reduced to the status of a "non sequitur."

Fortuitously (for immunologists, that is), it was at precisely this time (the early 1950s) that a number of discoveries took place which gave immunology a newly acquired respectability among the medically oriented disciplines. These were:

1. The discovery of immunologic tolerance.
2. The demonstration that autoimmune disease could indeed be induced consistently in the experimental animal, thus repudiating Ehrlich's dictum of "horror autoxicosis." This was followed by

3. The detection of autoantibodies in patients suffering from a number of diseases, thus laying the foundation for the field of autoimmune diseases.

4. The establishment of the allograft rejection reaction as an immunologic reaction, thus giving birth to the field of transplantation immunology.

5. The redefinition of clinical allergy as an illness resulting from the deleterious manifestations of an immune (mast cell-bound IgE antibody-allergen) reaction, rather than as a disease with an undefined etiology and pathogenesis. The study of the allergic response was thus recognized as a subspecialty in immunology.

6. The recognition, finally, of a role for the thymus, happily an immunologic role, and the demonstration of a state of immunoincompetence (mainly cell-mediated) following its extirpation in the experimental animal. This finding was quickly followed by

7. The detection of an immunoincompetent state in children born either euthymic or with an aplastic thymus. Thus was born the field of immunodeficiency diseases.

Interest in a discipline is often generated by the simultaneous appearance of a number of conditions which act, in unison, to stimulate activity designed to increase the knowledge and expertise in that discipline. There is no greater motivating force to explore and exploit a discipline than its anticipated utilization in the diagnosis and treatment of disease. At least three conditions must be met to achieve this objective and they presently exist with respect to immunology: (a) a high level of technology; (b) clinical conditions characterized primarily by a proven or suspected defect in, deficiency of, hyper- or inappropriate responsiveness of the immune response system; and (c) the failure of conventional modes of therapy—surgery, irradiation, and nonspecific chemotherapy—to achieve control or amelioration of these specific diseases and the expectation that the application of immunologic principles may provide clues, if not the means, to their regulation, prevention, or cure.

As a result of the discoveries referred to above, immunology expanded dramatically in the late 1960s, gaining converts by the hundreds every year as it was being touted as the discipline of the future, the veritable savior of mankind from a host of diseases, even from death itself. A radical fringe in the early 1960s purported to have identified hormones which would delay, indefinitely, the aging process. The early 1970s provided the stage for the new visionaries, the transplantation surgeons, to demonstrate their skills with heart, liver, and lung transplants. Unfortunately, they were found wanting. Their expectations were founded not on scientifically established facts but on beliefs, feelings, and intuitively derived inspirations. It was inevitable that the pendulum would swing back toward a more objective position.

Conditions now exist, in the early 1980s, for clinical immunology to demonstrate its applicability in both the diagnosis and therapy of a host of disease states. These can be categorized as follows: (a) malignant diseases, (b) autoimmune diseases, (c) immunodeficiency diseases, (d) allergic diseases, (e) iatrogenic diseases (complications resulting from the administration of immunosuppressive agents and other cytotoxic drugs aimed at preventing allograft rejection, the progression of certain suspected autoimmune diseases, or the amelioration of a malignancy).

Oncologists and transplantation surgeons have resorted to clinical trials with little understood chemical agents selected on a strictly empirical basis (a throwback to biochemistry research in the 1950s). The field trials provide a statistical basis for the utilization of these drugs. However, too often there is a failure to appreciate that statistics can only support and not replace knowledge based on scientific studies carried out in a systematic disciplined fashion. It is instructive to note that a number of drugs utilized for their purported "anticancer properties" are also utilized by transplantation surgeons to induce a state of immunosuppression (read temporary immunoincompetence) in the host in order to facilitate acceptance of the allograft. In the first instance the expectation is that these drugs will promote rejection of the malignancy, possibly via an immunologic mechanism, whereas in the second instance the expectation is that the drugs will suppress the host's immune response to the allograft. Obviously the same drugs cannot have totally diametrically opposed effects. This is just one example of our sadly deficient understanding of the mechanism of action of these agents. Many oncologists have turned to immunology and have resorted to what is referred to as "immunotherapy," which unfortunately, as it is generally practiced, is not really immunotherapy but adjuvant chemotherapy.

Similar criticisms may be leveled at the transplantation surgeons for considering that the rejection episodes could be controlled, if not prevented, by proper surgical technique and careful nonspecific management of the patient. However, a series of failures in their initial efforts at organ transplantation made it painfully obvious that a consideration of the immunologic role in allograft rejection was essential. Utilization of immunologic assays to predict and/or assess potential responses of the recipients to allografts has greatly improved the incidence and degree of "take"; further improvements have followed the introduction of immunosuppressant chemotherapy. However, the generally toxic properties of these drugs make them a last resort as therapeutic drugs. Transplantation rejection phenomena can be expected to be controlled once we learn to prepare transplantation antigens in forms which will induce a state of immunologic tolerance following their administration.

With regard to immunodeficiency diseases, the author anticipates progress in the reconstitution of immunocompetence by the administration of naturally occurring agents or hormones (i.e. thymosin) or superior synthetic analogues which will function to normally regulate the immune response by reestablishing normal numbers of T and B cells. Immunodeficiency disease may, in the future, be controlled much in the same way that diabetes can be controlled by the administration of exogenously derived insulin.

In the field of clinical allergy, a number of investigators, particularly Sehon and his colleagues, have demonstrated that a state of immunologic tolerance can be induced to the offending allergen irrespective of whether an IgE immune response had already taken place. What remains to be determined is the duration of the tolerant state and whether tolerance to the allergen can be reinstated should it break down. Unquestionably, the induction of a tolerant state specific to the allergen is the preferred, if not the ultimate, treatment of IgE-mediated allergic disease. The immune response to exogenous pathogens should not be affected. This form of treatment, although not strictly prophylactic, should result in the total and permanent amelioration of symptoms. It also obviates the need for pharmacologically very potent and often dangerous drugs. Hay fever and asthma, two of the most common non-life-threatening diseases in North America, afflicting literally millions of people every year, may become but a bitter memory of the past, much like polio is today.

It is likely that when the discipline will reminisce in the 1980s and 1990s as to its performance in the 1960s and 1970s, it will not consider the present era of applied immunology to have been one of its finer hours, nor the primitive attempts to alter, restrict, regulate, suppress, or reconstitute immune responsiveness with nonspecific, highly toxic agents as its more notable achievements. The author anticipates that once the results of current research in immunology are integrated with attainable objectives in terms of today's technology, drugs with a more selective action appropriately documented in terms of their mechanism of action will become available for the therapy and management of diseases with an immunologic etiology and/or pathogenesis. Selective augmentation or suppression of the particular immune system will be effected by the appropriate agent so as to enlist the immune system as an accomplice and an accessory rather than as an adversary. The discipline of immunology will then be well on its way to achieving the objective of providing not just sophisticated tools which can be used in the differential diagnosis of diseases but also the methodology to effectively treat these diseases.

Epilogue

It is always the objective of an author to write a book which will be considered to constitute the definitive textbook within the discipline for a finite period of time. Unhappily, that period of time is usually shorter than the time span which elapses between the publication of the book and the receipt of the first royalty cheque. Such an objective can today be realized in some disciplines but not, alas, in immunology. Contradictory findings, uncertainty, disorder, and controversy rule the day in several of the dynamic and most visible areas of contemporary immunology. The great proliferation of lymphokines and other mediators, suppressor cells, soluble regulatory factors, subclasses of hitherto homogeneous classes of immunocompetent cells, the profusion of immunodeficiency diseases, and the cellular mechanisms capable of mediating the lysis of target cells, are indicative of the absence of a comprehensive unified concept governing the immune system. The majority of recent and current investigations have been conducted under in vitro conditions, with the result that a large body of information has accumulated which is relevant only insofar as it may facilitate the elucidation of reactions investigated in the artifically contrived, nonphysiologic milieu of the test tube. The majority of in vitro findings cannot be extrapolated to in vivo situations. More disturbing is the trend toward increased sophistication of investigations utilizing in vitro systems while important questions raised by cellular immunologists more than a decade ago concerning the nature of the immunocompetent cells, the mechanism(s) of their interaction with antigen and with each other in vivo, their in vivo migration pathways, and organ(s) of maturation and/or localization, go unanswered and do not appear to arouse sufficient curiosity to initiate extensive investigations in vivo. The pressures on the investigators to "publish or perish" coupled with the ease with which one can "discover" new factors, agents, mediators, etc., utilizing a totally in vitro system have clouded the perspective of the discipline as a whole with only a few investigators daring to swim against the tide by carrying out research in vivo.

The objectives to provide clues or answers to puzzling clinical problems by calculated, systematic in vivo investigations in the experimental animal are skirted in the desire to accumulate data within the shortest period of time, which usually translates as the in vitro system. Long-term investigations are conducted with cells of highly inbred strains of rodents and much value is attributed to results obtained thereof, in spite of the fact that results obtained in one inbred strain cannot be verified in a second inbred strain, let alone be extrapolated to the human. Nevertheless, a high percentage of current immunologic investigations is centered about the rodent, the model which has displaced the prototype, the human, with the result that we have, collectively, a better understanding of some diseases of the rodent than we do of the counterpart diseases in the human for which the rodent was to provide the model.

The absurdity of the contemporary research scene is best illustrated by the fact that investigations in the rodent far outnumber those in humans in the current journals of cancer research. It is a delusion that more investigations on the rodent, or other nonprimates, will enhance the probability of a solution to human diseases. The persistent failure to put into practice, in the clinical setting, "major" discoveries of the past decade based on investigations in nonprimate systems has done nothing to assure an ever more suspicious lay public of our competence and skills. Indeed, we appear to be rather inept. To many outsiders, it appears as though the majority of immunologists have forgotten that the ultimate objective of research is to apply the new knowledge to the diagnosis, understanding, pathogenesis, and treatment of diseases in humans considered to have an immunologic etiology or pathogenesis and which require immunologic intervention.

The most visible of these diseases is cancer. Yet in spite of the hundreds of investigations being carried out yearly in nonprimates, the role of the immune response in the control or ablation of a malignant lesion in humans is clouded in abject uncertainty and confusion. One reason is that investigators are financially supported more for their efforts to study the life cycles of virally or chemically induced malignancies in the rodent than to evaluate the role of the humoral and cell-mediated immune responses in the cancer patient. The cancer research Establishment and the funding agencies must accept responsibility for this state of affairs in view of their consistent willingness to provide financial support for well-intentioned but scientifically unsupportable clinical trials in the hope of beneficial fallout in the short-term (better known as shotgun or slot-machine research) at the expense of long-term investigations aimed at understanding the largely biochemical lesions which characterize the malignant cell which permit uncontrolled proliferation. How else can one interpret the almost frantic atmosphere and frenetic efforts by the cancer Establishment to bring interferon into production, at a great expense, when in fact there is no assurance whatsoever from current investigations that interferon will provide any greater benefit than current therapy? In point of fact, the discipline is still in the process of identifying different species of interferon(s) and determining its (their) composition. The same is true with respect to the practice of immunotherapy in the treatment of cancer. We justify the injection of cancer-specific antigens into patients on the assumption that "immunity is always good for you" when nothing could be further from the truth. In fact, evidence to date would strongly suggest the opposite—only the cellular immune response appears to play a patient-protective role by providing enhanced resistance to tumor cells, whereas antibodies tend to protect tumor cells from interaction with and destruction by sensitized cells. However, in spite of the fact that the cancer-specific antigens have not yet been isolated or characterized and the immune responses by the patients to these antigens not quantitated, immunotherapy proceeds as usual. Such is the present state of the art.

It is essential that investigators pause and reflect upon the obvious lack of correlation between the many findings and few understandings which characterize the body research and recognize that a statement, irrespective of how often or in how loud a voice it is pronounced, does not confer validity or truth to it; only the results of an objective, systematic, and deliberate scientific investigation can do that.

We seem to be mystically guided by the principle that conventional wisdom must be obeyed and practiced. Unfortunately, the "conventional wisdom" is a contradiction in terms—if it is conventional, it is rarely wisdom; and if it is wisdom, it is more often than not highly unconventional. The discipline, by its own devices, now finds itself on the peak of a tall mountain and is only beginning to realize that the trail it followed took it to the peak of the wrong mountain. How the discipline will fare during the decade of the 1980s, as it attempts to descend from the "rodent" mountain and to ascend the "human" mountain, is a story which can only be told as it unfolds.

Recommended Reading

BASIC IMMUNOLOGY

Introductory Texts

1. *Textbook of Immunology* (Third Edition).
   Barrett, J.T.
   C.V. Mosby Company, 1978.
2. *Immunobiology.*
   Good, R.A. and Fisher, D.W., Editors.
   Sinauer Associates, Inc., 1973.
3. *The Immune System: A course on the molecular and cellular basis of immunity.*
   Hobart, M.J. and McConnell, I.
   Blackwell Scientific Publications, 1975.
4. *Immunology.* II.
   Bellanti, J.A.
   W.B. Saunders Company, 1978.
5. *Biology of the Immune Response.*
   Abramoff, P. and La Via, M.
   McGraw-Hill Book Company, 1970.
6. *Fundamentals of Immunology.*
   Weiser, R.S., Myrvik, O.N. and Pearsall, N.N.
   Lea and Febiger, 1969.
7. *Immunology and Serology.*
   Carpenter, P.L.
   W.B. Saunders, 1965.
8. *Fundamentals of Immunology.*
   Boyd, W.C.
   Interscience Publishers, 1966.
9. *Antibodies and Immunity.*
   Nossal, G.J.V.
   Basic Books, Inc., 1969.
10. *Understanding Immunology.*
    Cunningham, A.J.
    Academic Press, 1978.
11. *Immunology.*
    Bach, J.F., Editor
    John Wiley and Sons, 1978.

Advanced Texts

1. *Essential Immunology.*
   Roitt, I.M.
   Blackwell Scientific Publications, 1981.
2. *The Cellular Basis of the Immune Response.*
   Golub, E.S.
   Sinauer Associates, Inc., 1981.
3. *On the Origin and Fate of Immunocompetent Cells.*
   Nieuwenhuis, P.
   Wolters-Noordhoff Publishing Groninger, 1971.
4. *Defence and Recognition, Biochemistry Series One*, Vol. 10.
   Porter, R.R., Editor.
   Butterworths, 1973.
5. *The Antibody Molecule.*
   Nisonoff, A., Hopper, J.E. and Spring, S.B.
   Academic Press, 1975.
6. *Lymphocytes and Their Interactions.*
   Williams, Jr., R.C., Editor.
   Raven Press, 1975.
7. *Mechanisms of Cell-mediated Immunity.*
   McCluskey, R.T. and Cohen, S., Editors.
   John Wiley and Sons, 1974.
8. *Principles of Immunology.*
   Rose, N.R., Milgrom, F. and van Oss, C.J., Editors.
   MacMillan Publishing Company, Inc., 1979.
9. *T and B Lymphocytes.*
   Greaves, M.F., Owen, J.J.T. and Raff, M.C.
   Excerpta Medica, 1973.
10. *Cellular Immunity.*
    Burnet, Sir MacFarlane.
    Melborne University Press, 1969.
11. *Immunology: An introduction to molecular and cellular principles of the immune responses.*
    Eisen, H.N.
    Harper and Row, 1980.

12. *Delayed Hypersensitivity.*
Turk, J.C.
North-Holland Publishing Company, 1975.
13. *Mediators of Cellular Immunity.*
Lawrence, A.S. and Landry, M., Editors.
Academic Press, 1969.
14. *Advanced Immunochemistry.*
Day, E.D.
Williams & Wilkins Company, 1972.
15. *Ontogeny of Acquired Immunity.*
A Ciba Foundation Symposium.
Associated Scientific Publishers, 1972.
16. *Comparative Immunology.*
Marchalonis, J.J., Editor.
Blackwell Scientific Publications, 1976.
17. *Immunologic Tolerance.*
British Medical Bulletin, Vol. 32, # 2, 1976.
18. *B and T Cells in Immune Recognition.*
Loor, F. and Roelants, G.E., Editors.
John Wiley and Sons, 1977.
19. *Textbook of Immunology.*
Benacerraf, B. and Unanue, E.R.
Williams & Wilkins, 1980.

CLINICAL IMMUNOLOGY AND IMMUNOPATHOLOGY

1. *Fundamentals of Clinical Immunology.*
Alexander, J.W. and Good, R.A.
W.B. Saunders Company, 1977.
2. *Medical Immunology.*
Thaler, M.S., Klausner, R.D. and Cohen, H.J.
J.B. Lippincott Company, 1977.
3. *Essential Immunology*
Roitt, I.M.
Blackwell Scientific Publications, 1981.
4. *Basic Immunology and Its Medical Application.*
Barrett, J.T.
C.V. Mosby Company, 1976.
5. *Clinical Immunology.*
Freedman, S. and Gold, P.
Harper and Row, 1976.
6. *Basic and Clinical Immunology.*
Fudenberg, H.H., Stites, D.P., Caldwell, J.L. and Wells, J.V.
Lange Medical Publications, 1980.
7. *Immunological Diseases.*
Samter, M., Editor.
Little, Brown and Company, 1971.
8. *Introduction to Clinical Allergy.*
Feingold, B.F.
Charles C Thomas, 1973.
9. *Immunologic Disorders in Infants and Children.*
Stiehm, E.R. and Fulginiti, V.A.
W.B. Saunders Company, 1973.
10. *Immunodeficiency in Man and Animals.*
Bergsma, D., Editor.
Sinauer Associates, Inc., 1975.
11. *Immunology for Students of Medicine.*
Humphrey, J.H. and White, R.G.
Blackwell Scientific Publications, 1970.
12. *Immunology, Immunopathology and Immunity.*
Sell, S.
Harper and Row, 1980.
13. *Immunology in Clinical Medicine.*
Turk, J.L.
William Heineman Medical Books, Ltd., 1972.
14. *Clinical Aspects of Immunology.*
Gell, P.G.H., Coombs, R.R.A. and Lachman, P.J., Editors.
Blackwell Scientific Publications, 1975.
15. *Allergic Diseases. Diagnosis and Management.*
Patterson, R., Editor.
J.B. Lippincott Company, 1972.
16. *Immediate Hypersensitivity.*
Stanworth, D.R.
North-Holland Publishing Company, 1973.
17. *Biochemistry of the Acute Allergic Reaction.*
Austen, K.F. and Becker, E.L., Editors.
Blackwell Scientific Publications, 1971.
18. *Clinical Evaluation of Immune Function in Man.*
Litwin, S.D., Christian, C.L. and Siskind, G.W., Editors.
Grune and Stratton, 1976.

19. *Laboratory Diagnosis of Immunologic Disorders.*
Vyas, G.N., Stites, D.P. and Brecher, G.
Grune and Stratton, 1975.
20. *Atlas of Experimental Immunobiology and Immunopathology.*
Waksman, B.H.
Yale University Press, 1970.
21. *Textbook of Immunopathology.*
Miescher, P.A. and Muller-Eberherd, H.J., Editors.
Grune and Stratton, 1968.
22. *The Immunology of Malignant Disease.*
Harris, J.L. and Sinkovics, J.G.
C.V. Mosby Company, 1976.
23. *Humoral Aspects of Transplantation.*
Rubin, A.L. and Stanzel, K.H., Editors.
Grune and Stratton, 1976.
24. *Transplantation Today.*
Schlesinger, M., Billingham, R.E. and Rapaport, F.T., Editors.
Grune and Stratton, 1975.
25. *Transplantation.*
Najarian, J.S. and Simmons, R.L., Editors.
Lea and Febiger, 1972.
26. *The Reticuloendothelial System in Health and Disease: Functions and Characteristics.*
Reichart, S.M., Escobar, M.R. and Friedman, H., Editors.
Plenum Press, 1976.
27. *The Reticuloendothelial System in Health and Disease: Immunologic and Pathologic Aspects.*
Friedman, H., Escobar, M.R. and Reichart, S., Editors.
Plenum Press, 1976.
28. *The Pathogenesis and Treatment of Immunodeficiency. Monograph in Allergy*, Vol. 10.
Horowitz, S.D. and Hong, R.
S. Karger, 1977.
29. *Immunodeficiency.*
Hayward, A.R.
Edward Arnold (Publishers) Ltd., 1977.
30. *Autoimmnity: Genetic, Immunologic, Virologic and Clinical Aspects.*
Talal, N., Editor.
Academic Press, 1977.
31. *Comprehensive Immunology.*
Good, R.A. and Day, S.B., Editors.
(Volumes 1 to 5 published).
Plenum Press, 1977.
32. *Immunology in Medicine.*
Holborow, E.J. and Reeves, W.G., Editors.
Academic Press, 1977.
33. *Immunology of Human Reproduction.*
Scott, J.S. and Jones, W.R.
Academic Press, 1977.
34. *Immunology: An outline for students of medicine and biology.*
Weir, D.M.
Churchill Livingstone, 1977.
35. *Diagnosis and Treatment of Immuno deficiency Diseases.*
Ashepon, G.L., and Webster, A. D.B.
Blackwell Scientific Publications, 1980.

TEXTBOOKS WHICH STRESS METHODOLOGY

1. *In Vitro Methods in Cell-mediated Immunity.*
Bloom, B.R. and Glade, P.D., Editors.
Academic Press, 1971.
2. *Handbook of Experimental Immunology.*
Weir, D.M., Editor.
Blackwell Scientific Publications, 1973.
3. *Immunological Methods.*
Ackroyd, J.F., Editor.
Blackwell Scientific Publications, 1964.
4. *Methods in Immunology and Immunochemistry.*
Williams, C.A. and Chase, M.W., Editors.
Academic Press (Volumes I to V published).
5. *Methods in Immunology.*
Campbell, D.H., Garvey, J.S., Cremer, N.E. and Sussdorf, D.H.
W.A. Benjamin, Inc., 1970.
6. *Cell Separation: Methods in Hematology.*
Cutts, J.H.
Academic Press, 1970.

7. *The Antigens.*
Sela, M., Editor.
Academic Press (Volumes I to V published).
8. *Laboratory Diagnostic Procedures in the Rheumatic Diseases.*
Cohen, A.S., Editor.
Little, Brown and Company, 1975.
9. *Immunopathology: Clinical Laboratory Concepts and Methods.*
Nakamura, R.M.
Little, Brown and Company, 1974.
10. *Immunoelectrophoresis: Theory, Methods, Identification, Interpretation.*
Arguembourg, P.C.
S. Karger, 1975.
11. *In Vitro Methods in Cell-mediated and Tumor Immunity.*
Bloom, B.R. and David, J.R., Editors.
Academic Press, 1976.
12. *Manual of Clinical Immunology.*
Rose, N.R. and Friedman, H., Editors.
American Society for Microbiology, 1980.
13. *Experimental Immunochemistry.*
Kabat, E.A. and Meyer, M.M.
Charles C Thomas, 1971.
14. *Practical Methods in Clinical Immunology.*
Nairn, R.C., Editor.
Churchill Livingstone, 1980.
(Volumes I and II published).

GENERAL REFERENCE PERIODICALS

1. *Journal of Immunology.*
2. *Immunology.*
3. *European Journal of Immunology.*
4. *Scandinavian Journal of Immunology.*
5. *Journal of Experimental Medicine.*
6. *International Archives of Allergy and Applied Immunology.*
7. *Journal of Allergy and Clinical Immunology.*
8. *Journal of Clinical Immunology and Immunopathology.*
9. *Transplantation.*
10. *Clinical and Experimental Immunology.*
11. *Advances in Immunology.*
12. *Clinical Immunobiology.*
13. *Progress in Allergy.*
14. *Contemporary Topics in Immunobiology.*
15. *Contemporary Topics in Molecular Immunology.*
16. *Progress in Clinical Immunology.*
17. *Progress in Immunology.*
18. *Recent Advances in Clinical Immunology.*
19. *Comprehensive Immunology* (Series Editors: Robert A. Good et al.)
20. *Immunological Reviews.*

BOOKS OF A HISTORICAL NATURE

1. *Topley and Wilson's Principles of Bacteriology and Immunity.* (Sixth Edition).
Wilson, Sir G.S. and Miles, Sir A.
Williams & Wilkins Company, 1975.
(The chapters on immunology are not much changed from those in the editions published in the 1940s. That is all to the good as these chapters are among the best written in the English language. The early (pre-1920) work is discussed in detail and placed in perspective. These chapters and the book by Boyd (see below) should be mandatory reading for any individual seriously contemplating a career in academic immunology.)
2. *Fundamentals of Immunology.*
Boyd, W.C.
Interscience Publishers, Inc., 1966.
(Reprint of 1st Edition, 1943).
(This book has not been surpassed insofar as an in-depth and systematic approach to the basic principles of immunology is concerned.)
3. *Paul Ehrlich.*
Marquardt, M.
William Heinemann Medical Books, Inc., 1949.
(A fascinating insight into the life of a giant in medical research of all

time.)
4. *The Specificity of Serological Reactions.*
Landsteiner, K.
Dover Publications, Inc., 1962.
(A reprinting of the original published in 1936.)
5. *The Chemistry of Antigens and Antibodies.*
Marrack, J.R.
British Medical Research Council, 1938.
(The first attempt to define immunity in chemical terms.)
6. *The Production of Antibodies.*
Burnet, F.M. and Fenner, F.
MacMillan and Company, 1949.
(The first elucidation of the clonal selection theory.)
7. *Serum Sickness.*
von Pirquet, C.F. and Schick, B.
Williams & Wilkins Company, 1957.
(A translation of the original book entitled *Die Serumkrankheit*: von Pirquet, C.F. and Schick, A., Franz Deutick, 1905.)
(This book serves as an example as to how clinical research should be carried out. The only thing outdated about this book is its stated year of publication.)
8. *The Nature and Significance of the Antibody Response.*
Pappenheimer, Jr., A.M., Editor.
Columbia University Press, 1953.
(One of the first symposia held on immunology.)
9. *Experimental Immunochemistry.*
Kabat, E.A. and Mayer, M.M.
Charles C Thomas, 1948.
(A new edition was published in 1961.)
(An excellent introduction to the subspeciality of immunochemistry, in both the theoretical and practical approaches.)
10. *Principles of Pathology.*
Adami, J.G.
Lea and Febiger, 1908.
(This text and the following two texts should be compulsory reading for those of us who think that knowledge of a subject begins within the few years just preceding one's introduction to it.)
11. *Applied Immunology.*
Thomas, B.A. and Ivy, R.H.
J.B. Lippincott Company, 1915.
12. *Infection, Immunity and Inflammation.*
Gurd, F.B.
C.V. Mosby Company, 1924.
(A restatement of the role of inflammation in resistance and the immune response. A reaffirmation of concepts originally introduced by Virchow and Rockitansky in the 1880's.)
13. *The Clonal Selection Theory of Acquired Immunity* (The 1958 Abraham Flexner Lectures).
Burnet, Sir M.
Vanderbilt University Press, 1959.
(The various theories advanced to explain the mechanism of antibody formation and the mechanism whereby the immune system differentiates self (or endogenous) from nonself (or exogenous) antigens are discussed in clear and unambiguous terms by the originator of the clonal selection theory.)
14. *A History of Immunization.*
Parrish, H.J.
E. and S. Livingston, Ltd., 1965.
(The author presents an in-depth discussion of the history of immunization, which is really the history of immunology. He also places immunization procedures in perspective, pointing out their effectiveness. The author also modifies and rejects older unsupported beliefs and theories, which have served only to detract from and delay acceptance of results of contemporary investigations carried out by the scientific method and statistically validated.)

Index

Accelerated rejection, 249
Acetylcholine receptor antibodies, 195, 229
Acquired variable hypogammaglobulinemia 165, 179–182
Activated macrophage, 65
ADCC (*see also* Cytotoxicity), 111–112, 299
Adenosine deaminase, deficiency, 172–173
Adjuvant (*see also* Freund's adjuvant), 28–29
  anti-tumor action, 270–271
  depot effects, 28–29
  in immunization, 28–29
  macrophage activation and, 28–29
Adrenalin, in anaphylaxis, 225
Agammaglobulinemia, Bruton's X-linked, 163, 168–169
Agglutination reaction, 85–87
  difference between precipitation reaction and, 85–87
Aging and immunity, 200–207
Allergens, radioallergosorbent test (RAST), 227–228
Allergic alveolitis, 232–234
Allergic contact dermatitis, 240
Allergic drug reactions, 212, 239
  penicillin, 224–225, 239
  reagin dependent, 224–225, 239
Allergy
  definition, 1–3, 212
  mechanism, 214–216
  mediators, 215–216
  pathogenesis, 214–216
  treatment, 221–224, 226
  type I reaction, 212–227
  type IV reaction, 239
Allograft
  definition, 248–249
  rejection, 249–252
Allotypes, allotypic antigens of Ig, 17–18
Alpha-fetoprotein, 271–272, 295, 303–304
Alternate pathway of complement activation, 78–80
Aluminum hydroxide, as adjuvant, 29
Anamnestic response, 31–32
Anaphylactoid reaction to radiographic contrast media, 226–227
Anaphylatoxin(s), 79–82
  histamine release and, 79–80
  vascular permeability and, 79–80
Anaphylaxis, anaphylactic shock, 212–215, 218–221
  desensitization, 221
  IgE antibodies, 212–215, 223
  local immediate skin reaction, 116–118, 214
  mechanism, 218–221
  mediators, 220–221
  systemic, 218–221
  to local anesthetics, 226–227
Anemia
  hemolytic, autoimmune, 195, 209, 210
  intrinsic factor autoantibodies, 195
  pernicious, 209, 210
Angioneurotic edema, 83
Antibodies (Ab) (*see also* Immunoglobulins), 12–24
  allotype, 17–18
  antinuclear (ANA), 88, 90, 294
  antinucleolar, 88, 90
  binding sites, 13–14, 16–17
  cell stimulation by, 240
  concentration, 15, 24
  cytotoxic, 227–229
  detection of, 70–123
  four-peptide chain, 13–15
  heterogeneity, 15, 17–24
  homocytotrophic, 213
  idiotype, 17
  IgA, 20–22
  IgD, 23–24
  IgE, 23
  IgG, 18–19
  IgM, 19–20

Antibodies—*continued*
placental transfer of, 19, 166–167
specificity, 13–16
stimulation of cells by, 241
structure and composition, 13–15, 17–18
Antibody-dependent cell-mediated cytotoxicity (ADCC), 111–112, 299
Antibody formation
aging, 275–282
anti-idiotype antibodies, 126–127
bursectomy, 48–49
memory cells, 31, 34, 44, 47
mechanism(s), 51–55
morphologic changes, 35–38
nutrition, 200–207
primary response, 31–33
regulation by antibodies, 125–127
role of B cells, 38–40, 48–50
role of macrophages, 40–45
role of T cells, 38–40, 47–48
second signal triggering, 289–290
secondary response, 31–33
suppressor cells, 128–147
synthesis (organs), 33–38
thymectomy, 47–48
Antibody-forming cells
assay for the presence of, 97–100
B cells, 38–40, 43–47
identity, 38–40, 103–104, 149, 151
memory cells, 31, 34, 44, 47
plasma cells, 30, 34–38
Anti-DNA antibodies, 294
Antigen (Ag), 25–29
adjuvants, 28–29
antibody interaction, 71–77, 85–97
appendix-specific, 50
as template, 52
bone marrow (B cell) specific, 50
cancer
alpha-fetoprotein, 271–272, 295, 303–304
carcinoembryonic (CEA), 271–272, 295, 303–304
competition, 124
definition, 25–26
determinants, 25–26
hapten, 26–28
heterogeneity, 25
organ specific, 50
appendix, 50
bone marrow, 50
thymus (theta antigen), 50
presentation, 43–47
processing, 40–42, 44–45
reactive cell (ARC), 39
thymus dependent, 49–50
thymus independent, 49–50
thymus (T cell) specific, 50
tolerogenic, 41–42, 184–186, 256–257
transplantation or histoin-compatibility (HLA), 257–260
valency, 70
Antigen-binding fragment (Fab), 13–14
Antigen reactive cell (ARC), 39
Antigenic competition, 124
Antigenic determinants, 25–26
allotype, 17–18
carrier, 26
hapten, 26–28
idiotype, 17
Anti-histamines, 125
Anti-idiotype antibodies, 16–18, 126–127
Anti-lymphocyte globulin (ALG), 255–256
lymphocyte transformation, 240
Appendix specific antigen, 50
Armed macrophage, 65
Arthritis, rheumatoid, 195, 293–294
autoantibodies, 195, 293–294
autoimmune response to IgG, 195
Arthus reaction, 119, 229–231
mechanism of injury in, 119, 229–230
role of complement, 119, 229–230
role of neutrophils, 119, 229–230
Asthma, 209, 212, 225
Atopic diseases, 212–227
immunotherapy of, 221–223
drug treatment of, 225–226
Atopy, 212
Autoantibodies, 191–199
human disease and detection (table), 195
immunofluorescent tests, 87–90, 293–295

tests, diagnostic value, 302–303
Autoimmune disease, 191–199
etiology, 191–194
pathogenic mechanisms, 196–199
Autoimmune hemolytic anemia, 195, 209, 210, 227, 293
Azathioprin, 253

B lymphocyte
antigen binding, 33–35
deficiency, 168–169, 172–173
definition, 38–39, 103–104, 149, 151
identification, 103–106, 149–150
lymph node areas, 49–50
response to mitogens, 101, 300–302
rosettes, 103–106
spleen areas, 49–50
surface immunoglobulins, 300
surface markers, 103–106, 300
T-cell cooperation in immune response, 38–40
test of immunocompetence, 97–101, 286, 300–302
tolerance, induction and, 186–187
triggering, by T-independent antigens, 45–46
Blastogenic response, lymphocytes (*see* Mitosis)
Blocking antibody, 222–223
Bone marrow
antibody forming cells, 38–40
primary lymphoid organ, 38–40
Bruton's agammaglobulinemia, 168–169
Bursa of Fabricius, 48–50
Bursectomy, 48–50
antibody synthesis and, 48–50
neonatal, 48

C'1 esterase inhibitor, 82
Cancer
antigens, 265–267, 271–272, 295, 303–304
effect of immunodeficiency, 273–274
enhancing (or protecting) antibodies in, 269
immune response in, 269–271
immunological surveillance, 267
immunotherapy of, 270–271
radioimmunoassay, 271–272, 295
Candidiasis, chronic mucocutaneous, 175–176
Carcinoembryonic antigen (CEA), 265–267, 271–272, 295
Carrier, 26
Cell-mediated immune reactions
type IV, 237–240
type V, 240–241
type VI, 241–242
type VII, 241–242
Cell-mediated immunity, 58–69
Cell-mediated target cell lysis (*see* Cytotoxicity)
Cell stimulation, by antibodies, 240
Chediak-Higashi syndrome (CHS), 177–179
Chemotactic factors, 79–80
Chronic granulomatous disease, 174–175
Chronic mucocutaneous candidiasis, 176
Clinical immunology laboratory, 286–307
Clonal selection theory, 52–54
CMI (*see* Immunity, cell-mediated)
Complement, 77–85
activation, 77–80
alternative pathway, 78–80
cascade, 77–78
chemotactic factors, 79–80
classical pathway, 78–80
deficiency, 176–177
definition, 77
fixation test (CFT), 83–85
receptor for, 103–105
role in Arthus reaction, 119, 229–230
role in immune-complex reaction, 80
role in phagocytosis, 80
Cytotoxicity, cell mediated
antibody-dependent cell mediated (ADCC), 111–112, 299
mitogen-induced, cell-mediated (MICC), 114, 299
naturally occurring cell-mediated (NOCC), 112–113, 299

Delayed hypersensitivity (skin) reaction, 62, 118–119
Dermatitis, contact, 239
Dermatomyositis, 195

Desensitization
in allergy to pollens, 221–225
in allergy to drugs, 225–226
in anaphylaxis, 221
Diabetes mellitus, 195
Dick test, 123
DiGeorge syndrome, 170–171
Disodium cromoglycate (Intal), treatment in allergy, 225–226
Disseminated intravascular coagulation (DIC), 121
Double diffuse reaction in agar gel, 75–76
Drug reactions, allergic, 212, 225–227, 241–242

Edema, hereditary angioneurotic, 83
Electrophoresis, 12, 296–298
Endotoxin
as adjuvant, 29
complement activation, 79
shock, 81
Enhancing antibodies
in cancer, 270
in graft rejection, 187–188, 253
Enzyme-linked immunosorbent assay (ELISA), 95–97
Extrinsic allergic alveolitis, 213, 232–234

Fab, fragment of Ig, 13–14
$F(ab)_2$, fragment of Ig, 13–14
Farmer's lung, 213, 231–232
Farr technique, 91
Fc fragment of Ig, 13–14
Fluorescein, 87
Fluorescence microscopy, 87–90
Forbidden clones, 192
Freund's adjuvant
complete, 28–29
incomplete, 28–29

Gamma-globulin(s)
classes, classification, 12, 15
prophylactic use, 169, 171, 173
Gm groups, 18
Goodpasture's syndrome, 195, 228
Graft rejection
first and second set, 249–252
immunological basis, 249–253
immunological tolerance in, 188–189, 256
immunosuppressive drugs, 253–256
lymphocyte role, 251–252
prevention, 253–257
relation to autoimmune disease, 262
role of antibody, 249–251
tissue matching
mixed leukocyte reaction (MLR), 106–108, 305–306
lymphocytotoxicity assay, 295–296, 305–306
Graft versus host reaction, 173
Graves disease, 239–240
Guillain-Barré syndrome, 234

Hapten, 26
Hashimoto's thyroiditis, 194, 195, 209, 210
Hay fever, 213
Heavy chains, 13–16
Helper cell, 39, 154
Hemagglutination
BDB, 86–87
mechanism, 86–87
tanned red cell, 86–87
Hemolytic anemia, autoimmune, 195, 209, 210, 227, 293
Hemolytic disease of the newborn (erythroblastosis fetalis), 189–190
Hemolytic plaque assay, 97–100
Histamine, 80–81, 213–215, 220–221
anaphylaxis and, 220–221
mast cells and, 213–215
Histocompatibility antigens,
biologic significance, 257–261
immune response and, 258–261
microorganisms and, 260–261
recognition systems and, 260–261
Hypocomplementemia syndrome, 177
Hypogammaglobulinemia
acquired, 179–182
congenital, 168–169

Idiopathic thrombocytopenic purpura

(ITP), 195, 209, 210, 228, 293
Idiotypes, 17
Immediate skin reaction, 116–118, 213–214
Immune complex disease, 229–236
Immune response
antibodies (*see* Antibody formation)
cell-mediated, 58–69
role in immunity to infection, 59–61, 236–239
role of macrophage, 62–65
role of T cell, 63, 64, 65, 69
suppressor cells, 141, 144
thymectomy, 47–48
Immunity
aging, 275–282
essential fatty acids, 200, 202–203, 206
nonspecific mechanisms, 283–285
nutrition, 200–207
prostaglandins, 202, 205–206
trace metals, 200–206
vitamins, 200–206
zinc, 200–206
Immunoassays
agglutination, 85–87
complement fixation, 77–85
enzyme-linked immunosorbent assay (ELISA), 95–97
hemolytic plaque-forming cells, 97–100
immunoelectrophoresis, 76–77
immunofluorescence, 87–90
interfacial ring test, 71–73
nephelometry, 93–95
passive hemagglutination, 87
precipitin reactions, 73–76
in gel, 75–76
in liquid medium, 73–75
radioimmunoassay, 90–93
Immunodeficiency diseases, 161–182
acquired variable hypogammaglobulinemia, 179–182
Bruton's agammaglobulinemia, 168–169
Chediak-Higashi syndrome, 177–179
chronic granulomatosus disease, 174–175
chronic mucocutaneous candidiasis, 176
classification, 163–166
DiGeorge syndrome, 170–171
hypocomplementemia syndrome, 177
Nezelof syndrome, 171–172
primary, 168–179
secondary, 165–166
severe combined (Swiss type), 172–173
Wiskott-Aldrich, 173–174
Immunodiffusion, radial, 297
Immunoelectrophoresis, 76–77
Immunofluorescence, 87–90
direct test, 87–90
indirect (sandwich) test, 87–90
Immunoglobulin A (IgA)
antibodies, 20–22
biological properties, 15, 20–22
composition, 15, 18, 21–22
site of synthesis, 21–23
Immunoglobulin D (IgD) biological properties, 15, 23–24
Immunoglobulin E (IgE)
biological properties, 15, 23, 223
composition, 15, 18, 23
physiological role, 15, 23, 223
radioallergosorbent test (RAST), 225–226
Immunoglobulin G (IgG)
antibody synthesis, feedback inhibition on, 125–127
biological properties, 15, 18–19
blocking antibody, 222–223
composition, 15, 18
fragmentation by papain, 13–14
subclasses, 19
Immunoglobulin M (IgM)
antibody synthesis, feedback stimulation on, 125–126
biological properties, 15, 19–20
composition, 15, 18
Immunoglobulins
allotypes, 17–18
antigen binding sites, 13, 14, 16
biological properties, 15, 18–24
classes, 15
idiotypes, 17–18

Immunoglobulins—*continued*
serum levels, 15
structure, 15, 18
Immunological surveillance, 267
Immunological tolerance, 183–190
cancer and, 265
definition, 183
high dose (or zone), 184
in adult, 184
in newborn, 184
low dose (or zone), 185
mechanism, 185–188
suppressor cells, 185
Immunopathology
type I reaction, 212–228
type II reaction, 228–230
type III reaction, 230–237
type IV reaction, 237–240
type V reaction, 240–241
type VI reaction, 241–242
type VII reaction, 241–242
Immunosuppressive drugs, 253, 255–256
Immunotherapy of cancer, 270–271
Interferon, 63
Interpretation of
blastogenic responses, 300–302
electrophoretic analysis, 296–298
histocompatibility tests, 305–306
immunoelectrophoretic analysis, 296–298
precipitin tests, 304–305
Intrinsic factor, autoantibodies, 195
Islet cell antibodies, 195

J-chain, 18, 20, 21
Jerne hemolytic plaque assay, 97–100

LATS, *see* Thyroid
LD antigens
defined, 306
in MLR, 305–306
Leucocytes, migration inhibition, 109–110
Levamisole, 271
Lupus erythematosus, 141, 195, 210
suppressor cells in, 195
Lymph node
B-cell areas, 49–50
immune response and, 33–35
T-cell areas, 49–50
Lymphoid organs
primary, 49–50
secondary, 49–50
Lymphokines, 63–65, 109–111
chemotactic factor, 63, 109
definition, 63, 109
interferon, 63, 109
lymphotoxin, 63, 109
MAF, 63–65, 109
MIF, 63, 109–111
transfer factor, 63, 109
Lymphopenic agammaglobulinemia (Swiss-type agammaglobulinemia), 172–173

Macrophages
activating factor (MAF), 6, 65
"angry" or "armed," 6, 65
B- and T-cell cooperation and, 42–45
migration inhibition factor (MIF), 63, 65
Malnutrition, in cancer, 273–274
Mast cells
degranulation, 213–215
histamine release, 213–215
Maternal-fetal relationship, 262–265
Memory cells, 31, 34, 44, 47
Migration inhibition factor (MIF), 63, 109–111
Migration stimulating factor (MSF), 144
Mitogen-induced cell cytotoxicity (MICC), 114–116, 299
Mitogens
Concanavalin-A (Con-A), 101
defined, 101
phytohemagglutinin (PHA), 101
pokeweed (PWM), 101
Mitosis
induced by ALS, 240
induced by anti-Ig, 240
of B cells, 101, 300–302
of T cells, 101, 300–302
Mixed leukocyte reaction (MLR), 106–108, 305–306
one-way MLR, 106–107

two-way MLR, 106–108
Multiple myeloma, 240
Myasthenia gravis, 195

Naturally occurring cytotoxic cells, (NOCC), 112–113, 299
Nephelometry, 93–95
Nezelof syndrome, 171–172
Nude mice, 267
Null cells, 104, 150
Nutrition and immunity, 200–207

Ouchterlony double diffusion precipitation technique, 75–76
Ovalbumin, valency, 26

Pancreas, islet cell antibodies, 195
Papain, IgG fragmentation, 13, 14
Penicillin, allergy to, 224–225, 242
Pepsin, IgG fragmentation, 13, 14
Periarteriolar lymphoid sheath, 49
Pernicious anemia, 195, 209, 210
Physiologic hypogammaglobulinemia, 166–168
Plaques
direct, 97–100
indirect, 97–100
techniques, antibody detection and, 97–100
Plasma cells, antibody synthesis, 34–35
Platelets, 195, 209, 210
Poison ivy, 237
Polyarteritis nodosa, 195
Praüsnitz-Kustner (P-K) test, 222, 226
Precipitation, gel, 75–76
Precipitin reaction, 71–75
Pregnancy, maternal-fetal relationship and immune responsiveness, 262–265
Primary immune response to antigen, 31–33
Prostaglandins, 202–206
Protein, as hapten carrier, 26–28
Protein-calorie malnutrition effect on immune response in cancer, 273–274
Purpura, idiopathic, 195, 209, 210, 228
thrombocytopenic Sedormid induced, 228

Radioallergosorbent test (RAST), 226–227
Radioimmunoassay, 226–227
Ragweed allergy, 213
Reagin, 213
Rejection, of allograft, 249–252
Rheumatoid factor, 195, 294
Rhodamine, 87
Rosettes, 101–106
C′3 (B cells), 103
E(SRBC) (T cells), 103
Fc (null cells), 103

Sanarelli-Schwartzman reaction, 119–121
Schick test, 122–123
Schwartzman reaction, 120–122
SCID (severe combined immunodeficiency disease), 172–173
Scleroderma, 195
SD antigens
defined, 306
in MLR, 305–306
Secondary response to antigen, 31–33
Serotonin, 80–81, 213, 220–221
Serum sickness, 234–236
Severe combined immunodeficiency disease (SCID), 172–173
Shock
anaphylactic, 80–82, 218–220
cardiogenic, 81
endotoxin-induced, 80–82
IgE-induced, 81, 212, 226
immune complex-induced, 81
mediators, 81
Side-chain theory, 53–54
Skin-sensitizing antibody, 213
Skin test, detection of allergy, 116–118, 213–214
SLE (systemic lupus erythrmatosus), 193, 195, 210
Slow reacting substance of anaphylaxis (SRS-A), 215
Spleen
B-cell area, 49–50
immune response and, 33–35
T-cell area, 49–50
Stimulation of cells by antibodies, 240

Suppression of antibody response by
antibodies, 125–127
anti-idiotype antibodies, 126–127
suppressor cells, 128–140
suppressor factors, 124–125
Suppression of cell-mediated immune response by
suppressor cells, 141, 144
suppressor factors, 124–125
Suppressor cells, 128–147
Swiss-type agammaglobulinemia, 172–173
Systemic lupus erythematosus (*see* SLE)

T lymphocyte
antigen (T_3, T_4, T_5), 158–160
antigen receptor, 38–39, 42–43
B-cell cooperation in immune response, 38–40, 43–47
cell-mediated immunity, 47–48, 63, 64, 66–67
deficiency, 170–173
"helper" cell, 39, 154
lymph node areas, 49–50
rosettes, 101–103
spleen areas, 49–50
suppressor cells, 129–131, 134, 138–147
T_C cells, 156, 159
T_G cells, 156, 159
T_{G+C} cells, 156, 159
T_M cells, 156, 159
T_{M+C} cells, 156, 159
T_N cells, 156, 159
Tannic acid, red cell modification for passive hemagglutination, 87
Template theory, 51–52
Thymectomy
cell-mediated reaction and, 47–48
neonatal, 47–48
Thymosin, 51, 281
Thymus dependent cells (*see* T lymphocytes)
Thyroid
autoantibodies, 195, 209, 210
Hashimoto thyroiditis, 210
long acting stimulator (LATS), 239–240
stimulating antibody, 239–240
Thyroiditis, autoimmune (Hashimoto), 210
Thyrotoxicosis, 239–240
Tissue matching, for grafts
MLR, 106–108, 295–296, 305–306
lymphocytotoxicity assay, 295–296, 305–306
Tolerance (*see* Immunological tolerance)
Transfer factor, 63, 65, 174
Transplantation antigens, 257–262
Trophoblast, 264
Tumors (*see* Cancer)

Ulcerative colitis, 209
Unresponsiveness to cancer antigens, 266, 268
Urticaria, 216–218

Wasserman test, 83–85
Wiskott-Aldrich syndrome, 173–174

Xenograft, definition, 248